A quick reference to the surfaces of the heart as seen on the ECG, including ECG wave form abnormalities common to coronary artery occlusion

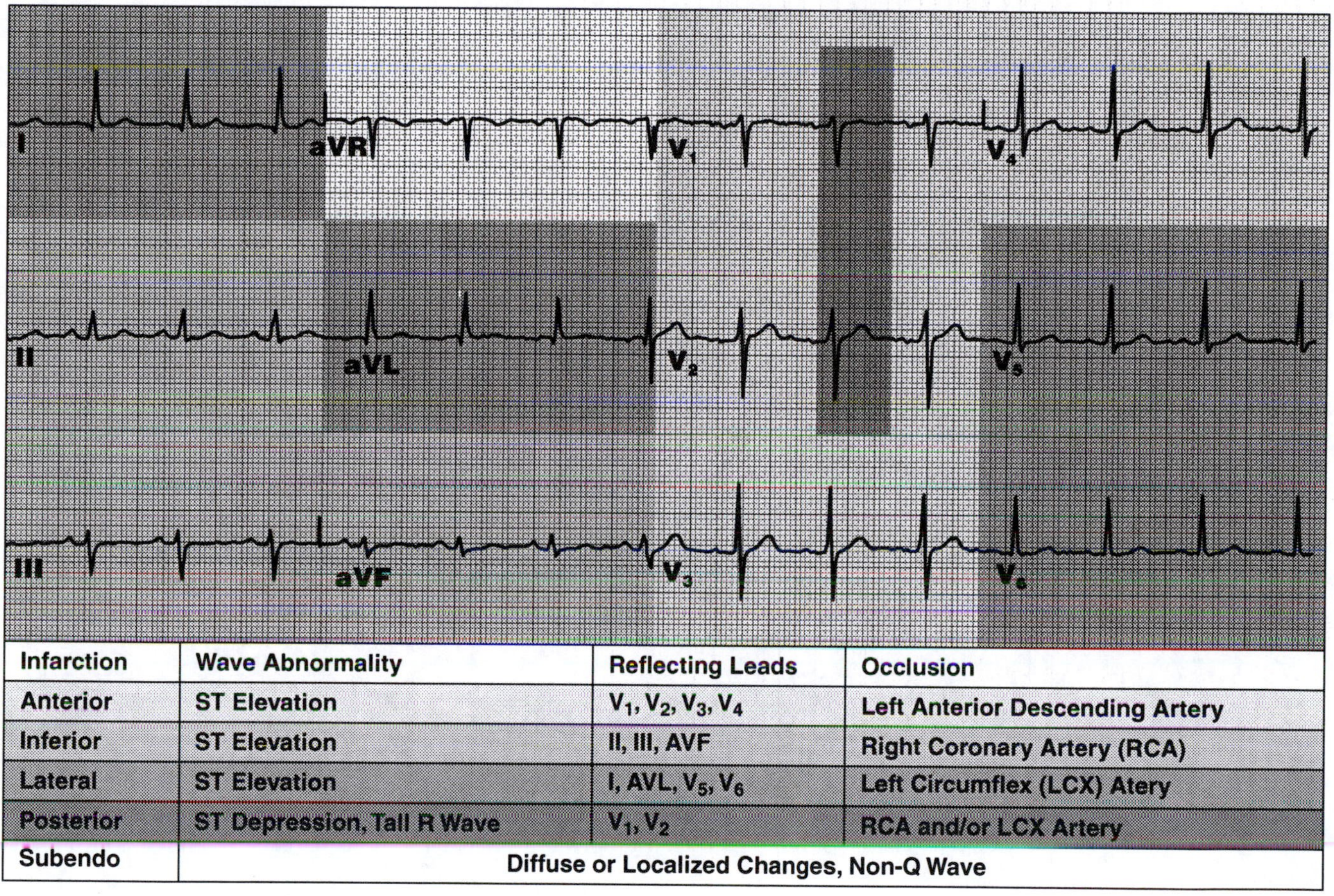

Infarction	Wave Abnormality	Reflecting Leads	Occlusion
Anterior	ST Elevation	V_1, V_2, V_3, V_4	Left Anterior Descending Artery
Inferior	ST Elevation	II, III, AVF	Right Coronary Artery (RCA)
Lateral	ST Elevation	I, AVL, V_5, V_6	Left Circumflex (LCX) Atery
Posterior	ST Depression, Tall R Wave	V_1, V_2	RCA and/or LCX Artery
Subendo	Diffuse or Localized Changes, Non-Q Wave		

Sensible Analysis of the
of the
12-Lead ECG

....

To my Ed–
Michelle and Mark

To my brother, Jady

Sensible Analysis of the 12-Lead ECG

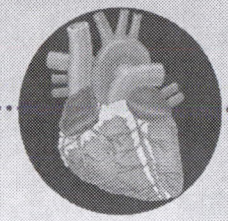

Kathryn Monica Lewis, RN, BSN, PhD

Phoenix, Arizona

Edited by

Kathleen A. Handal, MD, DABEM

Scottsdale, Arizona

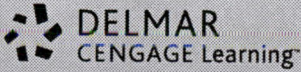

DELMAR
CENGAGE Learning

Australia • Brazil • Japan • Korea • Mexico • Singapore • Spain • United Kingdom • United States

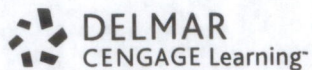
DELMAR
CENGAGE Learning

Sensible Analysis of the 12-Lead ECG
Kathryn Monica Lewis

Health Care Publishing Director:
  William Brottmiller

Development Editor: Darcy Scelsi

Executive Marketing Manager: Dawn Gerrain

Project Editor: Stacey Prus

Production Coordinator: John Mickelbank

Art and Design Coordinator: Mary Colleen
  Liburdi

Cover Design: TDB Publishing Services

For product information and technology assistance, contact us at
Cengage Learning Customer & Sales Support, 1-800-354-9706

For permission to use material from this text or product,
submit all requests online at **www.cengage.com/permissions**
Further permissions questions can be emailed to
permissionrequest@cengage.com

Library of Congress Control Number: 99-044880

ISBN-13: 978-0-7668-0524-8

ISBN-10: 0-7668-0524-7

Delmar
Executive Woods
5 Maxwell Drive
Clifton Park, NY 12065
USA

Cengage Learning is a leading provider of customized learning solutions with office locations around the globe, including Singapore, the United Kingdom, Australia, Mexico, Brazil, and Japan. Locate your local office at **international.cengage.com/region**

Cengage Learning products are represented in Canada by Nelson Education, Ltd.

To learn more about Delmar, visit **www.cengage.com/delmar**

Purchase any of our products at your local bookstore or at our preferred online store **www.ichapters.com**

Printed in the United States of America
1 2 3 4 5   15 14 13 12 11

FD052

Contents

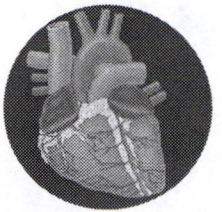

Foreword x
Preface xi

CHAPTER 1

The Heart's Conduction System 1

Introduction 1
The Electrical Conduction System 1
   The Sinus Node ● *2*
   The AV Junction ● *2*
   The Bundle Branch System ● *2*
   The Purkinje's Fibers ● *2*
Electrophysiology of the Heart 3
   The Phases of the Cardiac Cycle ● *3*
   Properties of the Specialized Cells ● *4*
Electrical Conduction 6
Pacemakers, Escape Rhythms, and Ectopic Foci 6
Summary 6
Self-Assessment Exercise 7

CHAPTER 2

The ECG and the 12-Lead System 9

Introduction 9
The ECG Leads: A Point of View 10
   Limb Leads ● *10*
   Augmented Leads ● *11*
   Precordial (Chest) Leads ● *12*
   Monitoring the Posterior Surface of the Heart ● *14*
   MCL Leads ● *15*
   Hazards of Improper Lead Placement ● *15*
Summary 15
Self-Assessment Exercise 17

CHAPTER 3

Rate, Rhythm, and Wave Forms 19

Introduction 19

Calculating Rate and Rhythm 20

Wave Forms, Complexes, and Intervals 23

P Waves ● *24*
PR Interval ● *25*
QRS Complex ● *25*
ST Segment ● *26*
T Wave ● *27*
QT Interval ● *28*
U Wave ● *29*

Abnormal Wave Forms 29

Abnormal P Waves ● *29*
Abnormal PR Interval ● *30*
Abnormal QRS Complexes ● *32*
Abnormal QT Interval ● *33*
Abnormal U Waves ● *34*

Alterations in ECG Wave Forms 35

Drug-Induced Changes on the ECG ● *35*
Hyperkalemia ● *36*
Hypokalemia ● *37*
Hypercalcemia ● *37*
Hypocalcemia ● *38*
Low-Voltage QRS ● *39*
Pericarditis ● *40*
Ventricular Aneurysm ● *42*
Hypertrophic Cardiomyopathy ● *42*
Increased Intracranial Pressure ● *42*
Pulmonary Embolism ● *44*

Summary 45

Self-Assessment Exercises 45

CHAPTER 4

Axis Determination and Implications 48

Introduction 48

Normal Axis 48

Axis Deviation 49

Right Axis Deviation ● *49*
Left Axis Deviation ● *50*

Calculating Axis 50

Normal and Abnormal Values 54

The Lewis Circle ● *55*

Summary 56

Self-Assessment Exercises 56

Sinus Rhythm and the Arrhythmias 63

Introduction 63

How to Look at and Analyze Wave Forms 64

Labeling the ECG ● 64

How to Assess a Monitor Pattern ● 65

Sinus Mechanisms 66

Sinus Tachycardia ● 66

Sinus Bradycardia ● 67

Sinus Arrhythmia ● 67

Sinus Arrest ● 67

Sinoatrial (SA) Block ● 68

Summary of Sinus Mechanisms 68

Junctional Mechanisms 69

Junctional Rhythm ● 70

Premature Junctional Complex ● 71

Accelerated Junctional Rhythm and Junctional Tachycardia ● 73

Atrial Mechanisms 73

Premature Atrial Complex ● 74

Atrial Tachycardia ● 76

Supraventricular Tachycardia ● 76

Atrial Flutter ● 78

Atrial Fibrillation ● 79

Summary of Atrial Mechanisms 80

Ventricular Mechanisms 83

Characteristics of a Ventricular Ectopic ● 83

Narrow Complex PVCs ● 84

Variations in PVCs ● 85

Ventricular Tachycardia ● 88

Intermittent Ventricular Tachycardia ● 88

Polymorphic Ventricular Tachycardia ● 88

Ventricular Fibrillation ● 90

Ventricular Escape: Idioventricular Rhythm ● 92

Accelerated Idioventricular Rhythm ● 93

Aberrant Ventricular Conduction ● 93

Asystole ● 95

AV Conduction Defects 98

Sinus Rhythm with First-Degree AV Block ● 98

Sinus with Second-Degree AV Block: The Intermittent Conduction Defects ● 98

Second-Degree AV Block: The Wenckebach Phenomenon (aka Type I AV Block) ● 99

Second-Degree AV Block with Wide QRS Complex (Type II) ● 101

Second-Degree AV Block: AV Block with 2:1 Conduction (aka Fixed-Rate Second-Degree AV Block ● *102*

Sinus with High-Grade (Advanced) AV Block ● *102*

Sinus with Complete AV Block ● *102*

Arrhythmias Due to Abnormal Conduction Pathways 104

ECG Wave Forms Affected by Preexcitation ● *106*

Degrees of Preexcitation ● *107*

Arrhythmias with Preexcitation ● *107*

Lown-Ganong-Levine Syndrome ● *110*

Wolff-Parkinson-White Syndrome ● *111*

Summary 113

Self-Assessment Exercises 114

CHAPTER 6

Myocardial Perfusion Deficits and ECG Changes

Myocardial Perfusion Deficits and ECG Changes 124

Introduction 124

Coronary Artery Perfusion 125

Pathophysiology of Acute Myocardial Infarction 126

Consequences of Coronary Artery Occlusion 128

Reflecting and Reciprocal Leads ● *129*

Monitoring Myocardial Ischemia, Injury, and Necrosis on the ECG 129

Changes in Wave Forms ● *131*

ECG Indicators of Perfusion Deficits ● *138*

Inferior Wall (Diaphragmatic) Myocardial Infarction 138

Clinical Implications of Inferior Wall Myocardial Infarction ● *140*

Anterior Wall Myocardial Infarction 140

Clinical Implications for Anterior Wall Myocardial Infarction ● *142*

Anteroseptal Myocardial Infarction 142

Anterolateral Myocardial Infarction 142

Clinical Implications of Anterolateral Wall Myocardial Infarction ● *143*

Lateral Wall Myocardial Infarction 143

Clinical Implications of Lateral Wall Myocardial Infarction ● *144*

Posterior Wall Myocardial Infarction 144

Clinical Implications for Posterior Wall Myocardial Infarction ● *146*

Right Ventricular Myocardial Infarction 146

Clinical Implications of Right Ventricular Wall Myocardial Infarction ● *148*

Non-Q Wave Myocardial Infarction 148

Pseudo-Infarction Patterns 150

Early Repolarization ● *151*

Nonclassic ECG Presentation of Acute Myocardial Infarction 151

Continuous ST Segment Monitoring 151

Summary 154

Self-Assessment Exercises 154

CHAPTER 7 Intraventricular Conduction Defects 163

Introduction 163

The Bundle Branches and Arterial Perfusion 164

Normal Sequence of Ventricular Depolarization
and the QRS Vector 165

ECG Changes in Bundle Branch Block 166

Right Bundle Branch Block ● *167*
Left Bundle Branch Block ● *170*

Fascicular Blocks 174

Left Anterior Fascicular Block ● *174*
Left Anterior Fascicular Block and RBBB ● *177*
Left Anterior Fascicular Block and Myocardial Infarction ● *177*
Left Posterior Fascicular Block ● *177*

Complete Left Bundle Branch Block 179

Trifascicular Block 179

Summary 181

Self-Assessment Exercises 182

CHAPTER 8 Chamber Enlargement and Hypertrophy 187

Introduction 187

Right Atrial Enlargement 187

Left Atrial Enlargement 188

Ventricular Hypertrophy 188

Right Ventricular Hypertrophy ● *189*
Left Ventricular Hypertrophy ● *190*
Ventricular Strain Pattern ● *195*

Summary 197

Self-Assessment Exercises 198

Appendix A
Answers to Self-Assessment Exercises 203

Appendix B
**Normal Ranges and Variations in Adults
in a 12-Lead ECG** 227

Appendix C
How to Interpret the 12-lead ECG 229

Glossary 231

Index 237

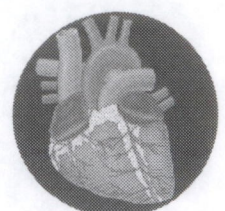

Foreword

This is the second book in the *Sensible ECG* series by Dr. Lewis and Dr. Handal. While the first text addressed rhythm problems and analysis, *Sensible Analysis of the 12-Lead ECG* expands on the clinical approach to the interpretation of 12-lead ECGs in various clinical situations.

Dr. Lewis, a nurse educator in the clinical and prehospital setting, and Dr. Handal, a seasoned emergency physician, bring a wealth of knowledge and clinical experience to the topic. They have written a pragmatic guide to issues surrounding ECG interpretation—at a time when the concept of "bringing the hospital to the patient" represents the current standard of care. They ground this book with over 40 years of combined clinical experience in a wide range of settings. Anyone with significant patient contact will benefit from their approach.

The real beneficiaries, however, will continue to be our patients. It is in the interest of their better health, as well as our own intellectual and professional development, that I invite you to continue with the *Sensible ECG* series.

Joanne M. Ceimo, MD, FACC
Scottsdale, Arizona

Preface

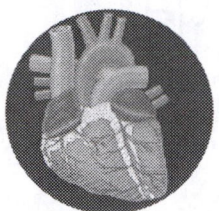

The purpose of this text is to introduce the clinician to the subject of the sensible analysis of PQRST wave forms using the 12-lead system. Importantly, this text was designed to give the clinician the information needed to understand an interpreted 12-lead ECG. *Sensible Analysis of the 12-Lead ECG* is written in a concise manner and supplemented with detailed ECG tracings taken from real-life patient scenarios. There are self-study questions that assess progress throughout the text.

In ECG rhythm identification, almost all ECG tracings studied use lead II. While there are many monitoring devices that are configured to observe a combination of leads, the 12-lead ECG remains the best tool for visualization of the surfaces of the heart, identification of sites of ischemia, injury, and infarction, as well as various intricate conduction abnormalities.

Sensible interpretation of ECGs using lead II and sometimes MCL_1 is considered basic and commonplace. The clinician learns and practices identification of normal wave forms, measurement, durations, and associated calculations to determine normal versus abnormal. This mastery requires organization, practice, and application of basic rules and is a necessary foundation for this text. The content is written and predicated on the knowledge and skills gained from the first text in this series, *Sensible ECG Analysis*.

The use of the 12-lead ECG requires the same diligent effort and a mastered, organized approach, adding nine or more leads. Many cardiac monitors offer a choice of one, three, or 12-leads in easily applied portable devices. Some electrocardiographic monitors are designed for and programmed to automatically generate a computerized interpretation. Often, these interpretations are skewed or incorrect. No matter how sophisticated the technology, the exacting effort and expertise of the clinician will never be replaced. The clinician, not the computer, has the ultimate responsibility for the interpretation.

Ischemia, injury, and necrosis may be obvious in some leads and not others. The patient with chest pain deserves the best possible visualization of all the heart's surfaces. Since time is so valuable, it is becoming increasingly more common to have 12-lead ECG application and transmission from the prehospital scene to a receiving hospital. Confirmation of myocardial changes within the short "window of opportunity" provides the patient with the best possible opportunity for reperfusion and survival.

Sensible Analysis of the 12-Lead ECG makes no pretense of enabling the reader to master the infinite intricacies of cardiac electrophysiology, pathology, and interventions. Nor is this an exhaustive treatise on the 12-lead ECG. Those who read, interpret, and monitor patients can make use of the ECG without the complexity of the physics involved.

The authors have exerted a great deal of diligence and effort to assure that medications and dosages set forth in this text are in accordance with current recommendations and practice at the time of this printing. In view of ongoing research and development in the laboratory and in clinical settings, the continual influx of knowledge and experiences, the reader has the ultimate responsibility for knowledge needed for the application of a proposed intervention technique or the administration of any medication.

The ECG reflects the heart and all its functions. It is a window to the magnificent process of electrical activation and subsequent life-sustaining pulses. This book is designed to help the practitioner read a 12-lead ECG and realize what that recording implies about the heart.

Sensible Analysis of the 12-Lead ECG is written for anyone who uses the 12-lead ECG as a tool in patient care. Anatomy, basic electrophysiology and timing techniques are explained. Each concept is described and accompanied by key terms, etiology, and clinical implications as they relate to interventions. A systematic approach to the analysis and interpretation of 12-lead ECG is explained. Helpful summaries of the characteristics for each of the concepts is provided. Practical self-assessments are included with detailed answer keys. There are references to provide the student with further insight and future study.

TO THE STUDENT

Accurate 12-lead ECG interpretation contributes to the differential diagnosis and overall care of the patient. The traditional ECG is a non-invasive tool that is vital to the identification and differential diagnosis of illness. Accurate interpretation of the 12-lead by the practitioner provides greater insight and a valuable contribution to the differential diagnosis.

We have written this text and designed the format to help you master the organized approach needed to accurately interpret a 12-lead ECG. The introductory chapters will provide baseline insight into the ECG configurations as they relate to cardiac electrophysiology. Wave forms and timing techniques are explained as they reflect the heart's function. Alterations in the wave forms and various arrhythmias are reviewed, described, and explained. Ventricular conduction defects are highlighted and the ECG characteristics for differential diagnosis of each are defined. Recognition and consequences of chamber enlargement and hypertrophy and the changes as seen on the ECG are presented.

Detailed attention to the pathophysiology and related ECG changes that occur with myocardial ischemia, injury, and infarction are defined and discussed. The significant ECG changes that contribute to the recognition of any of these conditions are specifically detailed. Clinical implications for each of these situations are addressed.

Many of the ECG tracings are taken from our clinical practices. These include patients whose clinical problems, signs, and symptoms are documented. We selected them because they realistically illustrate the content of each chapter. There are also many practice ECGs with detailed answers for your reference and simple, self-assessment exercises.

As you progress, you may be tempted to study directly from the answer key rather than come up with your own interpretation. Don't do this. The sample practice strips are an important part of the learning process—a step that should be followed carefully.

The key to mastering 12-lead ECG interpretation is consistent application of the steps to interpretation. Developing the foundation blocks of information is essential. Once you have completed *Sensible Analysis of the 12-Lead ECG*, you should be able to:

- help with decisions and care.
- correctly apply your skills.
- remember to always treat the patient, not the tool.

YOU are the critical link providing insight and clues vital to the care of the patient.

ACKNOWLEDGMENTS

The accumulation of knowledge and insight is never a solitary process. Since 1977, friends and family have stimulated and supported my efforts. Students have suffered through the various approaches to teaching and learning so we could all master these concepts. Dr. Leonard Caccamo gave me my first glimmer into the world of the ECG and patient assessment. Mary B. Conover fanned the flame all these years. Drs. S. Sridahr and Arthur Pelberg provided support through all the what-ifs and doubts; Dr. Friedman kept me organized and practical.

Arlene Copley, RN, patiently searched down the 12-lead ECGs and assured me that my teaching methods all these years had made a difference.

My boundless gratitude goes to the paramedic students who have demonstrated that all this information is truly applicable—they are indeed making a difference.

REVIEWERS

The authors and Delmar would like to acknowledge the following individuals who reviewed the manuscript and provided several valuable suggestions for improvement:

Shirley Jackson, MS, RN, CCRN

Susan Wood, PhD, RN

Ann Hudgins, RN, BSN, EMT-P

Richard Prentiss, MHM, RRT, C-PFT

The Heart's Conduction System

Premise ● Knowledge of the normal process of electrical conduction in the heart is key to interpreting electrocardiograms (ECGs).

Objectives

After reading the chapter and completing the Self-Assessment exercises, the student should be able to:

1. Identify the structures of the heart's electrical conduction system
2. Describe the process of electrical conduction
3. Describe the properties critical to electrical activity

Key Terms

absolute refractory period	ectopy	pacemaker
action potential	escape rhythm	refractoriness
automaticity	excitability	relative refractory period
conductivity	myocardial cells	repolarization
contractility	non-refractory period	specialized cells
depolarization		

Introduction

Electrical activity (depolarization) precedes mechanical activity (contraction). Electrical activation describes the events that result in the contraction and relaxation of cardiac muscle thus sustaining perfusion of the body and the heart itself. This electrical reaction causes chemical reactions and an electrical chain of events within cardiac muscle.

THE ELECTRICAL CONDUCTION SYSTEM

There are two types of cardiac cells. In combination, they are responsible for the mechanical and electrical activity of the heart. The **myocardial cells** make up the bulk of the heart's muscle. They are the actual contractile units of the heart, and

● **myocardial cells**

The bulk of the heart's muscle; the contractile units of the heart

specialized cells

Cells that make up the heart's electrical conduction system.

must be able to respond to electrical stimulus. **Specialized cells** make up the heart's electrical conduction system.

The heart's electrical conduction system consists of the sinus node, the AV junction, the bundle branch system, and the Purkinje fibers.

The Sinus Node

The sinus node governs the physiologic heart rate. The sinus node reaches potential more quickly than the rest of the cardiac tissue and is referred to as the "pacemaker." A **pacemaker** is a cell or group of cells that generates an impulse at a predictable rate of speed. The pacemaker normally generates electrical impulses at a rate of 60 to 100 per minute.

pacemaker

A cell or group of cells that generates an impulse at a predictable rate of speed.

The AV Junction

The AV junction consists of the AV node and the bundle of His down to where it begins to branch. The regions that constitute the AV junction are divided according to cell types: the atrial-nodal (AN) region, the nodal (N) region, and the nodal-His (NH) region. Impulses are delayed here before being transmitted to the ventricles

The Bundle Branch System

The bundle branch system consists of the right bundle branch and the left bundle branch. The right bundle branch extends down into the right ventricle. The left bundle branch divides into anterior and posterior fascicles and extends into the left ventricle.

The Purkinje's Fibers

The Purkinje's fibers are a network of conducting strands beneath the ventricular endocardium. They are responsible for the conduction of electrical impulses to both ventricles. Figures 1-1 and 1-2 illustrate the heart's electrical conduction system.

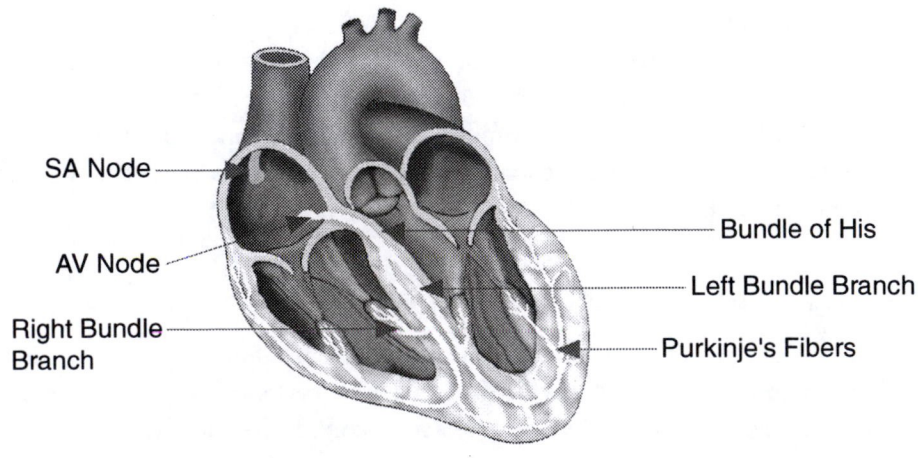

Figure 1-1 The position of the structures of the heart's electrical conduction system

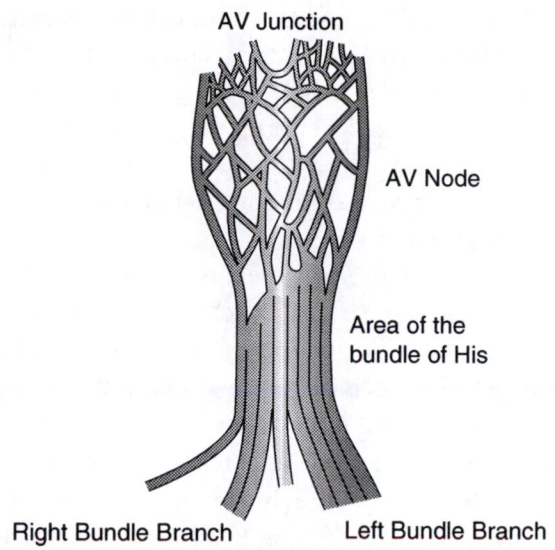

Figure 1-2 Schematic representation of the AV junction, demonstrating the entrance fibers into the AV node, orientation of the AV node to the bundle of His, and the entrance fibers into the interventricular septum

ELECTROPHYSIOLOGY OF THE HEART

The term **action potential** describes the electrolyte exchanges that occur across the cell membrane of the heart during depolarization and repolarization. **Depolarization** is the electrical activation of myocardial cells due to the spread of an electrical impulse. It is the process by which the inside of the cells become less negative. The following are mechanisms by which specific cells depolarize:

- in atrial and ventricular cells, there is a rapid influx of sodium into the cell;
- in the His-Purkinje system, there is a slow, time-dependent decrease in potassium permeability and an increase in sodium permeability; and
- in the sinus and AV nodes there is a slow inward flow of calcium.

Depolarization is an active process. Nevertheless, it is important to remember that ischemia can exist and not affect the wave forms that reflect depolarization. Unless an ischemic or injury process directly affects an electrical conduction pathway, it will not be apparent in a depolarization wave form.

Repolarization is the process by which the cells return to the resting level. Repolarization is rapid at first, until it reaches a plateau. Then, a longer, rapid surge occurs, until the resting state is achieved.

The Phases of the Cardiac Cycle

Phase 0, initial phase of the cardiac cycle, consists of rapid depolarization. As a change in cellular permeability occurs, sodium rushes into the cells making them more positive. This action produces the characteristic upstroke in the action potential.

During Phase 1, initial repolarization, a rapid influx of chloride inactivates the inward pumping of sodium. This serves to make the internal charge nearly equal to the external charge.

action potential

Term that describes the electrolyte exchanges that occur across the cell membrane of the heart during depolarization and repolarization.

depolarization

Electrical activation of myocardial cells due to the spread of an electrical impulse

repolarization

The process by which a cell, after being discharged, returns to its state of readiness

In Phase 2, the plateau, a slow inward flow of calcium occurs, while the flow of potassium is slowed considerably. The electrical charge remains nearly equal at this stage and contraction of the cardiac muscles begins.

Phase 3 consists of final rapid depolarization. During this phase there is a sudden acceleration of the rate of repolarization as the slow calcium current is inactivated and the outward flow of potassium is accelerated. Cells begin to regain their negative electrical charge at this stage.

In Phase 4, diastolic depolarization, there is a difference in activities of working cells and pacemaker cells. In pacemaker cells, there is a time-dependent fall in outward potassium current with a rapid sodium influx, causing self-initiated depolarization. Diastolic depolarization is extremely rapid in the cells of the sinus node, less rapid in the bundle of His, and quite slow in the terminal fascicles of the bundle branches. Nonpacemaker (working) cells remain in the steady state until their membranes are acted on by another stimulus. Figure 1-3A illustrates action potential and electrolyte movement, while Figure 1-3B illustrates the difference between action potential in pacemaker and working cells.

Properties of the Specialized Cells

The specialized cells of the heart's electrical conduction system have specific properties that govern their function: automaticity, excitability, conductivity, contractility, and refractoriness.

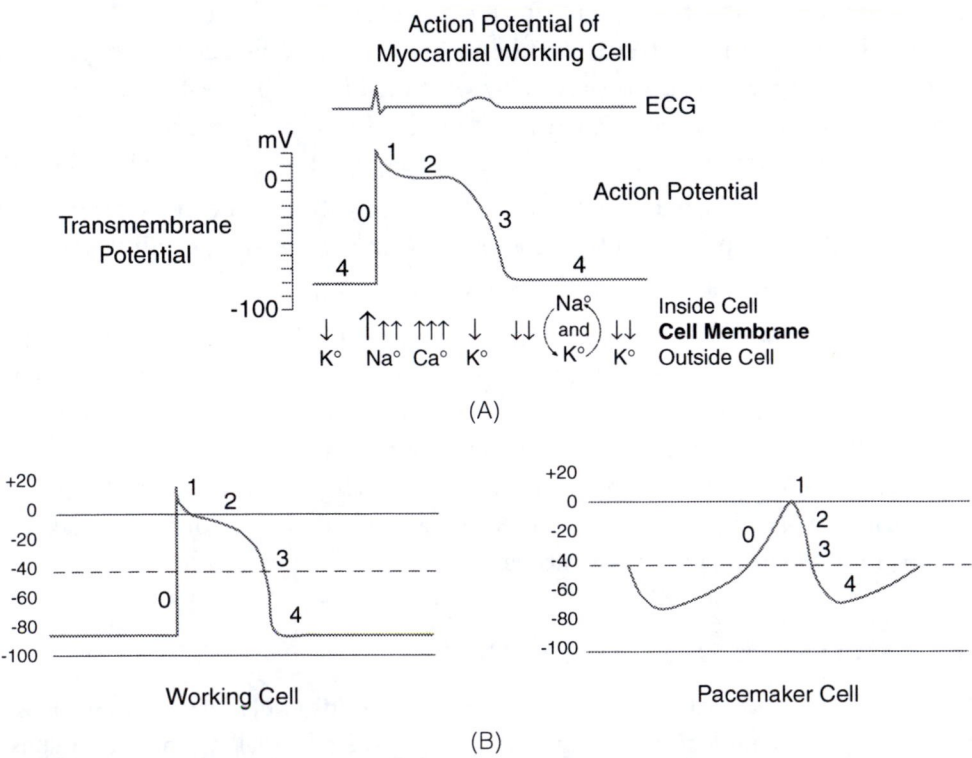

Figure 1-3 (A) Action potential of working myocardial cells; electrolyte exchanges occur across the cell membrane during action potential; (B) comparison of action potential in pacemaker and non-pacemaker (working) myocardial cells

Automaticity refers to the ability of a cell to reach the threshold needed to generate an action potential without being stimulated. This property is attributed to the pacemaker cells. In pacemaker cells there is a regular, predictable fall in potassium concentration during electrical diastole. It is this potassium leak, along with the increased permeability to sodium, that enables the cells to reach the threshold at which an action potential can occur at regular, usually predictable, intervals. The current is then transmitted along all the myocardial cells.

Excitability refers to the ability of a cell to reach threshold and respond to a stimulus. The smaller the amount of required stimulus, the more excitable the cell; if a cell requires greater stimulus, it is considered less excitable. Cardiac cells become "irritable" because of the difference in ion concentration. This degree of irritability determines their degree of excitability or responsiveness. Ischemia and hypoxia will enhance excitability and to some extent, promote premature, competitive behavior, called **ectopy.**

Conductivity describes the transmission or propagation of electrical impulses from cell to cell. Each cell has an inherent capacity for transmission, but there is a difference in the rate of transmission for atrial and ventricular cells.

For instance, from the time the sinus node discharges an impulse, preferential conduction through atrial tissue is roughly 0.08 second, followed by a delay of 0.12 to 0.20 second within the AV node. Subsequent activation of the bundle branch system takes place in only 0.02 second, while total ventricular activation is usually 0.10 second or less. These electrical events are translated to the ECG as specific wave forms.

The stimulation of cardiac cells is facilitated by the many lateral and end-to-end connections within the myocardial muscle fibers. Thus the electrical current can flow from cell-to-cell and laterally using these anatomical interconnections.

Contractility is the ability of cardiac muscle fibers to shorten and contract in response to electrical stimulation. In essence, it is the mechanical response to the other properties just described.

Refractoriness refers to the cells' ability to reject an impulse, or remain unresponsive to a stimulus. Refractoriness is divided into three phases:

1. The **absolute refractory period** is the time when the cells cannot respond to the stimulus. The term is synonymous with depolarization and is a protective mechanism that safeguards the heart from all other ectopic impulses.

2. The **relative refractory period (RRP)** is the time when only a strong stimulus can cause depolarization. The relative refractory period occurs when repolarization is almost complete and some cells can respond, although not entirely in a normal fashion. Some may therefore respond normally, while some may respond in a bizarre fashion, and still others may not respond at all. Serious life-threatening arrhythmias can occur if enough cells respond in a disorganized manner during the RRP.

3. The **non-refractory period** is the time when all cells are repolarized and ready to respond in a normal fashion.

The length of time for each of the refractory periods can vary among normal individuals, and also is affected by medications, recreational drugs, disease, electrolyte imbalance, myocardial ischemia, and myocardial injury.

⦿ **automaticity**

The property of cardiac muscles that describes the ability of a cell to spontaneously generate an impulse without being externally stimulated

⦿ **excitability**

The property of cardiac muscles that describes the capacity of a cell to respond to a stimulus

⦿ **ectopy**

Cells that possess automaticity in competition with pacemakers

⦿ **conductivity**

The property of cardiac muscle that describes the ability to transmit an impulse from cell to cell

⦿ **contractility**

The property of cardiac muscle that describes the ability of the heart to react to electrical conduction with an organized response; the mechanical response

⦿ **refractoriness**

The property of cardiac muscle that describes the cells ability to reject an impulse

⦿ **absolute refractory period**

Period of time in which cells cannot respond to a stimulus

⦿ **relative refractory period (RRP)**

Period of time when only a strong stimulus can cause depolarization

⦿ **non-refractory period**

Period of time when all cells are repolarized and ready to respond in a normal fashion

ELECTRICAL CONDUCTION

There is no recording on conventional ECG that represents SA node depolarization. Such depolarization can only be inferred from subsequent atrial activation. Following SA node depolarization, the atrial tissue is activated and is directed inferiorly to the AV node by preferential conduction, and from the right atrium to left atrium via Bachman's bundle. Preferential conduction also occurs in the left atrium.

The next area to be activated is the AV node, which is situated at the floor of the right atrium near the atrial septum. After physiologic delay at the AV node, the impulse is transmitted to the bundle of His. The bundle of His has two capabilities: one is simple conduction of the impulse as it comes through the AV node: the other is to generate an impulse forward to the ventricles and retrograde (backwards) up to the atria. An impulse that originates within the bundle of His is conducted through the ventricle bundle branch onward into the Purkinje system.

During the final stages of myocardial contraction, repolarization is initiated. In normal ventricular tissue, the wave of repolarization starts in the last area to be depolarized and travels in a direction opposite that of depolarization. The forces of repolarization move more slowly, and the magnitude of electrical potential at any given moment is considerably less than the forces of depolarization. Repolarization is a passive process and is greatly affected by ischemic and hypoxic tissue. As a result, the recordings of repolarization are smaller and wider than those of the depolarization wave front.

PACEMAKERS, ESCAPE RHYTHMS, AND ECTOPIC FOCI

◉ escape rhythm

The development of alternate pacemakers to stimulate the heart when there is sinus node slowing or arrest. The atria, AV junction, or ventricles may be the site of a single escape complex, or a sustained escape rhythm.

The sinus node is the primary pacemaker of the heart. If the sinus cannot fire, alternate slower pacemakers take over. The resulting rhythm is called an **escape rhythm.** The more common escape rhythms originate from the AV junction. The intrinsic rate for a junctional rhythm is 40 to 60 beats per minute. The intrinsic rate for a ventricular escape rhythm is 20 to 40 beats per minute.

If an irritable focus in heart muscle competes with the sinus node it is called ectopic. An ectopic focus may occur within atrial tissue, the AV junction, or within the ventricles, and is premature in the cardiac cycle.

Summary

Electrical conduction in the heart begins in the sinus node, then travels through the AV junction and into the ventricles. As a result of the path of this electrical current the cardiac cells experience phases of positive, negative, or neutral charges in response to the electrical stimulus. It is these charges that are recorded on the ECG.

Self-Assessment Exercise

● Matching

Find the definition in the right column that matches the numbered term in the left column. Then compare your answers with those found in the back of the book.

Term	Definition
____ 1. Automaticity	A. Ability to transmit an impulse
____ 2. Conductivity	B. Ability to respond to an electrical impulse
____ 3. Pacemaker	C. Electrical rest and recovery
____ 4. Depolarization	D. Ability to reject an impulse
____ 5. Ectopic	E. Generation of pacemaker cells when the sinus node slows or is in arrest
____ 6. Excitability	F. Ability to spontaneously generate an impulse without a stimulus
____ 7. Repolarization	G. Cells that generate an impulse at a predictable rate of speed
____ 8. Refractoriness	H. Activation of cells due to the spread of an electrical impulse
____ 9. Escape rhythm	I. Cells that generate an impulse in competition to pacemaker cells
____ 10. Action potential	J. Electrolyte changes that occur across cell membranes

References

Anderson, R. H. & Becker, A. E. (1995). Gross anatomy and microscopy of the conducting system. In W. J. Mandel (Ed.), *Cardiac arrhythmias: Their mechanism, diagnosis and management.* (3rd ed.). Philadelphia: Lippincott; 12-49.

Conover, M. B. (1996). *Understanding electrocardiography: Arrhythmias and the 12 lead ECG.* (7th ed.). St. Louis: Mosby-Year Book.

Conover, M. B. & Wellens, H. J. (1993). *The ECG in emergency decision making.* Philadelphia: W. B. Saunders.

Davigilus, M., Liao, W., Greenland, P., et al. (1999). Association of non-specific minor ST-T abnormalities with cardiovascular mortality. *Journal of the American Medical Association*; 281: 530-536.

Davis, D. (1992). *How to quickly and accurately master ECG interpretation.* (2nd ed.). Philadelphia: Lippincott.

Garson, A. Jr. (1993). How to measure the QT interval: What is normal? *American Journal of Cardiology*; 72:148-168.

Goldberger, E. (1982). *Textbook of clinical cardiology.* St. Louis: C.V. Mosby.

Goldberger & Goldberger. (1977). *Clinical electrocardiography.* St. Louis: C.V. Mosby.

Goldschlager, N. & Goldman, M. J. (1989). *Principles of clinical electrocardiography*; East Norwalk, CT: Appleton & Lange.

Hanrahan, J. P., Choo, P. W., Carlson, W., et al. (1995). Terfenadine-associated ventricular arrhythmias and QTC interval prolongation: A retrospective cohort comparison with other antihistamines among members of a health maintenance organization. *Annual Epidemiology*; 5:201-209.

Koepp, M., Schmidt, D. & Kern, A. (1995). Electrocardiographic changes in patients with brain tumors. *Arch Neurology*; 52:152-155.

Lemery, R., Kleinebenne, A., Nihoyannopoulos, P., et al. (1990). Q waves in hypertrophic cardiomyopathy in relation to the distribution and severity of right and left ventricular hypertrophy. *Journal of the American College of Cardiology*; 16:368-374

Lepeschkin, E. Physiological basis of the U wave. In R. C. Schlant & J. W. Hurst (Eds.). *Advances in electrocardiography.* New York: Grune and Stratton, 431-477.

Marriott, H. J. L. (1998). *Practical electrocardiography* (8th ed.). Baltimore: Williams and Wilkins.

Marriott, H. J. L. & Conover, M. B., *Advanced concepts in arrhythmias* (3rd ed.). St Louis: C. V. Mosby.

Michaelson, C. R. (Ed). (1983). *Congestive heart failure.* St. Louis: C. V. Mosby.

Mudge, G. H. (1986). *Manual of electrocardiography.* Toronto: Little, Brown.

Shapiro, E. (1980). The electrocardiogram and the arrhythmias: Historical insights. In W. J. Mandel (Ed.). *Cardiac arrhythmias: Their mechanism, diagnosis and management.* Philadelphia: Lippincott; 1-12.

Sokolow, M. & McIlroym M. B. (1979). *Clinical cardiology* (2nd ed.). Los Altos, CA: Lange Medical.

Sreeram, N., Cheriex, E.C., Smeets, J. L. R., et al. (1994). Value of the 12-lead electrocardiogram at hospital admission in the diagnosis of pulmonary embolism. *American Journal of Cardiology*; 73:298-303.

Surawicz, B. (1995). *Electrophysiologic basis of ECG and cardiac arrhythmias.* Baltimore: Williams & Wilkins.

Tartora, G. J. (1994). *Introduction to the human body: The essentials of anatomy and physiology.* New York, NY: HarperCollins.

Yan, G. X. & Anztelevich, C. (1996). Cellular basis for the electrocardiographic J wave. *Circulation*; 93:372-379.

CHAPTER 2

The ECG and the 12-Lead System

Premise ● The sensible interpretation of the ECG using the 12-lead system is not difficult if the clinician:

1. knows the normal ECG wave form configurations;

2. remembers which surfaces of the heart are best "seen" by which leads;

3. associates 12-lead analysis with patient presentation; and

4. assesses serial ECG tracings.

Objectives

After reading the chapter and completing the Self-Assessment exercises, the student should be able to:

1. Explain the difference between unipolar and bipolar leads

2. Describe the formation of limb leads

3. Identify the position of precordial leads

4. Identify the surface of the heart monitored by each lead

5. Identify the signs of incorrect lead placement

Key Terms

augmented leads

axis

bipolar leads

diphasic

early transition

frontal plane

horizontal plane

poor R-wave progression

precordial leads

R-wave progression

unipolar leads

Introduction

The electrocardiogram (ECG) traces the variation in voltage produced by the heart muscle during depolarization and repolarization. The standard ECG records depolarization and repolarization along designated paths called *lead systems*. This chapter provides a brief overview of the ECG lead systems and how they visualize the surfaces of the heart.

THE ECG LEADS: A POINT OF VIEW

The word *lead* can be confusing in ECG. Sometimes it means the wires that connect the ECG to the patient. Correctly, a lead or lead system is an electrical picture of a heart's surface. We will simply use the term *lead*. Each lead traces the electrical activity between two points called electrodes.

If an electrode faces the advancing wave of depolarization, a positive deflection will be produced. Conversely, if the wave of depolarization recedes away from that electrode a negative deflection will be produced. The magnitude of the voltage of the wave form depends on the direction of the flow of depolarization.

If the electrodes are parallel to the flow of current, the resulting wave forms will be clearly defined. However if the electrodes are not directly parallel to the flow of current, the magnitude will be smaller. Electrodes that are perpendicular (at right angles) to the flow of current will show both positive and negative deflections. The resulting waveform is called **diphasic**.

The standard 12-lead ECG system utilizes at least 5 electrodes; 1 for each limb plus a floating electrode on the chest wall. The system is divided into 3 lead systems: standard limb leads, augmented leads and precordial (chest leads).

The initial 6 leads—I, II, III, aVR, aVL, and aVF — are called the extremity or limb leads because they are derived from electrodes attached to the arms and legs. The precordial leads are derived from electrodes that are placed across the chest, from front to right or left lateral sites.

Limb Leads

Using a 12-lead ECG, the limb leads are formed by placing electrodes on the right and left arms and the left leg.

The direction of flow of electrical current as seen in the limb leads lies in the **frontal plane**—a flat plane parallel to the chest. The direct path between 2 electrodes or between an electrode and the reference point is called the **axis** of that lead (see Chapter 3).

There are 2 types of limb leads. **Bipolar leads** are leads that are composed of 1 positive and 1 negative electrode. The bipolar leads are I, II, and III. The bipolar leads record the difference in voltage between two extremities.

Unipolar leads are leads that are composed of one positive electrode and a neutral reference point. The unipolar limb leads are aVR, aVL, and aVF (the augmented leads). The unipolar precordial leads are V_1, V_2, V_3, V_4, V_5 and V_6 and V_{1R}, V_{2R}, V_{3R}, V_{4R}, V_{5R}, V_{6R}. In some clinical settings, V_7 and V_8, on the right and left sides, are evaluated.

Lead I In lead I, the ECG designates the left arm as the positive electrode and the right arm as the negative electrode. Lead I traces electrical activity from left to right across the chest, providing a view of the left lateral wall of the heart. When the flow of current is to the left an upright (positive) deflection will be written. Normally, the predominant direction of the flow of depolarization is towards the left, therefore positive deflections are seen in lead I.

If there is an alteration in depolarization so that the direction of flow is to the right, the receding flow of current will be seen as a primarily negative deflection in lead I.

● **diphasic**

Having positive and negative components

● **frontal plane**

A flat plane parallel to the chest

● **axis**

The direct path between two electrodes or between an electrode and the reference point; the direction of flow of depolarization

● **bipolar leads**

Leads that are composed of one positive and one negative electrode; leads I, II, and III

● **unipolar leads**

Leads that measure the electrical voltages at one location relative to a zero potential, rather than relative to the voltages of another extremity; leads aVL, aVR, aVF, V_1 through V_6.

Lead II In lead II, the negative electrode is on the right arm, and the positive electrode is on the left leg. Lead II provides a view of the inferior surface of the heart. Because the predominant direction of the flow of depolarization is inferior and to the left, positive deflections are generally seen in lead II. If there are deviations in the normal depolarization wave front—that is, superior and to the left—the wave form in lead II will be either diphasic or predominantly negative.

Lead III In lead III, the positive electrode is on the left leg and the negative electrode is on the left arm. Lead III provides a view of the right inferior surface of the heart. Lead III is usually a positive deflection.

Leads I, II, and III are typically represented by a triangle that depicts the spatial orientation of these leads. If the electrodes are placed correctly and the leads recorded simultaneously, voltage of the wave form in lead II should equal the sum of the voltages in leads I and III. In other words, lead I + lead III = lead II. If the R wave in lead II is not equal to the sum of lead I and lead III, this is a clue that the leads are not placed appropriately.

Augmented Leads

The "a" in leads aVR, aVL, and aVF stands for **augmented** or amplified, so named because these leads are automatically set to increase in size by 50 percent without any change in the configuration of the electrodes by the machine's property.

Lead aVL In lead aVL, the electrode on the left arm is positive while the electrode on the right arm and left leg determines the neutral reference point. Lead aVL visualizes the left lateral wall of the heart. Lead aVL is usually positive and sometimes diphasic.

Lead aVF Lead aVF is the third of the inferior wall leads. In aVF, the electrode on the left leg is positive while the electrode on the right and left arms determines the neutral reference point. Lead aVF is usually positive and sometimes diphasic.

Lead aVR In lead aVR, the electrode on the right arm is positive while the electrode on the left arm and left leg determines the neutral reference point. Lead aVR is sometimes called *no man's land* or the *orphan lead* because it stands alone and does not view any single surface of the heart as directly as other lead systems. The ECG complexes in lead aVR are usually negative because the mean flow of current and depolarization of the heart goes from right to left, superior to inferior. The majority of current goes away from the positive electrode in aVR, therefore, the summative changes in that ECG tracing are predominantly negative.

In most normal ECGs looking at lead aVR is an easy point of reference to help determine the proper placement of the limb lead electrodes. If the electrodes are placed correctly and the leads recorded simultaneously, the sum of the voltages in aVR, aVL, and aVF should equal 0. In other words, aVR + aVL + aVF = 0.

Figure 2-1 shows the position of leads I, II, III, aVR, aVL, and aVF in relation to the heart.

⬤ **augmented leads**
Leads that are automatically set to increase in size by 50 percent without any change in the configuration of the electrodes by the machine's property; leads aVL, aVR, and aVF

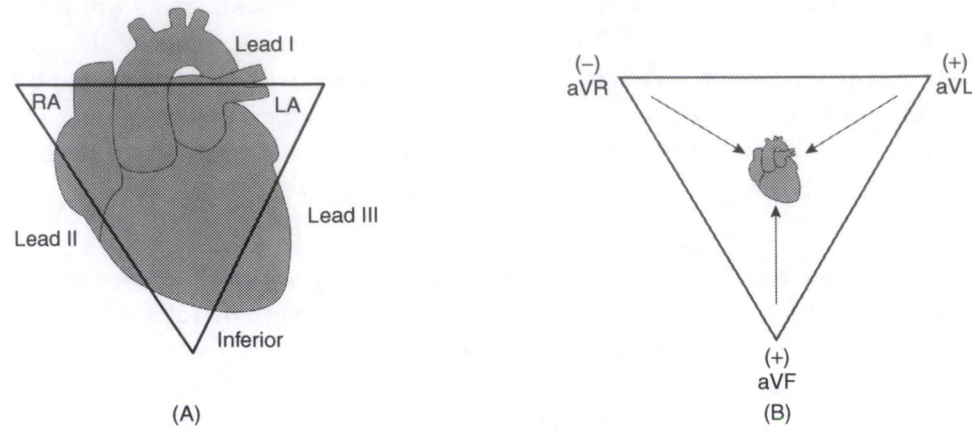

(A)

(B)

Figure 2-1 The surfaces of the heart are visualized from the point of view of the positive electrode in a specific lead. In (A), Limb leads I, II, and III are superimposed on the heart. (B) shows the augmented leads in relation to the heart's surface; note that leads II, III, and aVF face the inferior surface.

Precordial (Chest) Leads

🔵 **precordial leads**

Leads placed directly over the heart, on the anterior surface of the chest; also known as chest leads

🔵 **horizontal plane**

Plane perpendicular to the chest and frontal plane

The six **precordial leads**, also called *chest leads,* provide specific views of the heart's electrical activity. These leads are placed directly over the heart and encircle the precordium. The axes of the precordial leads lie in a **horizontal plane** perpendicular to the chest and to the frontal plane of the limb leads. The precordial leads are V_1 through V_6 and V_{1R} through V_{6R}. All precordial leads are unipolar. Proper and consistent placement of the precordial leads is essential for obtaining accurate ECG tracings. Serial ECG recordings are taken to determine the patient's progress, lack of progress, or change in the electrical conduction system. Consistent placement of the electrodes is critical to accurately determine trends in the patient.

Lead V_1 Lead V_1 is placed on the 4th intercostal space at the right sternal border. This lead provides a view of the anterior wall of the heart. V_1 will also display the activity of the intraventricular septum.

Lead V_2 Lead V_2 is placed on the 4th intercostal space at the left sternal border. This lead provides a view of the anterior wall of the heart. V_2 will also display the activity of the intraventricular septum.

Lead V_3 Lead V_3 is placed midway between V_2 and V_4. This lead monitors the activity occurring in the anterior surface of the heart.

Lead V_4 Lead V_4 is placed in the 5th intercostal space at the mid-clavicular line. This lead monitors the activity occurring on the anterior surface of the heart.

Lead V_5 Lead V_5 is placed on the 5th intercostal space (same level as V_4) at the left anterior axillary line. This lead monitors the left lateral wall of the heart.

Lead V₆ Lead V_6 is placed on the 5th intercostal space (same level as V_4) at the left mid-axillary line. This lead monitors the left lateral wall of the heart.

Lead V₁ᵣ Lead V_{1R} is placed on the 4th intercostal space at the left sternal border.

Lead V₂ᵣ Lead V_{2R} is placed on the 4th intercostal space at the right sternal border.

Lead V₃ᵣ Lead V_{3R} is placed midway between V_{2R} and V_{4R}.

Lead V₄ᵣ Lead V_{4R} is placed on the 5th intercostal space at the mid-clavicular line. This is the most useful of the right chest leads. It is used to assess patients for right ventricular wall involvement who present with inferior wall myocardial infarction.

Lead V₅ᵣ Lead V_{5R} is placed on the 5th intercostal space (same level as V_{4R}) at the right anterior axillary line.

Lead V₆ᵣ Lead V_{6R} is placed on the 5th intercostal space (same level as V_{4R}) at the right mid-axillary line.

Figure 2-2 illustrates the position of the electrodes for the precordial leads.

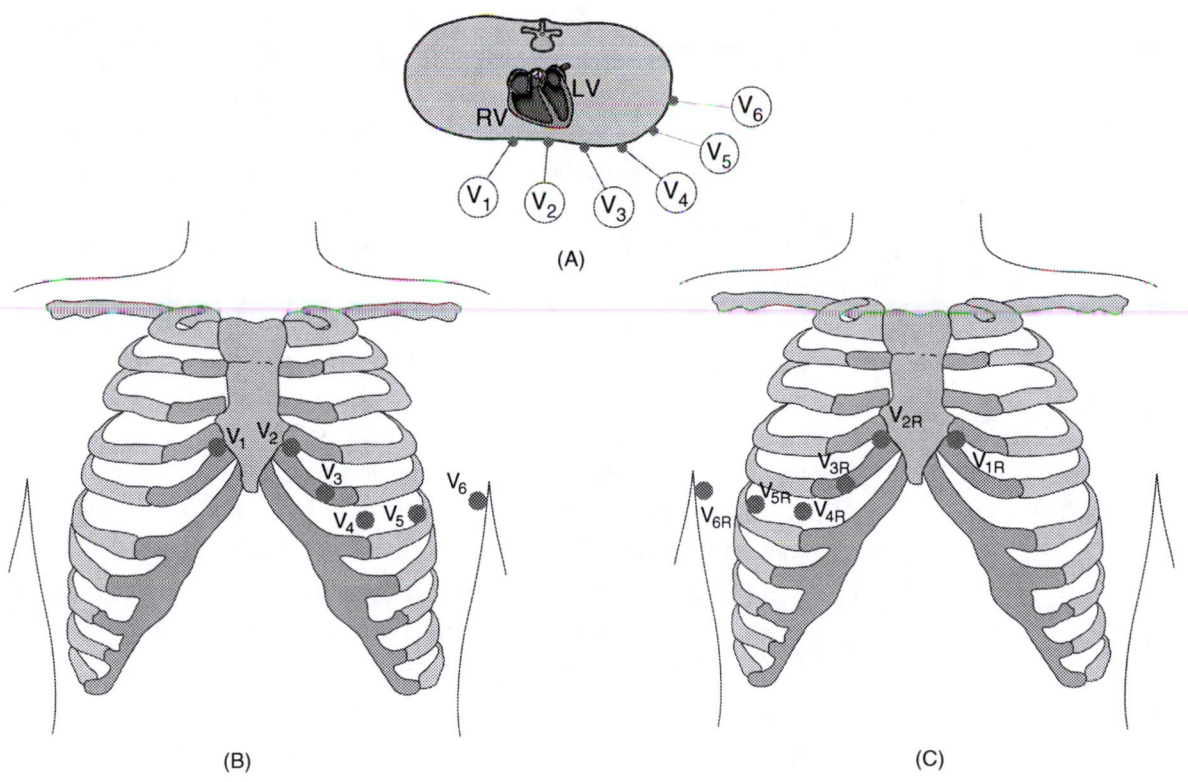

Figure 2-2 The placement of the precordial electrodes. (A) shows the precordial leads as they reflect the surface of the myocardium; (B) is the traditional left-sided placement of electrodes, and (C) is the placement of electrodes on the right side.

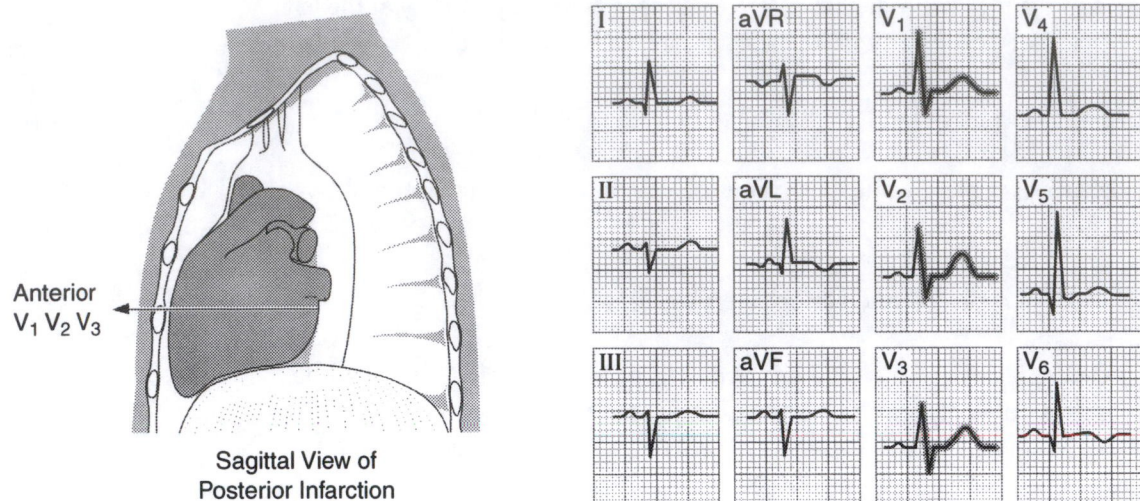

Figure 2-3 The position of the anterior precordial leads as they mirror the posterior surface of the heart. Leads V_1, V_2, and V_3 are more positive as they reflect depolarization away from the posterior surface in this patient with a posterior myocardial infarction.

Monitoring the Posterior Surface of the Heart

The posterior surface of the left ventricle lies in a plane parallel to the frontal plane. It is hidden from the precordial exploring electrodes by the anterior and septal surfaces. Infarctions of the posterior surface, usually by occlusion of the posterior descending coronary artery, may produce subtle ECG changes. Such damage will be primarily reflected in accentuation of depolarization forces over the anteroseptal surface, in V_1 to V_3, as a mirror image of the posterior surface. Figure 2-3 shows the position of anterior precordial leads as they mirror the changes in the posterior surface of the heart.

When assessing the precordial leads, the R waves become taller and the S waves become smaller as we move from right to left across the precordium. This is called **R-wave progression**. The precordial pattern can be summarized as follows:

- V_1 and V_2 depict an rS complex where a small R wave represents depolarization of the septum and right ventricle and the deeper S wave represents activation of the left ventricle. This is called the *right ventricular pattern*, because these leads lie over the surface of the right ventricle.

- V_3 and V_4 depict an RS complex. In these leads, the complex seems to be equiphasic; that is, the R and S waves are about equal in amplitude. This is called the *transition zone*.

- V_5 and V_6 depict a qR complex, in which a small q wave represents septal depolarization and the tall R wave represents ventricular activation. This is sometimes called the *left ventricular pattern*.

When the QRS complex does not become predominantly positive by lead V_4, or the R waves in V_1 and V_3 do not progressively increase in size, and transition is not seen until V_5 or V_6, this is called **poor R-wave progression**.

⬤ **R-wave progression**

The R waves become taller and the S waves become smaller as we move from right to left across the precordium

⬤ **poor R-wave progression**

The QRS complex does not become predominantly positive by lead V_4, or the R waves in V_1 and V_3 do not progressively increase in size, and transition is not seen until V_5 or V_6.

Early Transition occurs when the QRS complex becomes predominantly positive in V_1 or V_2. It can be a manifestation of posterior infarction or ventricular hypertrophy, or it may be simply a normal variant.

Reversed R-wave progression is possible with certain pathology (see Chapter 4). However, misplacement of the precordial leads can mimic reversed R-wave progression and cause confusion and misdiagnosis. Figure 2-4 illustrates the QRS complexes showing R-wave progression.

MCL Leads

MCL_1 is a popular bipolar chest lead that simulates V_1. In the 1960s Dr. Henry J. Marriott modified the placement of electrodes in the bipolar chest lead. He placed the positive electrode on the chest and the negative electrode on the left arm under the left clavicle. The modified chest lead in the V_1 position became known as *MCL_1*. Similarly, a positive electrode can be placed in the V_6 position for MCL_6.

The position of the electrodes for MCL_1 and MCL_6 is illustrated in Figure 2-5 and shows the position of the electrode at the right sternal border between the 4th and 5th intercostal spaces, the same as in precordial lead V_1. The negative electrode does not change from the original placement; recall it is indifferent in lead II, positive in lead I and now, negative in MCL_1. The lead selector must be adjusted to lead I. MCL_1 is a helpful tool in visualizing some wave forms, however, it should not be used as the sole differential in some tachycardias.

Hazards of Improper Lead Placement

Improper placement of leads can create misleading ECG patterns. The most common error is a switch between right arm and left arm leads. The resulting ECG mimics an anterolateral infarction pattern. Another common mistake, is switching right arm and left leg leads. The hazard here is that the resulting ECG tracing appears as characteristic of inferior wall myocardial infarction. Switching right arm and right leg leads creates diffuse, low voltage wave forms.

Summary

The standard ECG consists of 12 leads. Six leads—I, II, III, aVR, aVL and aVF—are the frontal plane leads, also called the limb leads. They provide information about the flow of current as it is directed toward the positive electrode in each lead.

Precordial, or chest leads, are the leads for the horizontal plane and provide information about the flow of current that is right, left, anterior, and posterior. The precordial leads extend from the right chest, at the sternal border from V_1 to the left midaxillary line. A mirror image of these leads on the right chest, from V_1 and extending to the right midaxillary line is the placement for right precordial leads.

The bipolar leads I, II, and III are common to many monitoring systems. The axes of these limb leads form a triangle about the heart. The axis for the unipolar limb leads—aVR, aVL, and aVF—are from the positive electrode on the limbs, aVR (right arm), aVL (left arm), and aVF (left leg). Some monitoring systems provide lead I or II in combination with a precordial lead, usually V_1.

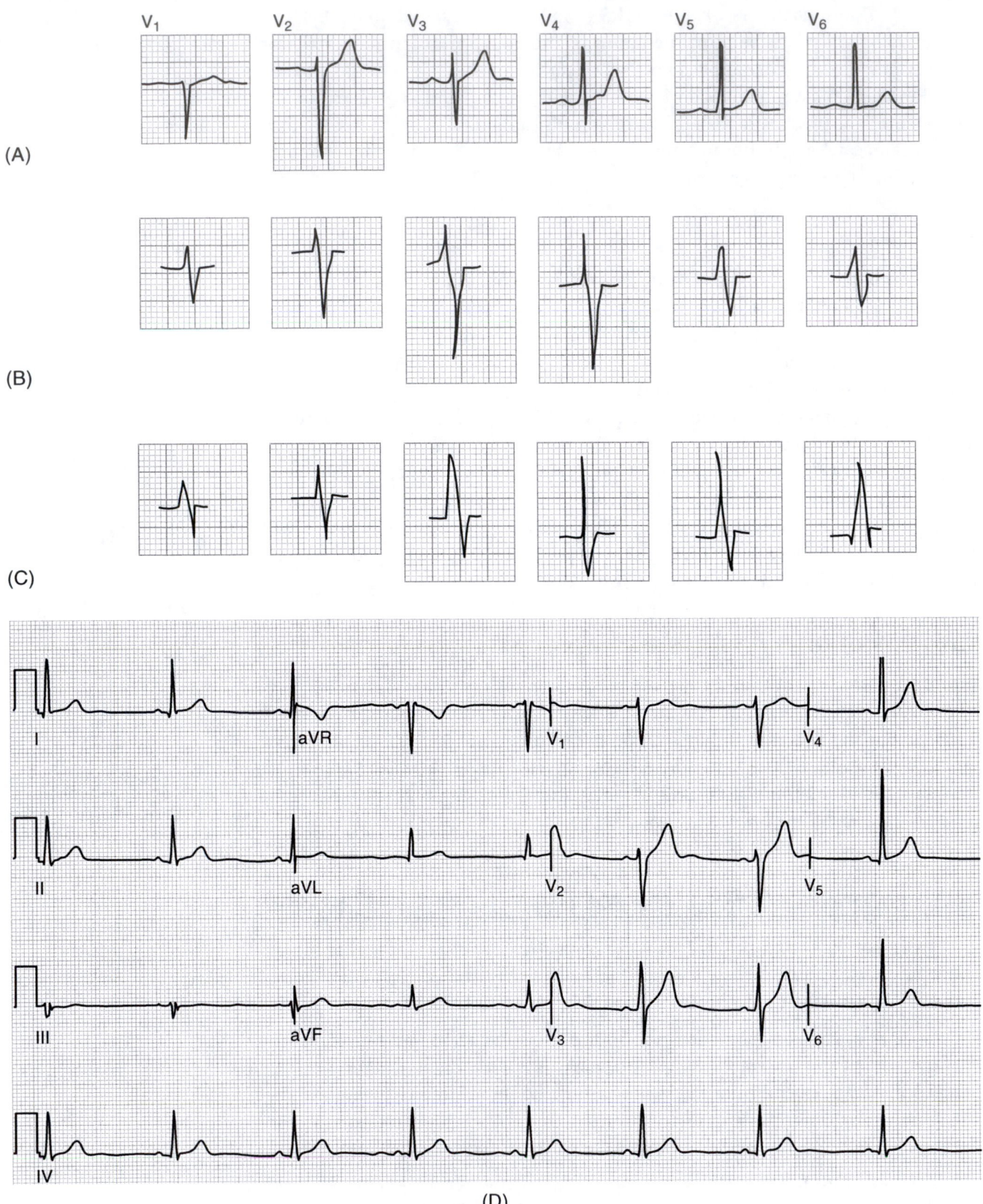

(A)

(B)

(C)

(D)

Figure 2-4 Illustrations of QRS complexes with (A) normal R-wave progression, (B) poor R-wave progression, note the transition occurred late in V_5 and V_6; (C) early transition seen in V_1 and V_2, and (D) a 12-lead ECG with normal R-wave progression.

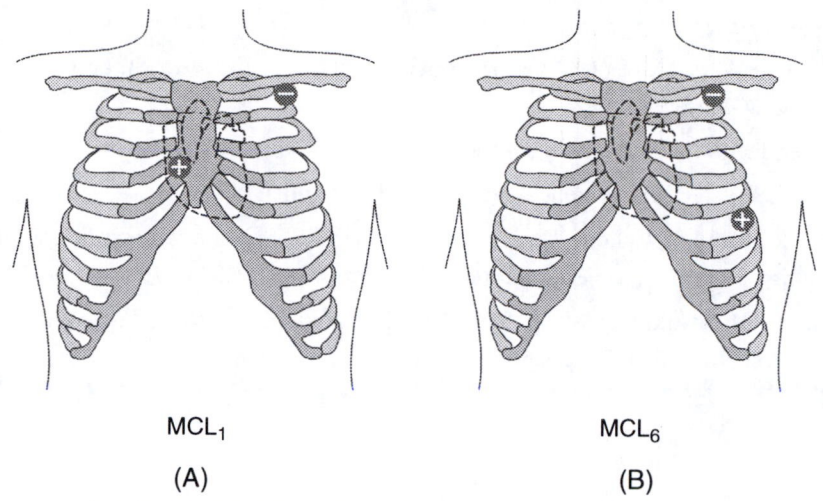

MCL₁ MCL₆

(A) (B)

Figure 2-5 The position of the electrodes for the MCL leads. (A) For MCL$_1$, the negative electrode is under the left clavicle, the positive at the level of V$_1$. (B) For MCL$_6$ the placement of the negative electrode is unchanged, and the exploring (+) electrode is in the V$_6$ position.

Proper lead placement is critical to accurate ECG interpretation. Each of the leads offers a perspective of the heart's electrical activity from the point of view of the positive electrode in that lead. No one lead is 100 percent demonstrative of the heart's electrical activity. The clinician must learn the surfaces of the heart as seen by each lead and the groupings that best provide information for analysis and diagnosis.

Self-Assessment Exercise

● Fill in the Blanks

Complete the statements and then compare your answer with those at the back of the book.

1. Lead I visualizes the _____.

2. Lead II visualizes the _____.

3. Lead III visualizes the _____.

4. Lead V$_1$ visualizes the _____.

5. Lead V$_2$ visualizes the _____.

6. Lead V$_3$ visualizes the _____.

7. Lead V$_4$ visualizes the _____.

8. Lead V$_5$ visualizes the _____.

9. Lead V$_6$ visualizes the _____.

References

Berne, R. M. & Levy, M. N. (1981). *Cardiovascular physiology* (4th ed.). St. Louis: C. V. Mosby.

Goldberger, E. (1982). *Textbook of clinical cardiology.* St. Louis: C. V. Mosby.

Topol, E. (1998). *Textbook of clinical cardiology.* Philadelphia: Lippincott-Raven.

Feola, M., Ribichini, F., Gallone, G., et al. (1994). Analysis of right electrocardiographic leads in 195 normal subjects. *Giorno Italian Cardiology,* 24:375-379.

Goldschlager, N. & Goldman, M. J. (1989). *Principles of clinical electrocardiography* (13th ed.). East Norwalk, CT: Appleton-Lange.

Rate, Rhythm, and Wave Forms

> **Premise** ◉ Estimating heart rate and evaluating duration and amplitude of wave forms are critical tasks in assessing the ECG. Clinicians need to understand wave forms as they relate to the cardiac cycle, and be able to identify abnormalities and recognize their implications.

Objectives

After reading the chapter and completing the Self-Assessment Exercises, the student should be able to

1. Calculate rate and rhythm
2. Identify the normal ECG wave forms, complexes, and their measurements.
3. Identify the changes in ECG measurements that may indicate electrolyte imbalance.
4. Identify the changes in the ECG that may occur with specific medications.
5. Identify clinical syndromes that cause alterations in the ECG.

Key Terms

bradycardia
delta wave
digitalis effect
hypercalcemia
hyperkalemia
isoelectric line
J point
low-voltage
nadir T wave
P mitrale
P pulmonale
P wave

pericardial effusion
pericarditis
PR interval
Q wave
QRS complex
QT interval
R wave
RR interval
S wave
ST segment
T wave
tachycardia
U wave

Introduction

Depolarization and repolarization are displayed on the ECG as wave forms and complexes that can be measured and assessed. A wave of depolarization that moves toward a positive electrode will record an upright deflection on the ECG, whereas a depolarization moving toward a negative electrode will record a negative deflection. When a wave of depolarization is moving perpendicular to the exploring electrode, a diphasic wave is recorded. The deflection of the wave of repolarization should be similar to that of depolarization. Because the heart is a three-dimensional structure, forces of depolarization must be viewed using multiple exploring electrodes that reconstruct the various dimensions of depolarization. Knowledge of ECG wave forms and the implications of the changes in those wave forms provide the basis for many patient care decisions; this is the exciting part of ECG analysis.

CALCULATING RATE AND RHYTHM

ECG monitors run at a standard rate and use paper with standard squares. Each small square is equal to 0.04 second. Each large square is made up of 5 small squares equal to 0.20 second. There are 5 large squares per second and 300 per minute. So, an ECG event occurring once every large square is occurring at a rate of 300 per minute.

Amplitude, or voltage, is measured on the vertical and each of the smallest blocks represents 0.1 millivolt (0.1 mV). The same small block measures height, with each block representing 1 millimeter (1 mm). Diagnostic ECG devices should be standardized so that 1 mV is equal to 10 mm. Figure 3-1 shows the large ECG square with the minimum units of measurement highlighted: 0.04 second, 1 mm, and 0.1 mV.

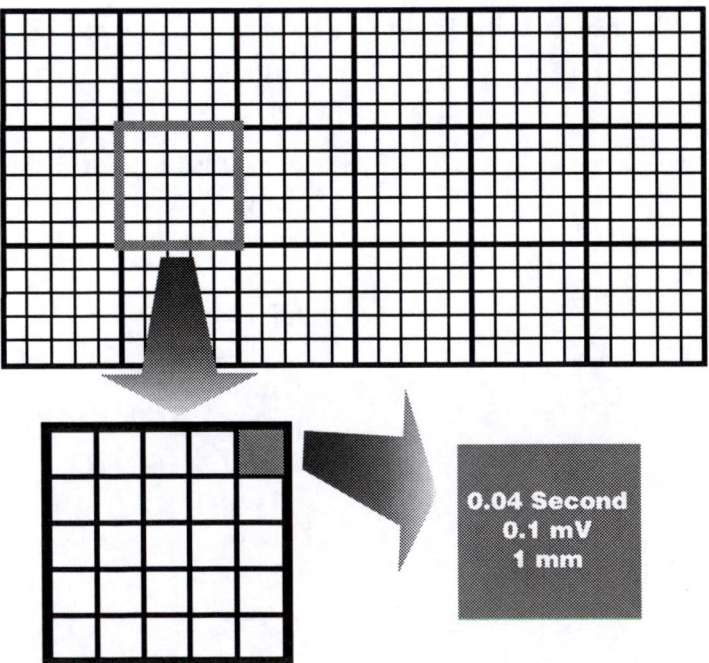

Figure 3-1 ECG monitoring paper with the blocks enlarged to illustrate the minimum units of measurement. The smallest of the blocks has 3 values: 0.04 second in duration (horizontal measurement); 0.1 mV in amplitude (vertical measurement), and 1 mm in height (also a vertical measurement).

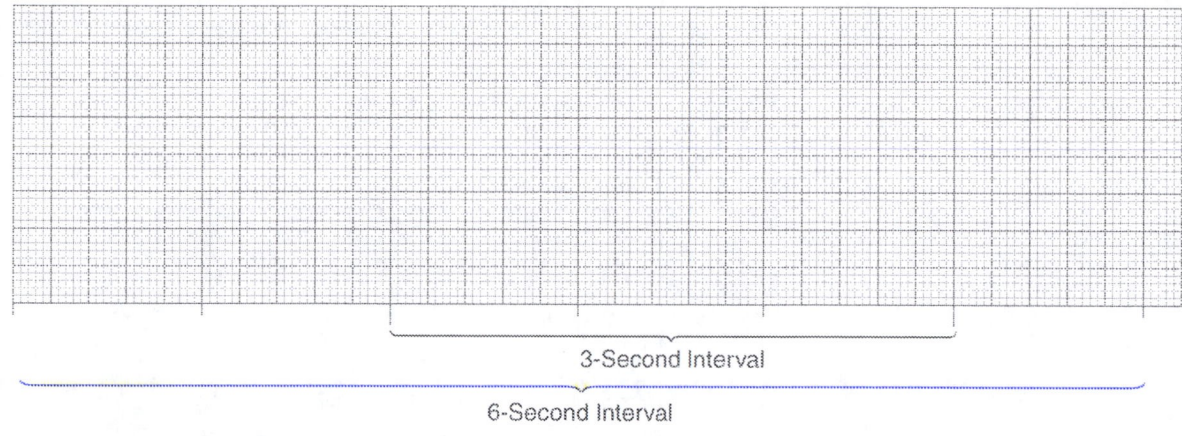

Figure 3-2 ECG monitoring paper showing markers indicating 3- and 6-second intervals. There are 15 blocks in 3 seconds, and 30 blocks in 6 seconds.

There are small vertical lines on the upper or lower margin of most ECG paper. There are 15 of the larger blocks between these margin lines; therefore they are placed 3 seconds apart—0.20 x 15 = 3 seconds and 0.20 x 30 = 6 seconds. In Figure 3-2, ECG paper shows the markers indicating 3- and 6-second intervals.

Time is measured on the electrocardiograph moving from left to right across the ECG paper. We use the ECG paper as a guide to calculate heart rate. When possible, use a QRS that is on a heavy line. First, count the number of large blocks between 2 consecutive QRS complexes, then divide that number into 300 to calculate the estimated heart rate. With very rapid rhythms, count the number of very small blocks and divide into 1,500. This method of calculation is shown in Figure 3-3 with ECG paper and an ECG rhythm. Table 3-1 and Table 3-2 provide guides for calculating rate.

Under normal conditions, the sinus node is the pacemaker for the heart. A heart rate that falls below 60 beats per minute is called sinus **bradycardia**. When heart rate increases to greater than 100 beats per minute, it is called sinus **tachycardia**.

bradycardia
Heart rate below 60 beats per minute

tachycardia
Heart rate greater than 100 beats per minute

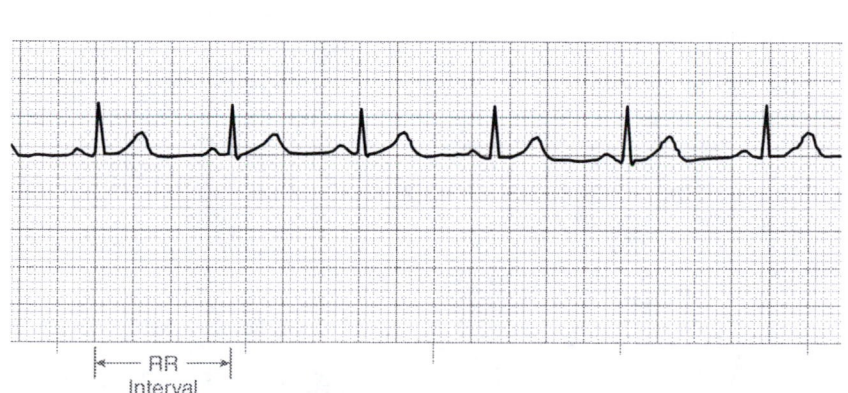

Figure 3-3 ECG recording with markers denoting the number of large squares (blocks) between the QRS complex (RR interval).

Table 3-1 Calculating heart rate by counting the numbers of large squares between 2 consecutive QRS complexes and dividing into 300.

Distance Between 2 QRS Complexes (No. of Large Boxes)	Estimated Rate per Minute
1	300
1-1/2	200
2	150
2-1/2	125
3	100
3-1/2	86
4	75
4-1/2	67
5	60
5-1/2	55
6	50
6-1/2	46
7	43
7-1/2	40
8	37
8-1/2	35
9	33
9-1/2	32
10	30
20	15

Table 3-2 Calculating heart rate by counting the numbers of small squares between 2 consecutive QRS complexes and dividing into 1,500.

Distance Between 2 QRS Complexes (No. of Small Boxes)	Estimated Rate per Minute
4	375
5	300
6	250
7	214
8	187
9	166
10	150
11	136
12	125
13	115
14	107
15	100
16	94
17	88
18	83
19	79
20	75

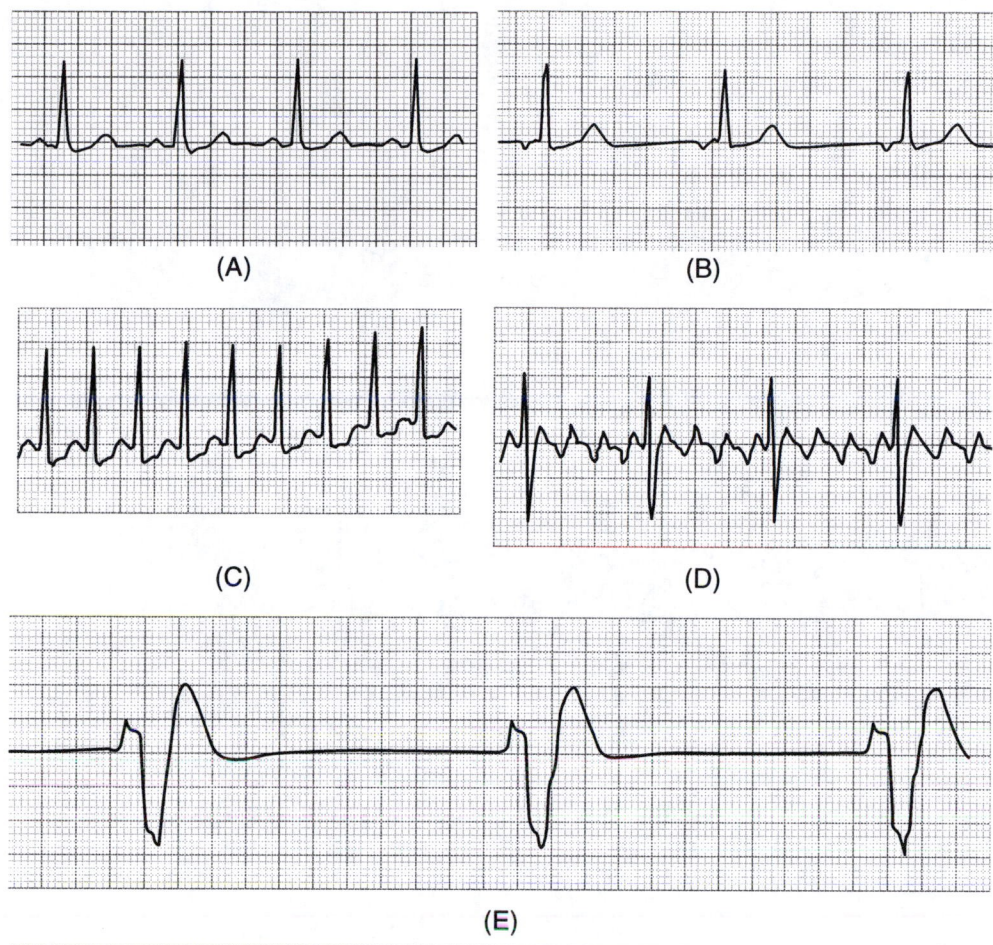

(A)

(B)

(C)

(D)

(E)

Figure 3-4 ECG tracings depicting regular rhythms: (A) shows the regular RR intervals with a sinus rhythm of 86 per minute; (B) shows a junctional rhythm of 55 per minute; (C) shows supraventricular tachycardia at 214 per minute; (D) shows an atrial flutter at 75 per minute; and (E) shows an idioventricular rhythm at 27 per minute.

Regular rhythms imply regular **RR intervals**—the period of time between two QRS complexes. A regular rhythm doesn't always mean normal sinus rhythm, however. Regular ectopic rhythms such as atrial tachycardia, some cases of atrial flutter, rhythms from the AV junction (junctional rhythm), or rhythms from a focus within the ventricles (idioventricular rhythm) may also produce a regular rhythm pattern. Figure 3-4 is an example of various rhythms that have equal RR intervals.

In the case of an irregular rhythm, the rate range should be calculated—first, the widest (slower) of the RR intervals, then the narrowest (faster) of the RR intervals. The calculated rate range is then reported. An irregular rhythm can be seen with sinus arrhythmia, atrial fibrillation, and in some cases of atrial flutter. Figure 3-5 depicts examples of irregular rhythms.

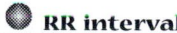 **RR interval**

The period of time between consecutive QRS complexes

WAVE FORMS, COMPLEXES, AND INTERVALS

The ECG tracing records the wave forms that represent various stages of myocardial depolarization and repolarization. The association of the wave forms to each other—assessing size, configuration, and duration—is the core of ECG analysis. The following is a brief review of the ECG wave forms and complexes.

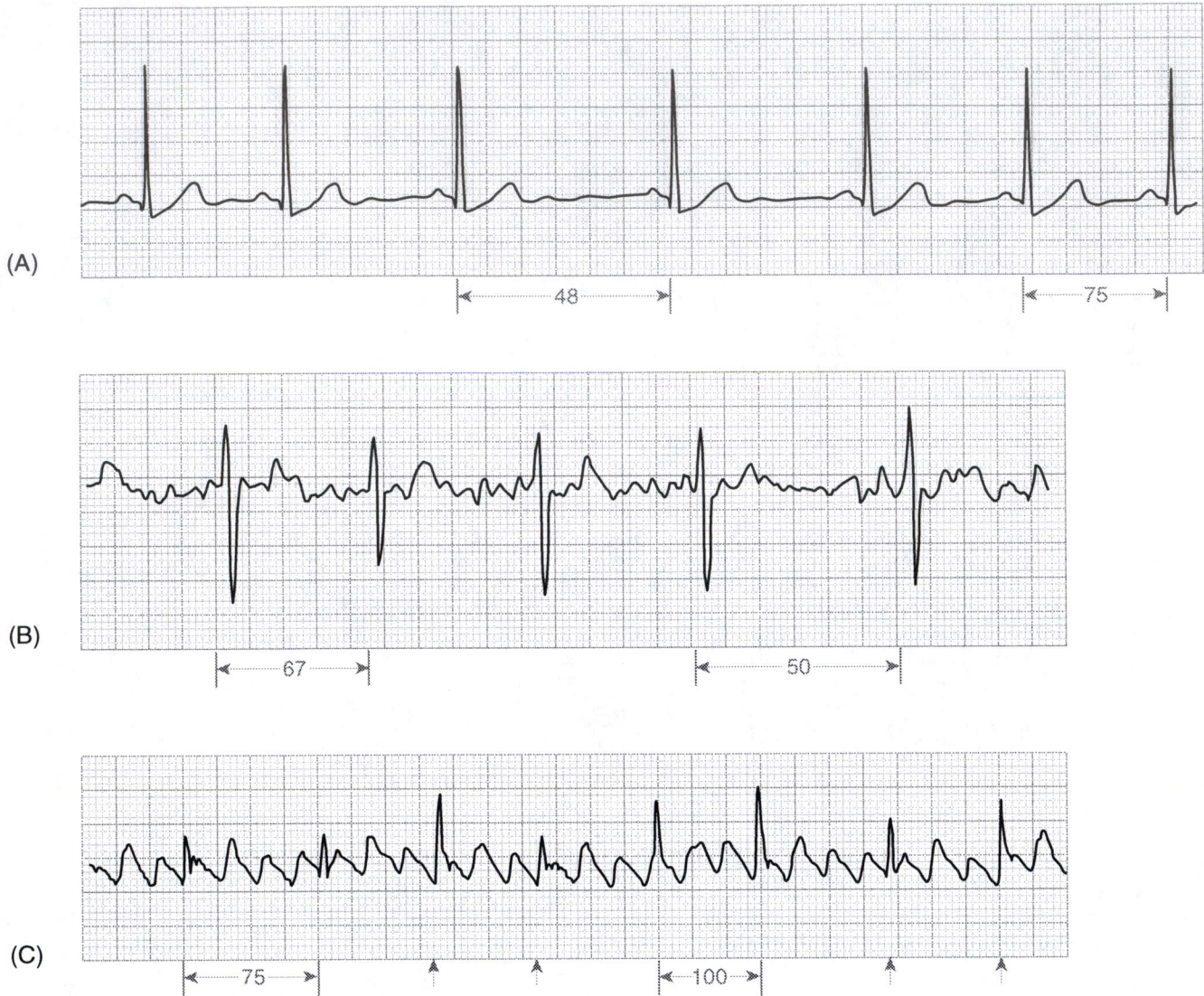

Figure 3-5 (A) is an example of an irregular rhythm. The ECG tracing shows sinus arrhythmia at 48-75 per minute. Calculate the widest and narrowest RR interval for the rate range. (B) shows atrial fibrillation with an irregular ventricular response of 50-67 per minute. (C) shows atrial flutter with an irregular ventricular response of 75-100 per minute.

P Waves

⬤ **P wave**

The wave form representing atrial depolarization; can be positive (+) when generated by a sinus and most atrial ectopic foci; is usually negative (-) when the atria are depolarized in a retrograde fashion from the AV junction

The **P wave** represents atrial depolarization. When the sinus node is in control, there should be a P wave for each and every QRS complex. The shape, duration, and amplitude of the P waves should be noted. The P wave usually measures 0.08 second and no more than 0.02 to 0.03 millivolts (mV) in amplitude.

Typically, sinus P waves do not plot through an ectopic from atrial tissue, since premature atrial depolarization will reset the sinus cadence. This is called a premature atrial complex (PAC). Sinus P waves usually plot through a premature ventricular ectopic complex (PVC) unless there is concealed retrograde atrial conduction. Figure 3-6 provides examples of premature complexes and the resulting changes in configuration and rate.

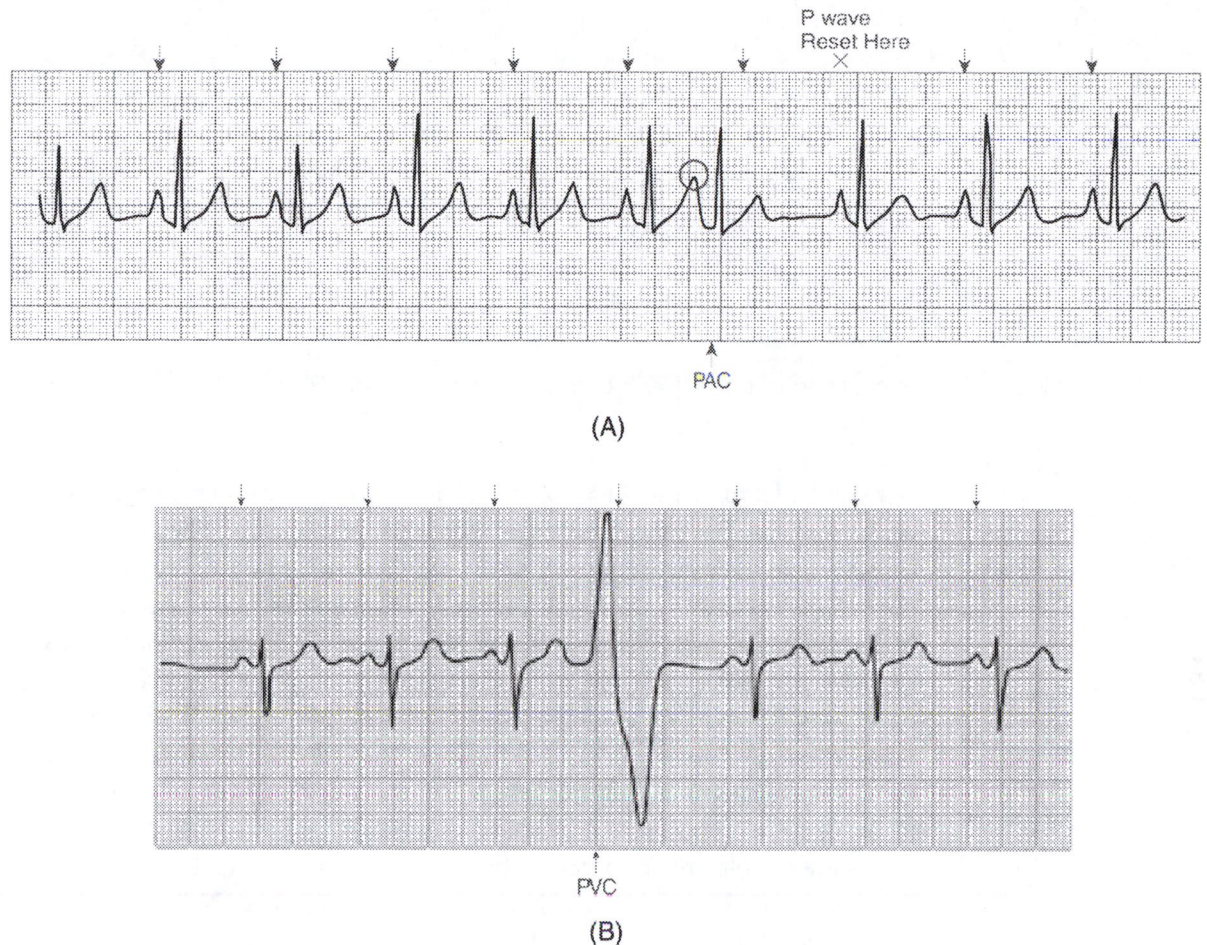

Figure 3-6 (A) is an example of a PAC (arrow). Plotting P waves through the PAC demonstrates the change in sinus cadence. (B) is an example of a PVC (arrow). Plotting P waves through the PVC shows no change in sinus cadence.

PR Interval

The **PR interval** represents the time the impulse initiated by the sinus node travels through the atria to the ventricular conduction system. The PR interval is measured from the beginning of the P wave to the beginning of the QRS complex. A normal PR interval ranges from 0.12 to 0.20 second. The PR interval may vary with heart rate, age, and the patient's physique. There are instances where the PR interval is inversely related to heart rate; in other words, the faster the heart rate, the shorter the PR interval. If a PR interval is greater than 0.20 second, look carefully to determine if there is a distortion to the P wave or if the PR segment is prolonged. Figure 3-7 provided ECG examples of the PR interval.

QRS COMPLEX

The **QRS complex** represents the ventricular depolarization. It can be comprised of any combination of 1, 2, or 3 wave forms. The **Q wave** is the first downward, or neg-

● PR interval
Period of time from the beginning of atrial depolarization (P wave) to ventricular activation (the QRS)

● QRS complex
That portion of cardiac cycle corresponding to depolarization of the ventricles; made of any combination of the Q, R, and S wave forms

● Q wave
Initial negative deflection of the QRS complex shown on the ECG. Q waves are considered pathologic when they they are new to the patient, and/or greater than 0.04 second.

PR Interval

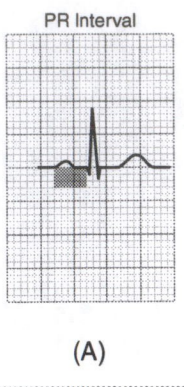

(A)

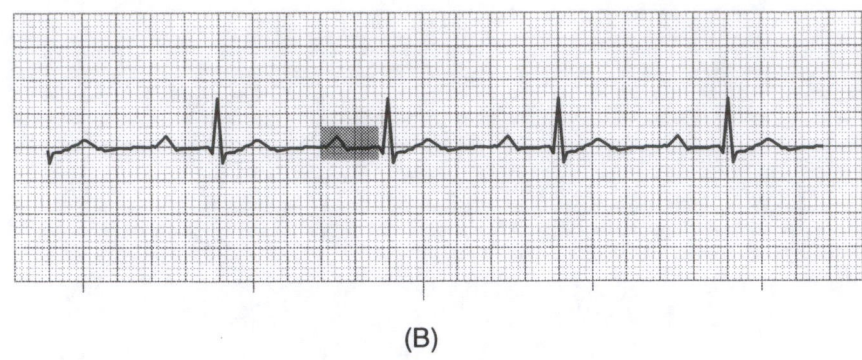

(B)

Figure 3-7 (A) shows a PR interval of normal duration, while (B) shows a prolonged PR interval.

⬤ **R wave**

The first positive deflection of the QRS complex shown on the ECG

⬤ **S wave**

The last negative deflection of the QRS complex shown on the ECG; represents completion of ventricular depolarization; usually less than 0.04 second in duration and less than 5 mm in depth

ative, wave form of the QRS complex. The **R wave** is the first positive, or upward, deflection. The R wave can occur with or without a Q wave. The next negative wave form is a downward deflection called the **S wave**. Multiple positive or negative deflections that follow the Q wave are called R prime (R′) or S prime (S′) respectively. Regardless of morphology—that is, whether a QRS, QR, R, RS, or QS is depicted—the complex is referred to as the QRS. Uppercase letters are usually used to denote a QRS complex. A mix of upper and lowercase letters is used to describe the relative size of the wave forms that make up the QRS; for instance, when describing the QRS complex as it is affected by fascicular conduction defects. (See Chapter 1 for more detail.) Larger wave forms are denoted by uppercase letters, smaller wave forms are denoted by lowercase letters. Therefore, rS means there is a small R wave in relation to the deep (greater than 5 mm) S wave. Figure 3-8 illustrates the relative size of wave forms and the use of upper and lowercase letters.

The normal duration of a QRS complex is about 0.10 second. There are wide limits to the amplitude of the QRS, but it generally ranges from 5 mm or the 0.5 mV to 15 mm or 1.5 mV depending on the lead. The duration of the Q wave should not exceed 0.04 second and the depth should be less than 5 mm. Q waves are not normally present in all leads; however, small Q waves can be normal in Leads I, aVL, aVF, V_5 and V_6. Once Q waves are seen, the challenge is to determine how recently they have appeared. If Q waves are new or just evolving in the patient, the clinical presentation and/or patient history will assist in the diagnosis of infarction.

The height of an R wave is usually proportional to the percentage of the heart's depolarization that occurs toward a given lead. The depth of an S wave represents the portion of depolarization that moves away from the positive electrode in a given lead.

ST Segment

⬤ **ST segment**

The line between the QRS and the T wave that represents early ventricular repolarization

⬤ **J point**

The point where the QRS ends

⬤ **isoelectric line**

Flat ECG line found between wave forms or cycles; for example, between the T wave and the next wave

The **ST segment** represents the window between ventricular depolarization and repolarization. The ST segment is an extremely sensitive visualization tool. If there are ischemic or injury processes within the heart, they will be seen in the ST segment in the lead facing the affected area.

The ST segment extends from the end of the QRS (the **J point**) to the beginning of the T wave. The ST segment is normally at baseline, that is, at the **isoelectric line**. One way to estimate deviation from the baseline is to draw a line from the PR segment, extending it through the T wave.

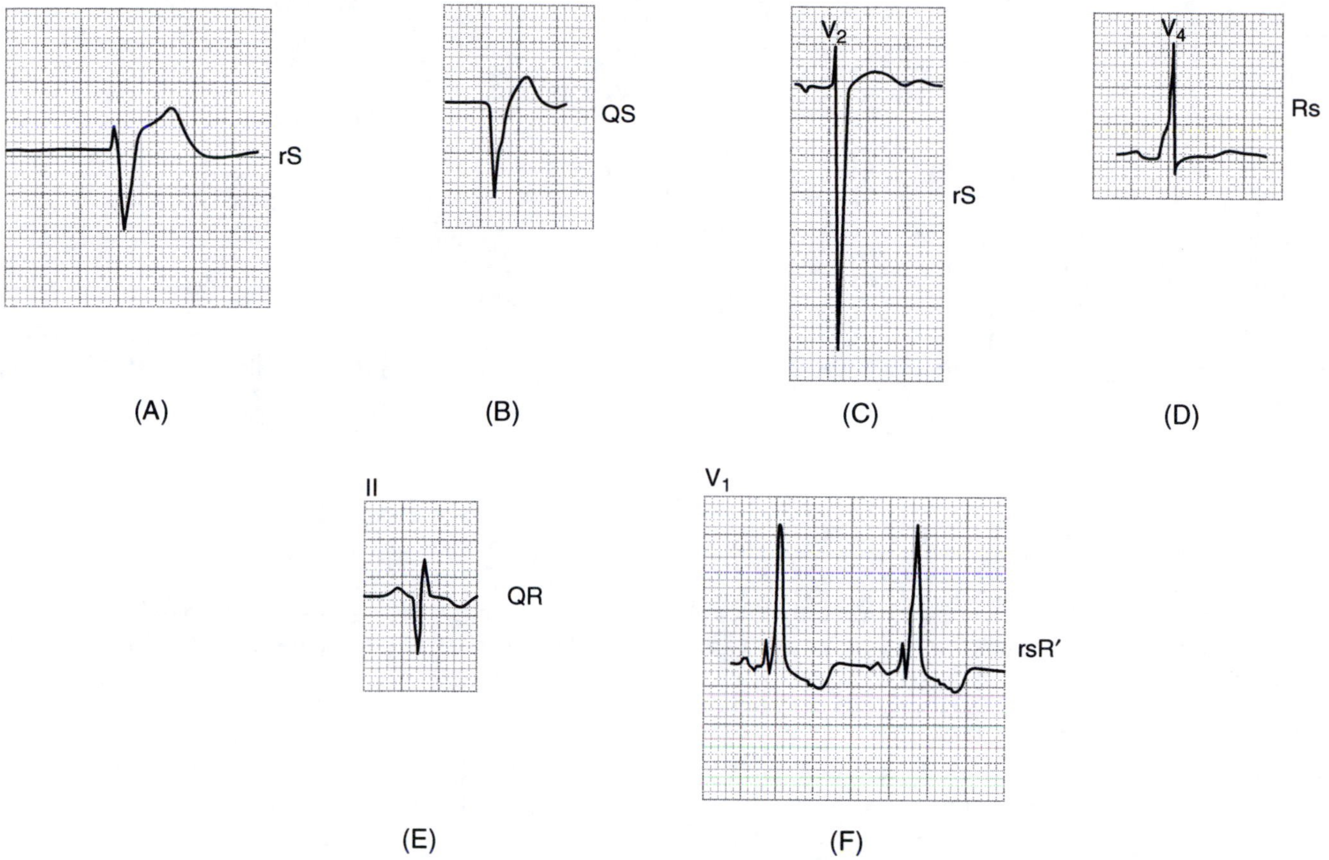

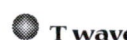

Figure 3-8 Upper and lowercase letters are used to describe the variations in sizes of the wave forms in QRS complexes. (A) an rS complex; (B) a QS complex; (C) an rS complex; (D) an Rs complex; (E) a QR complex; (F) an rsR' composite of the QRS complex.

The ST segment may be elevated or depressed with myocardial injury, ischemia, ventricular aneurysm, and with some medications. A normal ST segment may be elevated (above the baseline) for 1 to 2 mm, however, elevation greater than 1 mm in a symptomatic patient with chest pain is highly suspicious of hypoxia, ischemia, or injury in the myocardial surface exhibited by the lead facing that surface.

The J point and ST segment may be elevated up to 2 mm in the precordial leads in normal persons. ST segment elevation greater than 4 mm in the lateral precordial leads is rarely considered normal. During exertion a normal person's ST segments will become isoelectric. ST segment elevation seen in normal persons represents early repolarization of a portion of the ventricular myocardium. Figure 3-9 provides an example of ST segments. A straight or horizontal ST segment above or below the baseline is highly suggestive of ischemia. Significant changes also occur with the ST segments in hypothermia.

T Wave

The **T wave** represents ventricular repolarization. Usually a normal T wave is rather asymmetrical and low in amplitude, not exceeding 5 mm in the limb leads or 10 mm

⬤ **T wave**

The wave form corresponding to ventricular repolarization

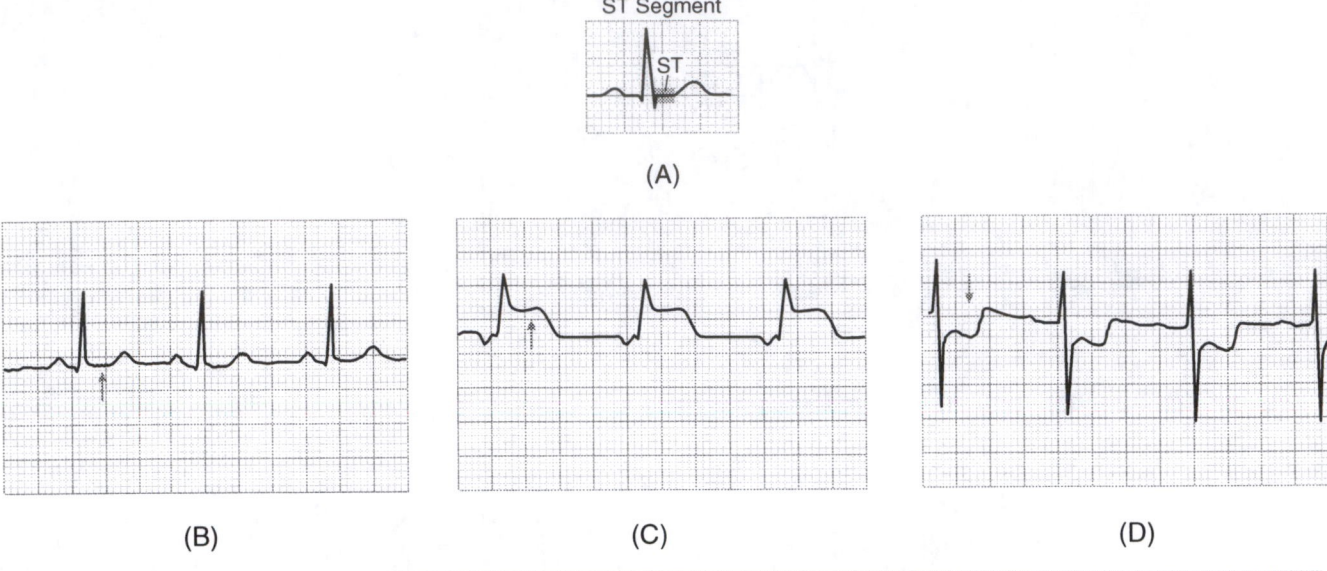

Figure 3-9 (A) is an ST segment at baseline highlighted within a cardiac cycle. Note the variations in the ST segments in (B), which is normal at baseline; (C)which has a 3 mm ST segment elevation; and (D), which has a 3 mm ST segment depression.

● **nadir T waves**

Symmetrical, negative T waves, greater than 5 mm in depth; considered to be an acute sign with a high degree of suspicion of coronary artery deficit

● **QT interval**

The period from start of the QRS complex until the end of the T wave; the time from ventricular depolarization to repolarization

in the precordial leads. T wave inversion greater than 5 mm and symmetrical is termed a **nadir T wave**, which can be an acute sign often indicating ischemia and/or injury. Figure 3-10 is an illustration of variations in the T wave.

QT Interval

The **QT interval** indicates the time from ventricular depolarization to repolarization. It is measured from the beginning of the QRS to the end of the T wave. The duration of the QT interval will vary depending on several factors including heart rate, gender, age, disease, obesity, and medications.

It is sometimes difficult to accurately measure the QT interval where there are low-amplitude T waves. Sometimes T waves will merge with subsequent isoelectric lines or with U waves. Several leads should be compared. The longest clearly visi-

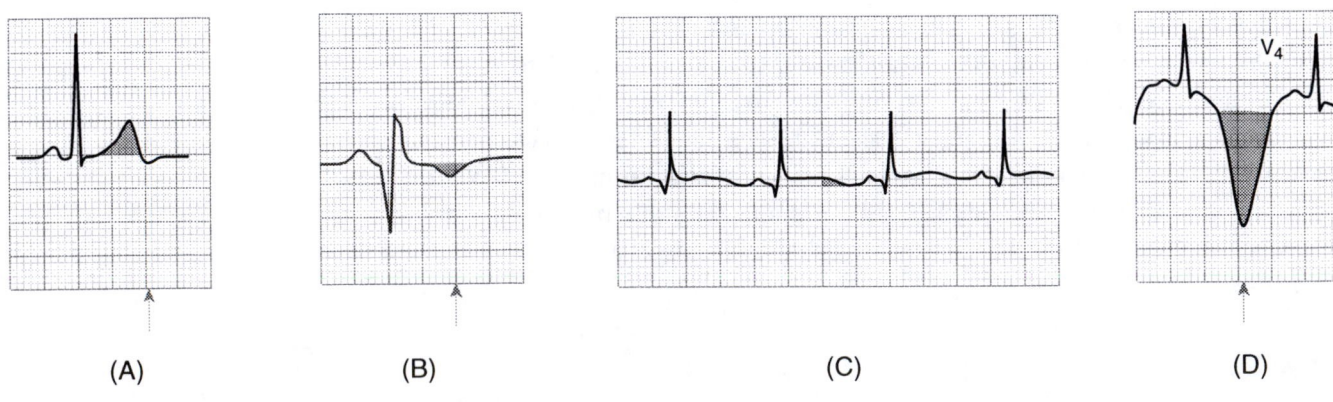

Figure 3-10 The normal PQRST complex, (A) highlighting the normal T wave; (B) highlighting T wave inversion; (C) highlighting flattened T waves; and (D) highlighting a nadir T wave.

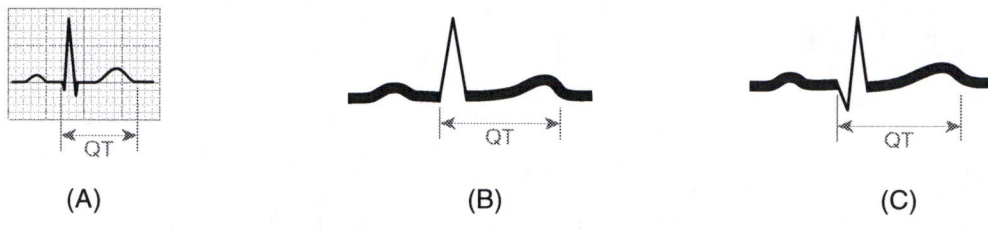

(A) (B) (C)

Figure 3-11 (A) The QT interval highlighted within the cardiac complex; (B) and (C) show the measurement of the QT interval based on the wave forms that make up the QRS complex.

ble QT interval should be the measurement reported. QT intervals should not exceed 50 percent of the RR interval. The importance of measuring a QT interval is to determine whether it is prolonged. A prolonged QT interval reflects an extended period of ventricular vulnerability to life-threatening arrhythmias. Figure 3-11 illustrates the measurements of the QT interval.

U Wave

There are many theories about the generation and importance of **U waves**. One is that they represent recovery of the Purkinje system or repolarization of papillary muscles. Recent electrophysiologic studies suggest that U waves represent repolarization of a population of subepicardial cells with unique activation properties. Conditions that favor U waves occurring include electrolyte abnormalities, left ventricular hypertrophy, and myocardial ischemia. When visible, U waves are recognized in leads V_2 and V_3.

It is not necessary to see U waves in all leads. Prominent U waves are frequently seen in patients with hypokalemia, with slow heart rates, and in patients who are taking certain medications including digitalis and beta-blockers. Generally U waves are the same polarity as the preceding T wave. A negative U wave following a positive T wave may be indicative of myocardial ischemia. Figure 3-12 illustrates the wave forms of the cardiac complex showing P wave, QRS complex, ST segment, and T and U waves. Table 3-3 provides a summary of the various wave forms and their characteristics.

ABNORMAL WAVE FORMS

Abnormal P Waves

A peaked P wave may indicate enlargement of the right atrium (RAE). This pattern is sometimes called **P pulmonale** because it is often associated with conditions such as pulmonary stenosis, pulmonary hypertension, hypertensive heart disease, and chronic obstructive pulmonary disease (COPD). P pulmonale is most evident in lead II.

Notching of a P wave in lead II may indicate left atrial enlargement (LAE). This is sometimes referred to as **P mitrale** because it is often associated with disease of the mitral valve such as mitral stenosis. In V_1, notching of the P waves and a negative

⬤ **U wave**

An ECG wave sometimes observed following the T wave; thought to be related to late repolarization of the ventricles

⬤ **P pulmonale**

Peaked abnormal P waves

⬤ **P mitrale**

Notched abnormal P waves

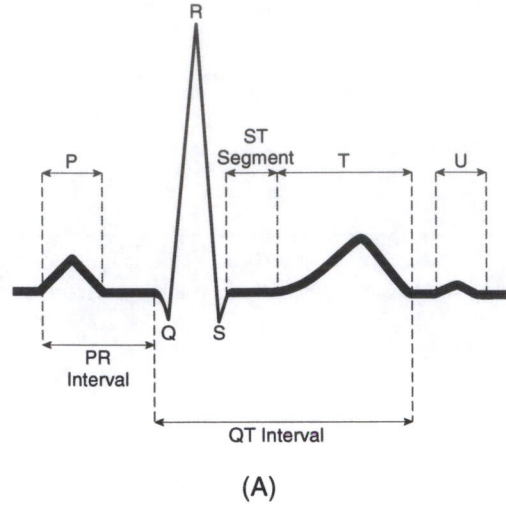

(A)

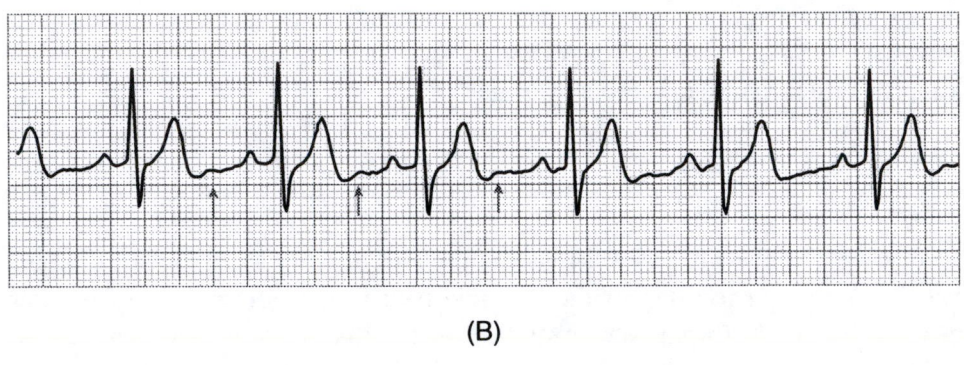

(B)

Figure 3-12 (A) Wave forms showing P wave, QRS complex, ST segment, T and U waves; (B) is an ECG tracing of a sinus rhythm with U waves (arrow).

deflection in the terminal part of the P wave deeper than 1 mm and lasting longer than 0.04 second may indicate LAE. The LAE pattern is particularly common in mitral regurgitation and certain myocardial lesions. LAE is also commonly seen with hypertensive heart disease. Figure 3-13 illustrates the variation in P waves.

Abnormal PR Interval

A PR interval longer than 0.20 second can be a normal variation or an effect of drugs such as digitalis, certain calcium channel blockers, and some antiarrhythmic medications. It is also commonly associated with aging, and may be the first indicator of underlying conduction system disease.

A shortened PR interval (less than 0.12 second) may be a normal variant of preexcitation or may occur when the electrical complex is promulgated along accessory tracts. Rhythms that originate in the high AV junction will have an inverted P wave prior to the QRS with a PR interval less than 0.12 second. Figure 3-14 illustrates the variations in the PR interval.

Table 3-3 Summary of ECG Wave Forms and Measurements

P Wave

- Represents atrial depolarization
- Measures 0.08 second and 2 to 3 mm in amplitude
- Shape is usually symmetrical and upright
- May be notched in appearance
- P' (P prime) indicates atrial depolarization from an atrial or junctional source.

PR Interval

- Total supraventricular activity; activation of the His-Purkinje system
- Measures 0.12 to 0.20 second
- PR segment represents AV nodal delay and measures about 0.12 second

QRS Complex

- Represents ventricular depolarization
- When supraventricular in origin, it is less than or equal to 0.10 second and 1 to 1.5

    mV in amplitude
- When ventricular in origin, it usually measures greater than 0.10 second and the amplitude is often greater than the normal QRS, and the QRS will be opposite in direction from the T wave

ST Segment

- Represents early ventricular repolarization
- Measures less than or equal to 0.12 second and may be angular, depressed, or elevated
- Deviations may reflect ischemia

T Wave

- Represents completed ventricular repolarization
- Measures less than or equal to 0.12 second and 5 to 6 mm
- May be positive or negative
- Rarely distorted or notched (Atrial repolarization may distort the T wave; this is referred to as *Ta distortion* where "T" means repolarization and "a" denotes the atria.
- Asymmetrical

QT Interval

- Total ventricular activity, 0.24 to 0.38 second
- Affected by ventricular rate and certain medications and electrolytes

U Wave

- Positive or negative deflection following the QRS
- Most often flat and unseen

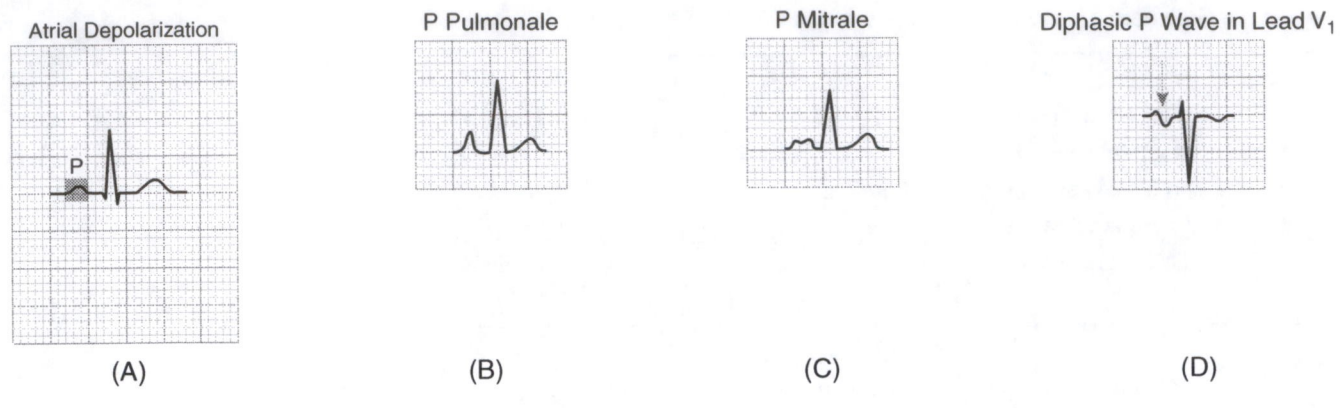

Figure 3-13 Normal and abnormal P waves: (A) normal P Wave, (B) peaked P wave called P pulmonale; (C) notched P wave called P mitrale; (D) diphasic P wave.

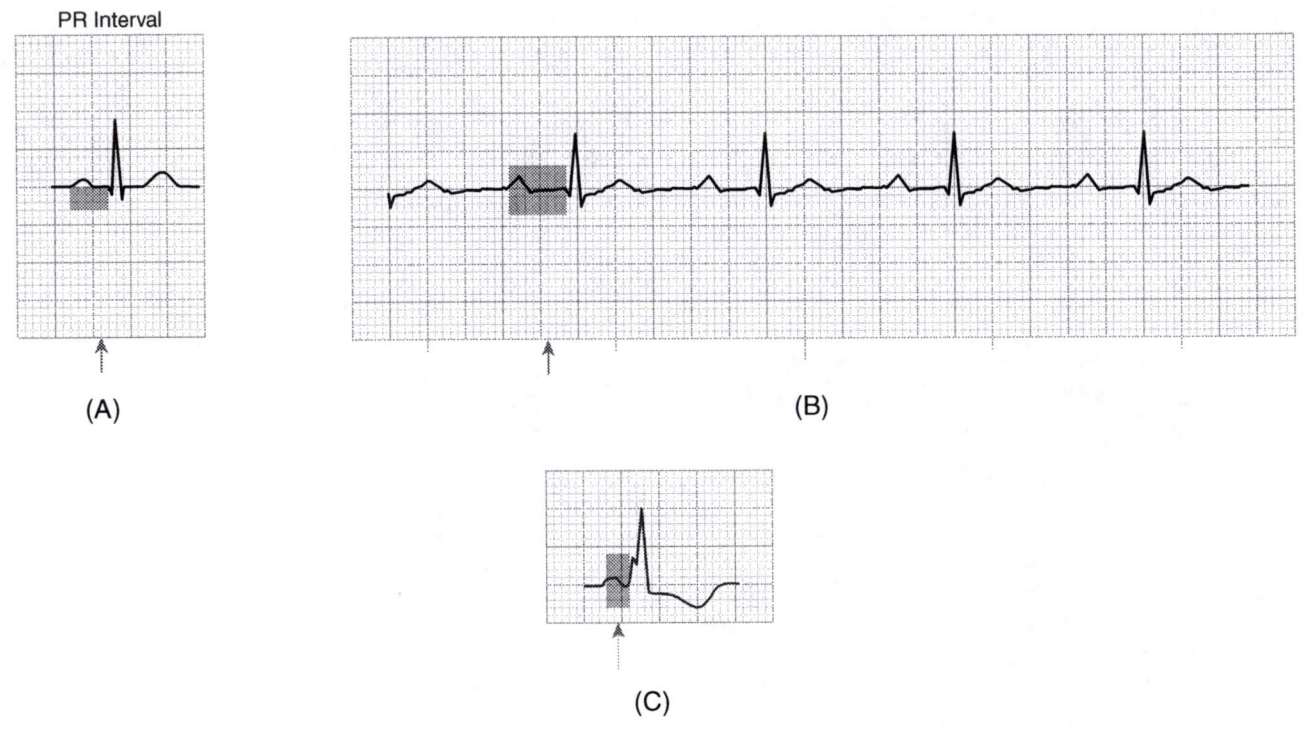

Figure 3-14 (A) Normal PQRST complex with a PR interval of normal duration; (B) a PR interval greater than 0.20 second; and (C) a PR interval less than 0.12 second.

Abnormal QRS Complexes

QRS complexes greater than 0.10 second may indicate abnormal intraventricular conduction. Prolongation itself is not the definitive diagnosis of the defect. Change in the amplitude of the QRS coupled with prolongation of the QRS duration may indicate abnormalities and specific fascicles of the ventricular conduction system. For instance, if the left anterior fascicle is obliterated or delayed, ventricular depolarization will be seen on the ECG as a small R and deep S waves, noted as an rS complex. (These are discussed in detail in Chapter 7.)

When the QRS bulges on the upslope or on the downslope it is said to be *slurred*. Slurring of the QRS can occur with abnormal ventricular conduction or if there is conduction using an accessory pathway. Notching of the QRS can occur with no evidence of pathology, however, notching is uncharacteristic and therefore suspicious of intraventricular conduction defects when the duration is greater than 0.10 second. Consequently, there are two items to look for; if the QRS is greater than 0.10 second and if the QRS complex has an uncharacteristic jagged look. These two conditions together may indicate a problem with intraventricular conduction. Again, the duration is the first and most important consideration.

Delta waves makes the QRS appear slurred. When this occurs, they represent preexcitation of the ventricle using an accessory atrioventricular pathway. The QRS takes on a more rounded shape and is usually associated with a short PR interval. A delta wave does not have to be visible in all leads. Figure 3-15 illustrates the variations of the QRS complex.

● **delta wave**

Initial slurring of the QRS complex

Abnormal QT Interval

A prolonged QT interval (greater than 0.38 second) indicates a delay in ventricular repolarization caused by the ST segment and T waves. Prolongation of the QT interval is a predictor of cardiovascular mortality even in the absence of overt heart disease. Prolonged QT intervals may be caused by:

- hypertrophic cardiomyopathy
- hypocalcemia
- hypokalemia
- hypothermia
- cerebral hemorrhage
- myocardial ischemia or infarction
- congenital
- medications
- obesity

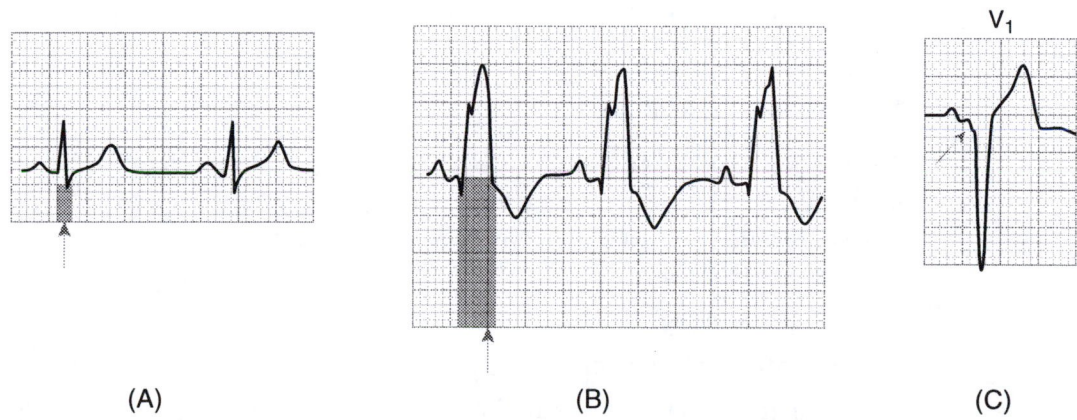

(A) (B) (C)

Figure 3-15 Variations in the QRS complex: (A) a normal QRS complex; (B) wide-notched QRS complex; and (C) slurring of the QRS complex, called a delta wave.

Prolongation of the QT interval is a potentially dangerous side effect of many antiarrhythmic medications. The antibiotics, erythromycin and ketoconazole, the antihistamine agents, astemizole and terfenadine, the phenothiazines, and terodiline,(a drug used to treat incontinence) have been associated with prolonged QT and QT intervals, Torsades de Pointes and sudden death. Prolongation of the QT interval can occur suddenly. The autonomic dysfunction that occurs commonly in diabetics and alcoholics may show up as prolonged QT intervals. Shortening of the QT interval is caused by hypercalcemia and hyperkalemia. Figure 3-16 illustrates normal and abnormal QT intervals.

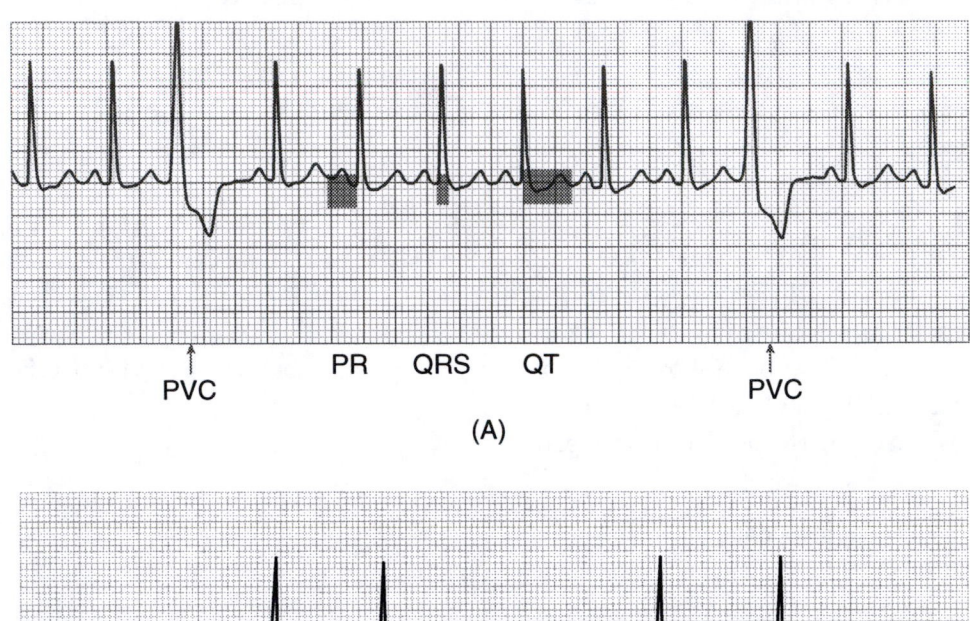

Figure 3-16 (A) normal QT interval; (B) prolonged QT intervals

Abnormal U Waves

U waves should be the same polarity as the preceding T waves. Negative U waves that follow positive T waves suggest ischemia and/or ventricular hypertrophy. Enlarged U waves (greater than 1 mm in amplitude) may be caused by:

- hypercalcemia
- hypokalemia
- intracranial hemorrhage
- left ventricular hypertrophy
- physical exercise

Figure 3-17 is a 12-lead ECG depicting U waves.

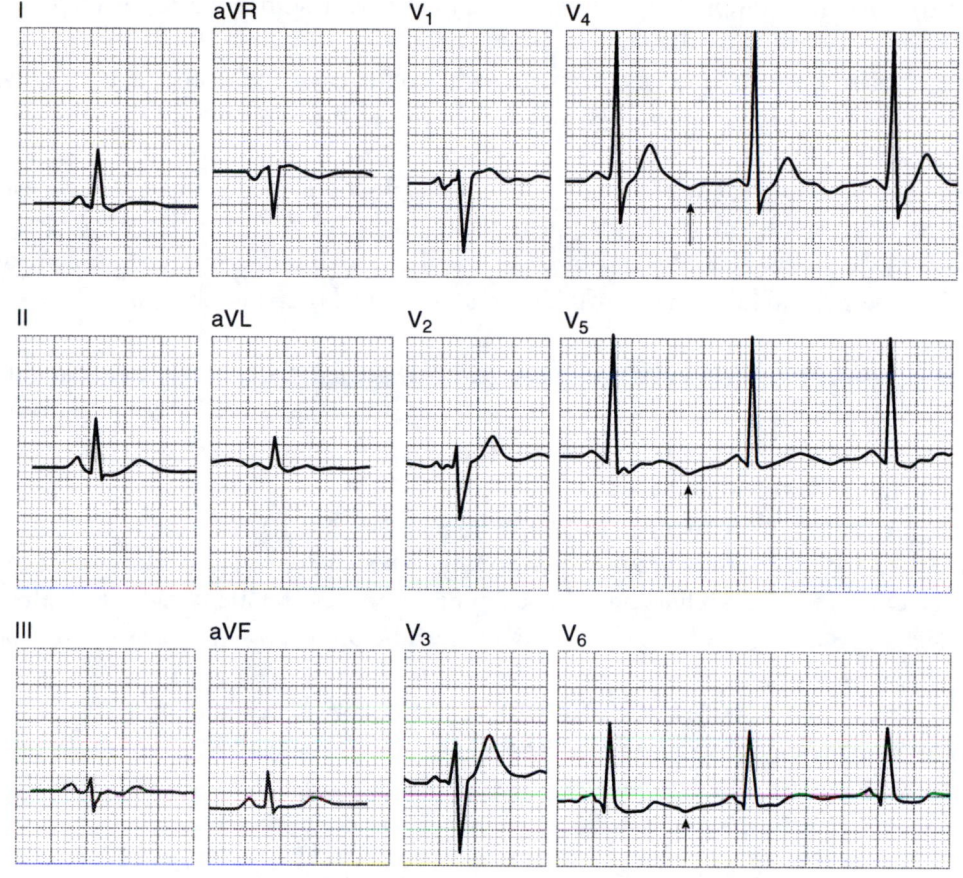

Figure 3-17 A 12-lead ECG where U waves are more obvious in some leads than others. Negative U waves are evident in V_4 through V_6. (Adapted from *Principles of Clinical Electrocardiography* by N. Goldschlager and M.J. Goldman, 1989, Stamford, CT: Appleton and Lange.)

ALTERATIONS OF ECG WAVE FORMS

Electrolyte imbalance and numerous medications can influence the heart's electrical function, causing changes in duration and amplitude of ECG wave forms. Similarly, ST segment elevation, depressing, and coving can be induced by medications and certain pathological conditions. The clinician does well to recognize the changes, but clinical correlation is critical. The following section discusses the changes that occur with electrolyte imbalance, cardiac medications and certain clinical diseases.

Drug-Induced Changes on the ECG

Many medications can affect the ECG wave forms. While most are nonspecific, many antiarrhythmic medications produce distinct changes on the ECG wave forms and measurement. Also, as characteristic as the variations are, they may not be present in all ECG leads.

Antiarrhythmic medications can cause a prolongation of ventricular repolarization, which extends the QT interval. The ST segment of the QT interval usually lengthens first. In later stages, with persistent ingestion of the drugs, ventricular depolarization will be prolonged and the QRS complex will increase beyond 0.10

second. There is no predictable incremental increase in either the ST or the QRS. The increases may be subtle but persistent, or sudden and dramatic. These changes may herald the development of polymorphic ventricular tachycardia, specifically, Torsades des Pointes. Antiarrhythmic medications, most commonly digitalis, will produce prominent U waves with a pattern similar to hypokalemia.

It is also important to remember that antiarrhythmic medications used to treat noncardiac conditions will still reflect changes in the ECG tracing. Such drugs include the use of beta-blockers for migraine therapy, timolol eye drops for control of glaucoma, and calcium channel blockers for control of hypertension.

Digitalis. Digitalis preparations (Lanoxin™, Digoxin™) are used to treat patients with heart failure and certain arrhythmias. One of the effects of digitalis is to shorten ventricular repolarization. This results in a reduction of the QT interval, specifically the ST segment and T wave.

● **digitalis effect**

A negative scooping or slurring of the ST segment seen in patients on a digitalis preparation; not to be interpreted as digitalis toxicity

A more typical change affected by digitalis is the characteristic ST segment change, that is, a negative coving or scooping. This change is sometimes called the **digitalis effect**. This characteristic scooping of the ST segment reflects digitalis effect and *does not* imply toxicity. Toxicity must be proven by lab analysis and clinical presentation.

When the digitalis effect is seen on the ECG, the ST segment and T wave are often fused so that clear distinction between the two is impossible. Figure 3-18 provides ECG tracings of changes in ST segments and T waves from patients with digitalis effect. Note the bradycardia that may be an effect of digitalis.

Hyperkalemia

● **hyperkalemia**

Condition in which there is an excessive amount of potassium in the blood; serum levels greater than 6.0 mEq/L

Hyperkalemia is a condition in which there is an excessive amount of potassium in the blood. Increased serum potassium levels greater than 6 mEq/L cause a narrowing and peaking of the T wave. There is a characteristic *tenting* of the T wave as the amplitude increases. Tall tented T waves by themselves may not reflect hyperkalemia. The combination of prolonged PR interval and decreased amplitude of the P waves are better evidence of suspected hyperkalemia.

In clinical persistent hyperkalemia, such as seen with renal failure, the increased QRS complex duration will manifest intraventricular conduction delay. As this change occurs, the QRS becomes distorted and takes on an undulating appearance. Figure 3-19 provides an ECG tracing showing changes in the QRS complex, ST segments, and T waves from a patient with hyperkalemia.

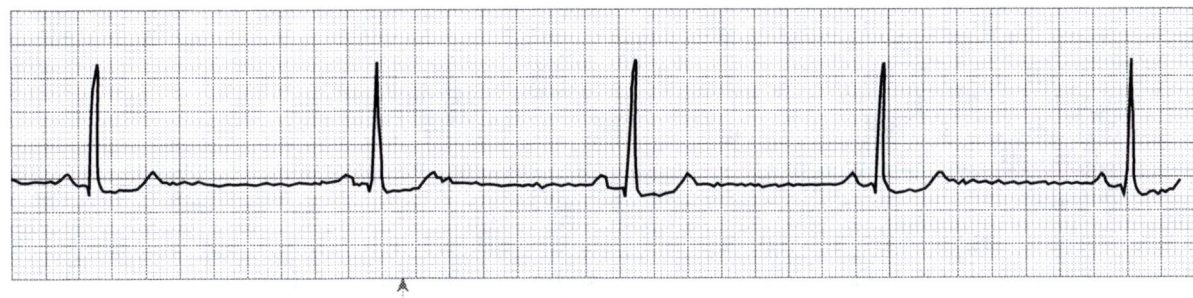

Figure 3-18 ECG tracing showing sinus bradycardia and ST segment depression characteristic of a patient on digitalis.

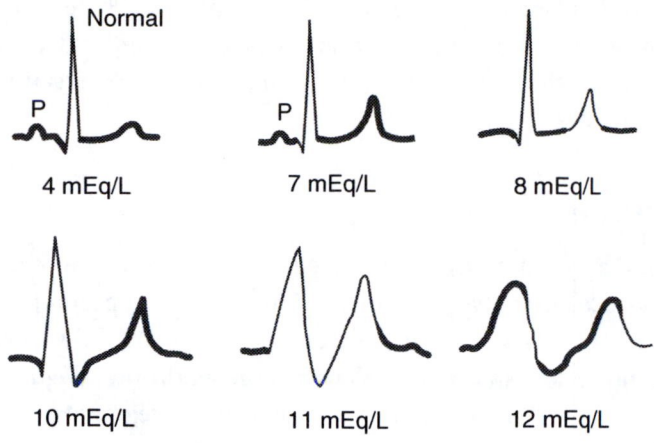

Figure 3-19 ECG tracing in a patient with documented hyperkalemia. Note the progressive changes in QRS complex associated with specific serum potassium levels.

Hypokalemia

Hypokalemia is a condition in which there is decreased concentration of potassium in the blood, that is, serum potassium levels less than 3 mEq/L that produce ST segment depression. U waves may also occur. The U waves may merge with the T waves making the QT interval appear prolonged. T waves also may flatten and U waves increase to a size greater than the amplitude of the T waves. The most common cause of hypokalemia is diuretic therapy without concurrent use of potassium supplements. Prolonged bouts of emesis, gastric suctioning, and diarrhea may also produce hypokalemia. Figure 3-20 provides an ECG tracing showing changes in the QRS complex, ST segments, and T waves in a patient with documented hypokalemia.

Hypercalcemia

Hypercalcemia is a condition in which there is an excessive amount of calcium in the blood. Serum calcium levels greater than 3.5 mEq/L cause decreased ventricular

● **hypokalemia**

Condition in which there is an extreme lack of potassium in the blood; serum levels less than 3.0 mEq/L

● **hypercalcemia**

Condition in which there is an excessive amount of calcium in the blood; serum levels greater than 3.5 mEq/L

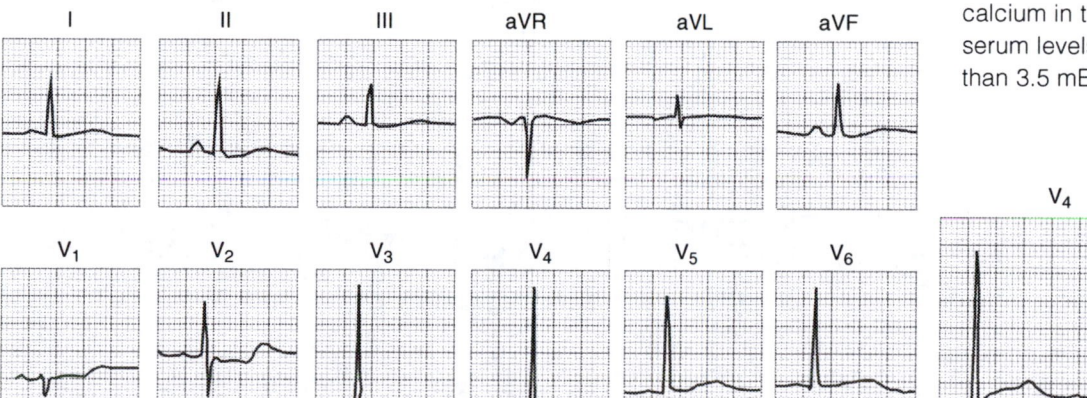

Figure 3-20 ECG tracing in a patient with documented hypokalemia of 2.2 mEq/L. Note the progressive changes in T and U waves. (Adapted from *Clinical Electrocardiography* by Goldberger and Goldberger, 1977, St. Louis: C.V. Mosby)

repolarization and subsequent decrease in the QT interval. Hypercalcemia is associated with multiple myeloma and hyperparathyroidism, and may be seen in cancer patients, particularly those with breast and lung cancer. Hypercalcemia can cause seizure, coma, and death in severe cases.

Hypocalcemia

● **hypocalcemia**

Condition in which there are abnormally low levels of calcium in the blood; serum levels less than 3.5 mEq/L

Hypocalcemia is a condition in which there is an abnormally low level of calcium in the blood. Serum calcium levels less than 3.5 mEq/L cause prolongation of the QT interval. Common causes include pancreatitis, renal failure, hypoparathyroidism, malnutrition, and certain intestinal malabsorption syndromes. Figures 3-21A and B provide ECG tracings of changes in the QRS complex, ST segments, and T waves from patients with hypocalcemia and hypercalcemia. Table 3-4 summarizes changes in ECG wave forms and complexes associated with certain medications and electrolyte imbalance. These changes must be correlated with clinical history and serum levels.

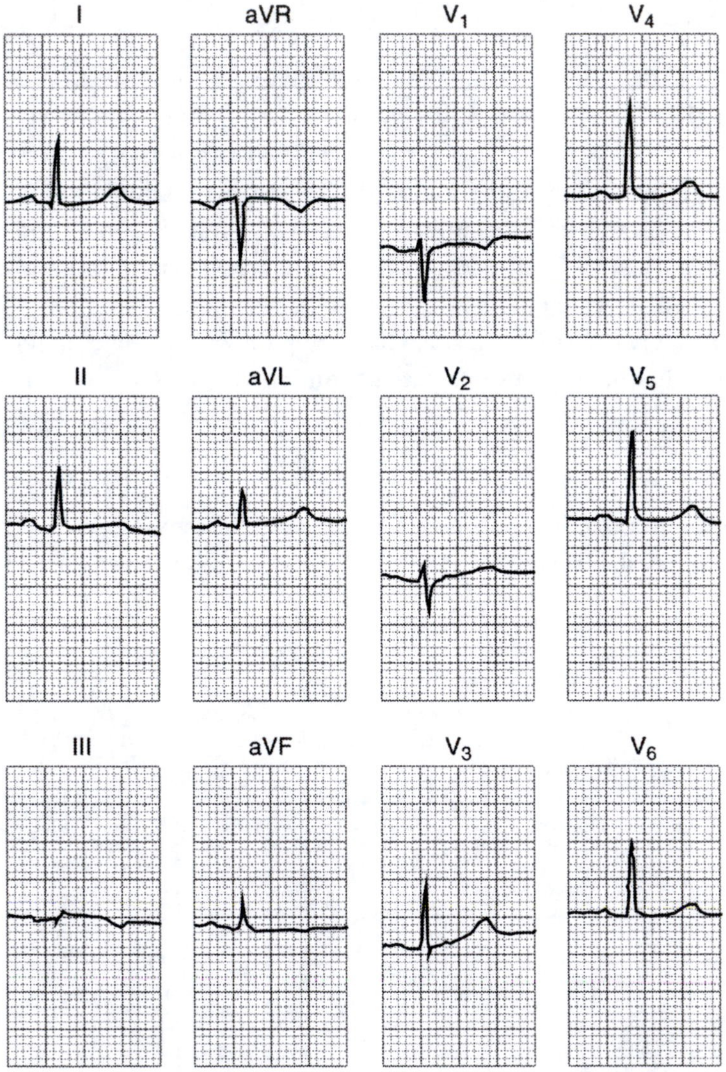

Figure 3-21A An ECG tracing of a patient with documented hypocalcemia; note the long ST segment

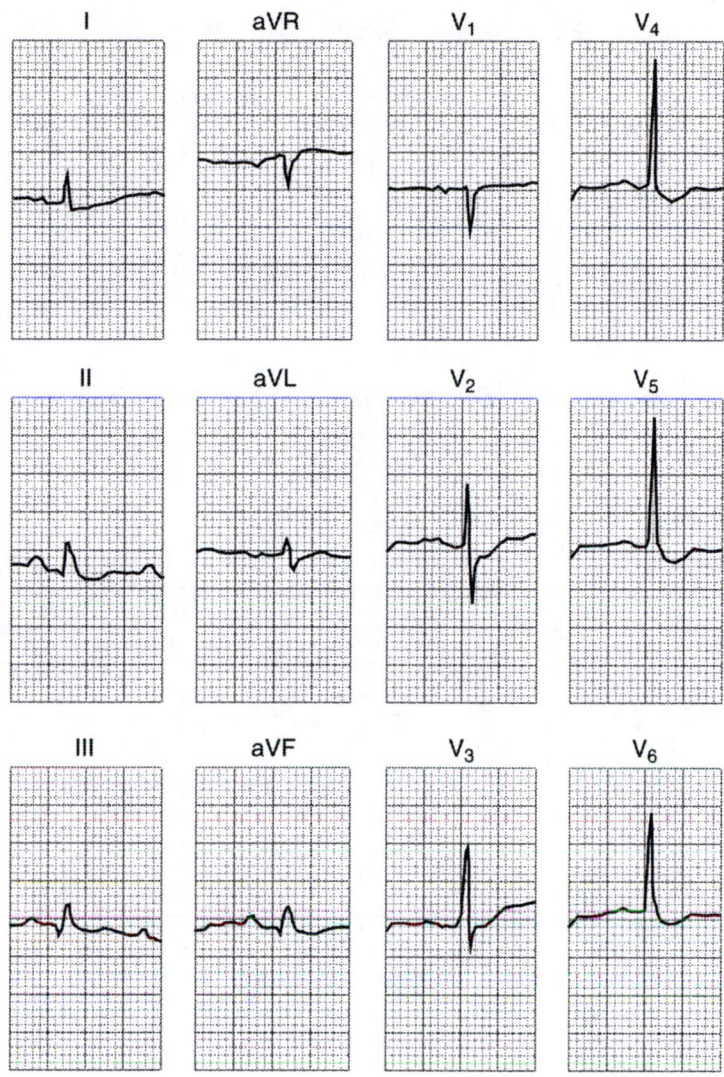

Figure 3-21B An ECG tracing of a patient with documented hypercalcemia; notice the short ST segment. (Adapted from *How to Quickly and Accurately Master ECG Interpretation*, 2nd ed. by D. Davis, 1992, Philadelphia: J.B. Lippincott.)

Low-Voltage QRS

Low voltage describes the diminished amplitude (less than 5 mm) of the QRS complex in all the extremity leads: I, II, III, aVR, aVL, and aVF. A common ECG sign of pericardial effusion is low-voltage QRS complexes due to the diminished conduction through the fluid surrounding the heart.

In emphysema, the accumulation of trapped air acts as a deterrent to the flow of current. In pericarditis, low-voltage QRS is seen in the precordial leads. Low-voltage QRS may also be a normal variant. Other conditions that can result in low-voltage QRS are:

- amyloidosis
- hypothyroidism
- heart failure
- myocardial fibrosis

low voltage

Lower than normal amplitude (less than 5 mm) for a given wave form at normal standard calibration

Table 3-4 Summary of ECG Changes Induced by Some Medications and Electrolyte Imbalance

ECG Wave Forms/ Complexes	Medication*	Electrolyte Imbalance
P wave amplitude↓		hyperkalemia
P wave notched	quinidine	
PR interval greater than 0.2 second	digitalis procainamide quinidine verapamil	hyperkalemia
QRS complex greater than 0. 10 second	disopyramide procainamide quinidine	hyperkalemia
ST segment↓	digitalis quinidine	hypokalemia
T wave amplitude↓	digitalis procainamide	hypokalemia
T wave amplitude↑	quinidine	hyperkalemia
T wave↓	digitalis procainamide	hypokalemia
U wave amplitude↑		hypokalemia hypomagnesemia
QT interval↓	hypercalcemia	
QT interval↑ (may be a normal variant)	hypocalcemia	

*The ECG measurements are sensitive to many drugs with antiarrhythmic potential, including medications taken for other reasons; for example, calcium channel blockers for hypertension and beta-blockers for angina. This list is not all inclusive.

Pericarditis

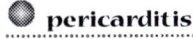

pericarditis

Inflammation of the pericardial sac

Pericarditis is an inflammation of the pericardial sac caused, for example, by viral or bacterial infection, metastasis, infarction, or uremia. Pericarditis of any etiology may show localized ST segment elevations and subsequent T wave inversion and is easily mistaken for acute myocardial ischemia.

Early in Stage 1 of pericarditis there is diffuse concave ST elevation in all the leads except for aVR. In aVR the ST segment is depressed and the PR segment is elevated. The term global is used to describe when these changes are present in all the leads. Usually, there are no convex ST segments and no reciprocal changes.

ST segment elevation in pericarditis usually represents general involvement of the ventricular subepicardium. Localized involvement of only the subepicardium is rare. If that is the case, ST elevation will occur in only a few leads with reciprocal ST depression. Q waves are not always associated with pericarditis. If Q waves are present they may suggest evolving or causative pathology. T waves are generally upright, while the PR interval is classically depressed except in lead aVR, where it is elevated. The segment between the end of the T wave and beginning of the P wave, the so-called TP segment, is a more accurate baseline for measuring ST segments.

Pseudonormalization occurs in Stage 2. *Pseudonormalization* is a term that describes when the ECG looks normal. ST segments return to baseline and may even be isoelectric; T waves are upright. The PR interval may be depressed, but is usually close to baseline.

In Stage 3 of pericarditis, the T waves change. T wave inversion is now present in the leads that previously had concave ST segment elevation; the ST segment itself is isoelectric. This pattern may last for days to weeks.

Stage 4 involves resolution. The PQRST complex resumes its original shape. In the early phases, ST segment elevation can be seen due to the inflammation of the epicardium. However, there is never Q wave formation with pericarditis, and the resolution of the ST segment and T wave changes takes place over a much longer period of time. The ST segment changes are usually seen in all leads, as opposed to myocardial infarction, where the acute changes of Q waves, ST elevation, and T wave inversion are seen in the leads facing the localized infarcted myocardial tissue. Remember there are no reciprocal changes with pericarditis. Figure 3-22 provides ECG tracings of changes in the ST segments and T waves in patients with pericarditis.

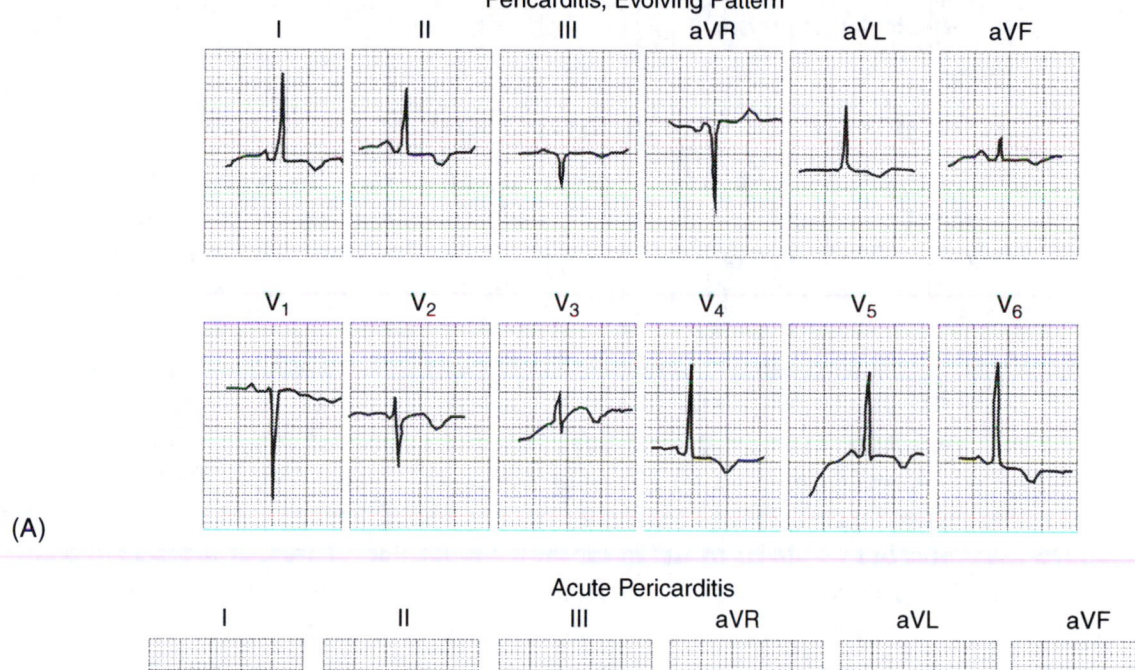

(A)

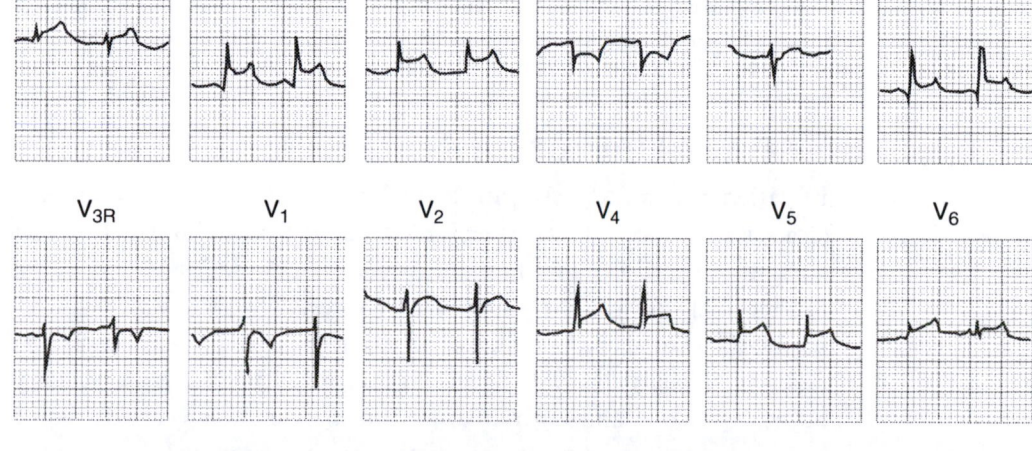

(B)

Figure 3-22 ECG tracings from patients with (A) evolving, and (B) documented acute pericarditis

● **pericardial effusion**
Condition in which there is abnormal accumulation of fluid within the pericardial sac

Pericardial Effusion. **Pericardial effusion** refers to abnormal accumulation of fluid within the pericardial sac. In most cases this is a complication of pericarditis, but can occur with hypothyroidism, uremia, and other systemic pathologies. The clinical significance of pericardial effusion is dependent on the rapidity with which the fluid accumulates. The tension created by the accumulation of fluid can cause progressive decrease in ventricular filling to the point of pericardial tamponade. In tamponade, the heart becomes so restricted, due to the high intrapericardial pressure, that effective contraction cannot occur.

Ventricular Aneurysm

Left ventricular aneurysm resulting from extensive infarction may cause persistent ST segment inversion over the damaged muscle. This ST segment elevation may be present for years and may be confused with acute necrosis. Such ST segment elevation and aneurysm formation may hide subsequent ischemic episodes. Figure 3-23 shows ECG tracings of changes in the ST segments and T waves in a patient with ventricular aneurysm.

Hypertrophic Cardiomyopathy

Inappropriate myocardial hypertrophy, often with the septum showing more involvement than the free ventricle wall, is common to hypertrophic cardiomyopathy (HCM). In up to 70 percent of HCM cases have familial patterns of occurrence with autosomal dominant inheritance. In children and adolescents, the ECG may be a more sensitive marker of early disease than an echocardiogram.

Patients with HCM often (25 to 50 percent) have significant Q waves on their ECG. Rather than infarction, these Q waves represent hypertrophied asymmetric ventricular muscle with distortion of normal depolarization patterns. Giant negative T waves in mid-precordial leads may be seen. "Voltage criteria" for left ventricular hypertrophy (LVH) in association with repolarization abnormalities is also common, but isolated increases in voltage without ST and T wave changes are infrequent (see Chapter 6). A pseudo-infarction pattern should always be suspected when the clinical setting and laboratory data do not correlate with electrocardiographic findings. Figure 3-24 shows ECG tracings of changes in the ST segments and T waves in a patient with hypertrophic cardiomyopathy.

Increased Intracranial Pressure

In patients with increased intracranial pressure (ICP), QT prolongation may occur along with deep T wave inversion and sometimes abnormal U waves. This is an almost universal ECG finding in this patient population. With sudden increases in intracranial pressure there may also be dramatic alterations to the T waves and ST segments. These changes do not reflect a primary myocardial problem, but rather changes in repolarization due to enhanced sympathetic nervous system activity. Supraventricular and ventricular arrhythmias, as well as conduction abnormalities, have been well documented in patients with cerebral hemorrhage and increased

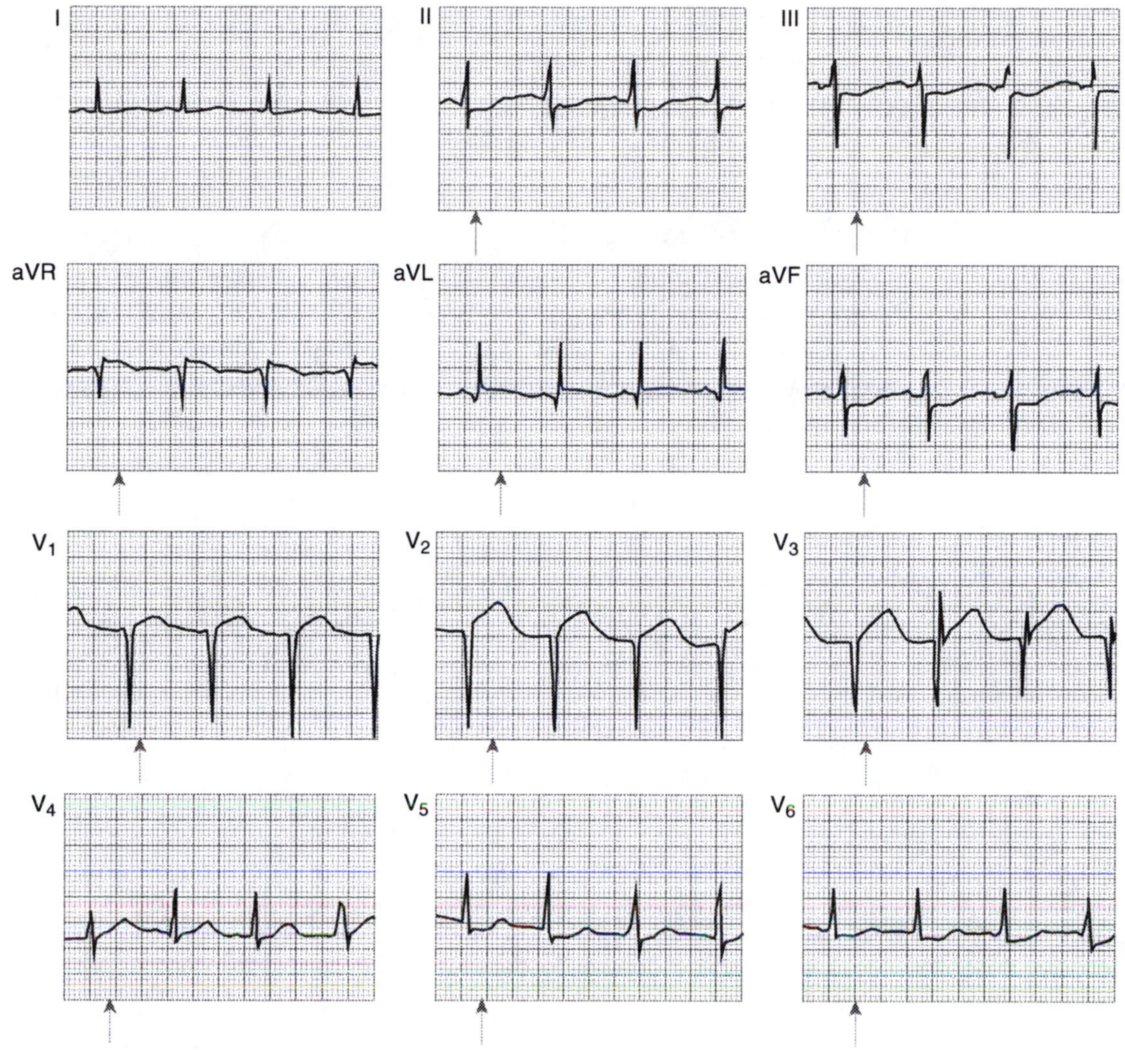

Figure 3-23 ECG tracing in a patient with documented anterior wall ventricular aneurysm. Note Q waves in V_1, V_2, V_3, and aVL and ST depression in II, III, and aVF.

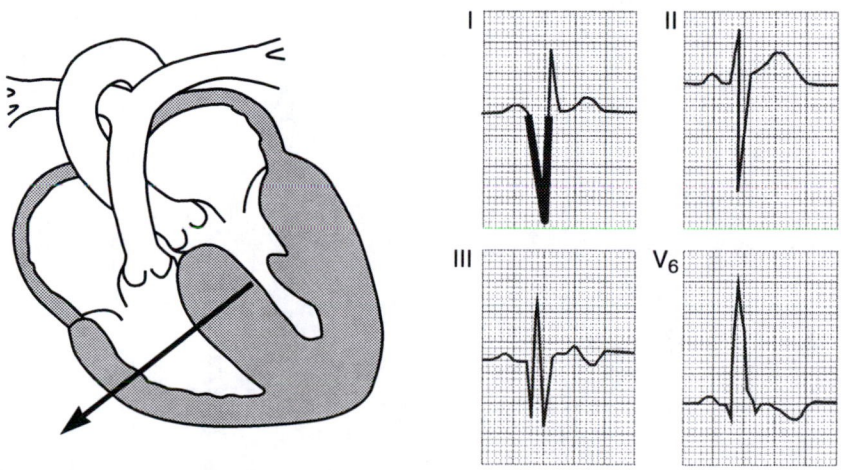

Figure 3-24 (A) Illustration of hypertrophic cardiomyopathy (B) An ECG tracing in a patient with hypertrophic cardiomyopathy; note the highlight Q wave in lead I.

intracranial pressure. Severe life-threatening arrhythmias in patients with subarachnoid hemorrhage include Torsades de Pointe in the setting of marked prolonged QT interval. Figure 3-25 provides a 12-lead ECG from a patient with increased intracranial pressure showing "cerebral" T waves.

Pulmonary Embolism

An embolism can occur and obstruct the pulmonary artery causing a sudden change in the ECG. Acute pulmonary embolism may cause right ventricular dilation and strain which is seen on the ECG as T wave inversion in the precordial leads, V_1 through V_4, and new right axis deviation may also be seen. New right bundle branch block may also be the sequelae to a massive pulmonary embolism.

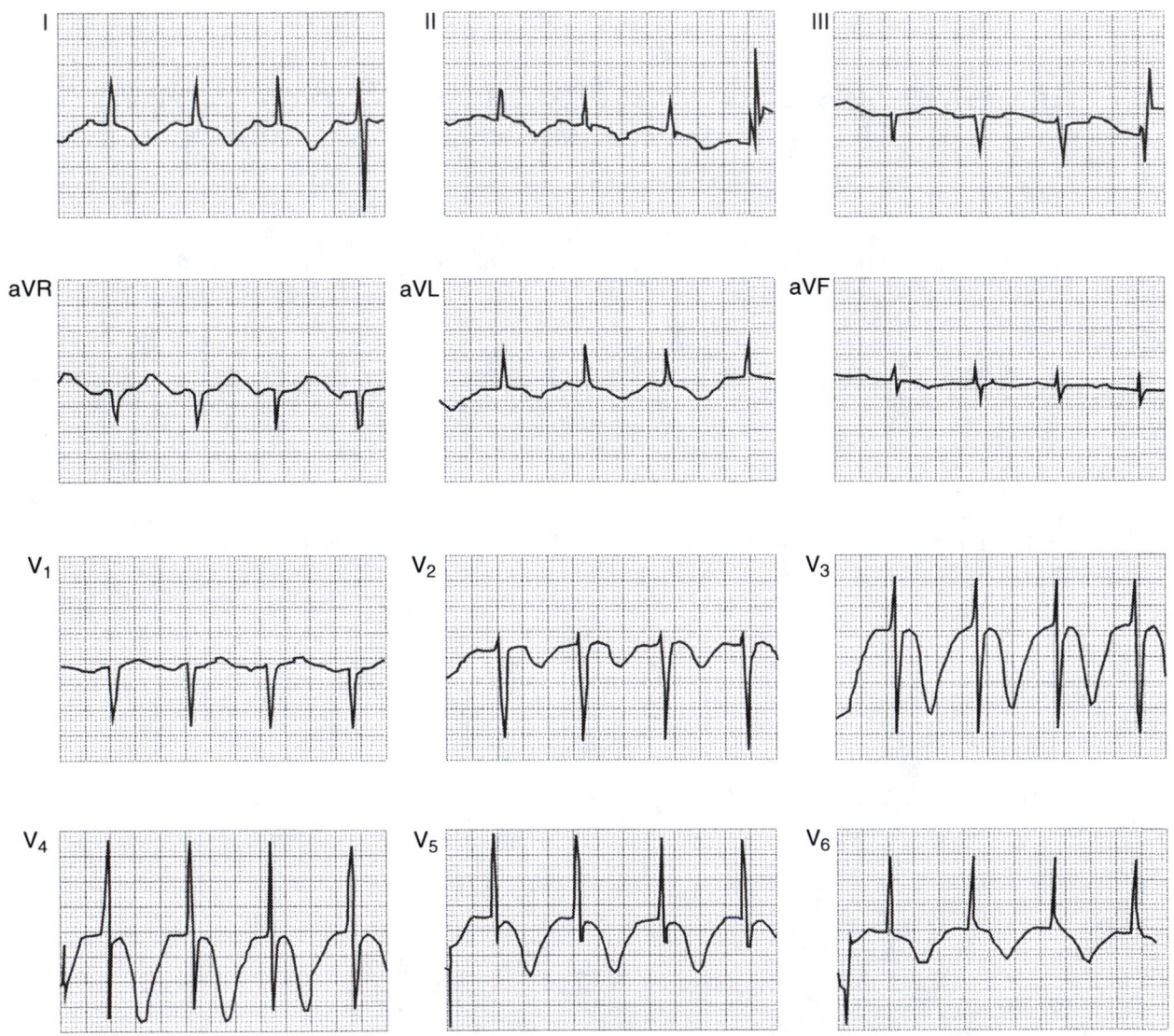

Figure 3-25 A 12-lead ECG from a patient with increased intracranial pressure. Note the QT interval of 0.48 second and the amplitude of the T waves in the precordial leads. (Adapted from *Manual of Electrocardiography*, 2nd ed., by G. H. Mudge, 1986, Toronto: Little, Brown and Company.)

Acute Pulmonary Embolism

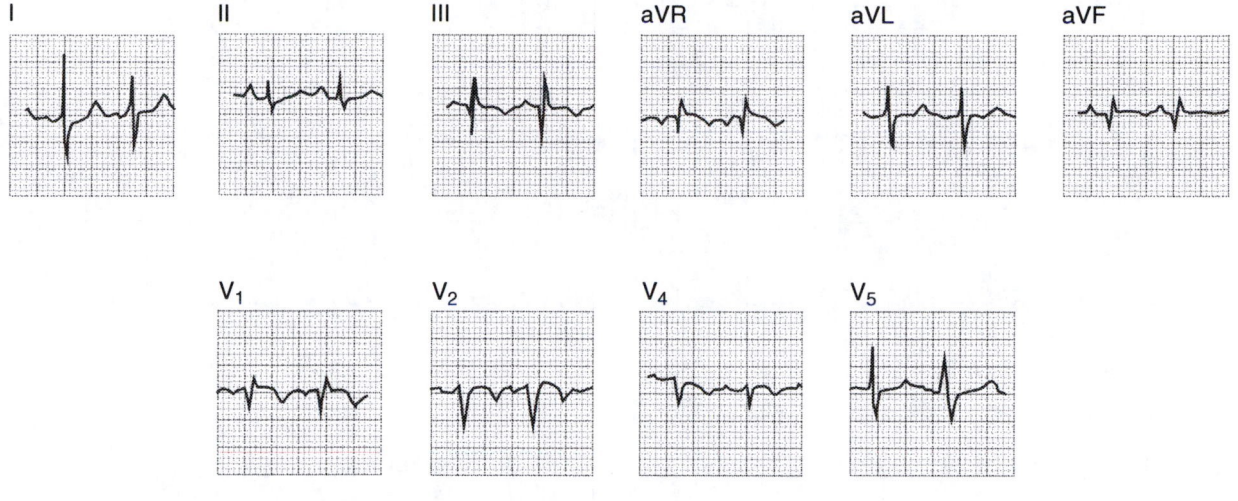

Figure 3-26 ECG tracing from a patient with documented pulmonary embolism.

Also, S waves in lead I and new Q waves in lead III with T wave inversion may occur. Referred to as an $S_1Q_3T_3$ pattern, this also is seen with inferior wall myocardial infarction. With pulmonary embolism, there is right axis deviation and the QRS is often greater than 0.10 second and the ventricular rate is often greater than 100 beats per minute. This is not the case in acute myocardial infarction. Figure 3-26 provides ECG tracings of changes in the ST segments and T waves from a patient with pulmonary embolism.

Summary

In this chapter we have reviewed ECG wave forms and how they relate to electrical conduction. We have identified some of the causes and resulting changes on the ECG. Deviation in the ECG wave forms could have clinical implications. Variations must be corroborated with clinical presentation and appropriate diagnostic studies.

Self Assessment Exercises

● ECG Rhythm Identification Practice

For the ECG practice rhythms,

1. Identify the P, Q, R, S, T (and U waves if evident).

2. Calculate the measurement and rates asked for in each strip.

3. When complete, compare your answers with those in the back of the book.

Figure 3-27

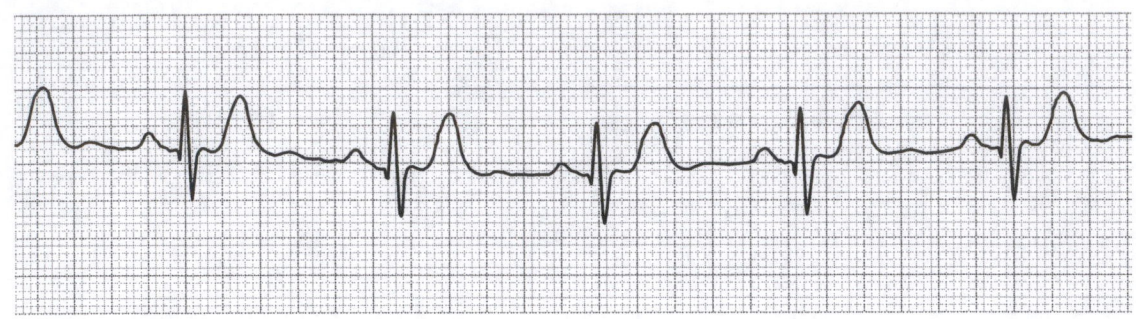

1. Can you identify P, Q, R, S, T, U waves?
2. Look to the left of the QRS, and identify each P wave.

   Is the P wave positive or negative? _____

3. QRS (ventricular) rate/rhythm _____
4. P (atrial) rate/rhythm _____
5. PR interval _____

Figure 3-28

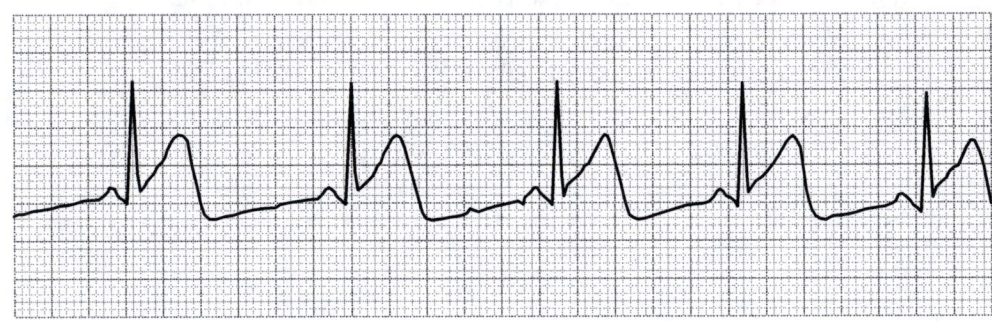

1. Can you identify P, Q, R, S, T, U waves?
2. Look to the left of the QRS, and identify each P wave.

   Is the P wave positive or negative? _____

3. QRS (ventricular) rate/rhythm _____
4. P (atrial) rate/rhythm _____
5. PR interval _____

References

Conover, M. B. (1996). *Understanding electrocardiography: Arrhythmias and the 12-lead ECG* (7th ed.). St. Louis: Mosby-Year Book.

Lemery, R., Kleinebenne, A., Nihoyannopoulos, P., et al. (1990). Q waves in hypertrophic cardiomyopathy in relation to the distribution and severity of right and left ventricular hypertrophy. *Journal of American College of Cardiology;* 16:368-374.

Marriott, H. J. L. & Conover, M. B., *Advanced concepts in arrhythmias* (3rd ed.). St Louis: C. V. Mosby.

Shapiro, E. (1980). The electrocardiogram and the arrhythmias: Historical insights. In Mandel, W. J. *Cardiac arrhythmias: Their mechanism, diagnosis and management.* Philadelphia: Lippincott; 1-12.

Wagner, G. S., (Ed.). (1994). *Marriott's practical electrocardiography.* (9th ed.). Baltimore: Williams & Wilkins.

Axis Determination and Implications

> **Premise** ● Calculating axis allows clinicians to understand the flow of electrical current as it reflects the heart's electrical conduction system.

Objectives

After reading the chapter and completing the Self-Assessment exercises, the student should be able to:

1. Identify the leads used in calculating axis
2. Determine normal axis
3. Determine left and right axis deviation
4. Explain the pathology associated with axis deviation

Key Terms

axis   right axis deviation
left axis deviation   vector
normal axis

Introduction

The average direction of the spread of the depolarization wave front through the ventricles as seen in the frontal plane is called the cardiac axis, and is useful in deciding whether the wave front is flowing in a normal direction. The axis is derived from the QRS complex as seen in leads I, II, and III, and is sometimes simply called the *net area* of the QRS. Figure 4-1 shows examples of the net area of QRS complex and the reciprocal values of leads I and III.

● **axis**

The direct path between two electrodes or between an electrode and the reference point; the direction of flow of depolarization

NORMAL AXIS

● **normal axis**

The flow of electrical current downward from right to left in the heart

Normal axis means that the depolarizing wave is spreading toward leads I, II, and III; therefore, the net area of the QRS is seen as primarily positive. Since normal depolarization flows primarily inferior and to the left, the most positive wave form would be lead II. Figure 4-2 shows the normal axis as seen in leads I, II, and III.

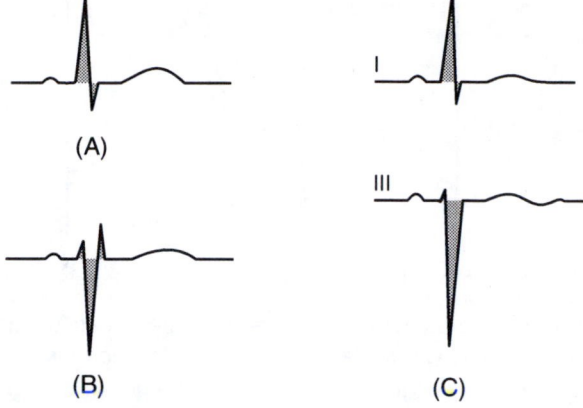

(A)

(B)   (C)

Figure 4-1 View A is the positive net area of a QRS complex; the shaded area of the QRS above the isoelectric line is more positive than the area below the line. View B is the negative net area of a QRS complex; the shaded area of the QRS below the isoelectric line is more negative than the area above the line. View C is the positive net area in lead I and the negative net area in lead III. Lead III is a mirror image of lead I; therefore, the current is directed away from lead III.

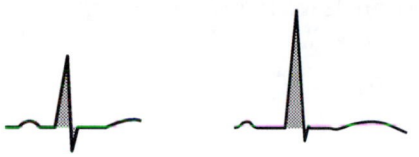

Figure 4-2 The net areas of leads I, II, and III are positive, with the greatest positive net area in lead II.

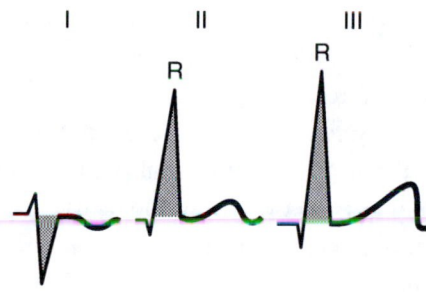

Figure 4-3 A negative net area in lead I and positive net areas in leads II and III, with lead III showing the greatest positive net area, is characteristic of right-axis deviation.

AXIS DEVIATION

Axis deviation may occur as a normal variant, but its presence should alert the clinician to assess for intraventricular conduction defects and ventricular hypertrophy.

Right Axis Deviation

If the flow of depolarization swings toward the right of normal, the QRS deflection in lead I is negative and lead III is positive; this is called **right axis deviation.** Figure 4-3 compares a negative net area in lead I with positive areas in leads II and III. Note that lead III is more positive than lead II.

⬤ **right axis deviation**

The flow of depolarization is inferior and toward the right of normal.

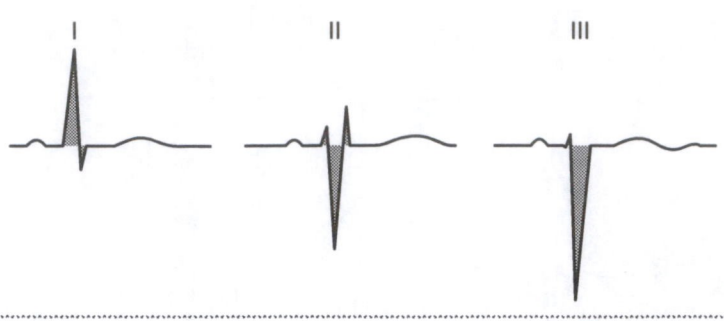

Figure 4-4 A positive net area in lead I and negative net areas in leads II and III, with lead III showing the greatest negative net area, is characteristic of left-axis deviation.

Left Axis Deviation

Similarly, when the flow of depolarization swings toward the left of normal, so the QRS deflection is positive in lead I, equiphasic in lead II, and extremely negative in lead III, **left axis deviation** exists. Figure 4-4 illustrates a net area in lead I that is very positive. In comparison, leads II and III are negative; note that lead III is more negative than lead II.

CALCULATING AXIS

Calculating the mean axis determines the predominant direction of the flow of electrical current in the heart. This is usually measured during ventricular depolarization (QRS) and uses the morphology of the QRS complexes in the limb leads. Calculating axis is one tool used to determine fascicular block. (See Chapter 7.) Calculating the mean flow of current (axis) can be done in several ways. Since not all QRS complexes are clearly different in polarity or configuration, the clinician would do well to learn several methods.

The hexaxial reference system—an intersecting pattern of 6 limb leads—is used to determine the axis of the heart in the frontal plane; in other words, this system refers to the flow of current as it occurs within the heart's conduction system. This is important clinically because deviation from normal can aid in differential diagnosis of many cardiac conditions and pathology within the heart's conduction system.

To apply the hexaxial system, the clinician must first understand the concept of vectors. A **vector** is the direction of force of electrical energy within the heart. The mean cardiac vector is a representation of the flow of electrical current during a cardiac cycle. To understand the hexaxial system, first imagine the triangle formed by leads I, II, and III. As those lines intersect, they create the skeleton for the hexaxial system. Next, add the position for aVR, aVL, and aVF, which also will intersect, producing 3 additional lines of reference. You would now see 12 lines as they visualize the heart's electrical system. Figure 4-5 illustrates building the hexaxial reference system.

Recall that, in the normal heart, the flow of electrical current usually travels downward from right to left. This generates what is called the normal axis of the heart. Figure 4-6 illustrates the mean flow of current in a heart with normal conduction.

Calculating the mean flow of current—or axis—can be done in several ways. The common two-step method is as follows:

1. Identify the equiphasic QRS.

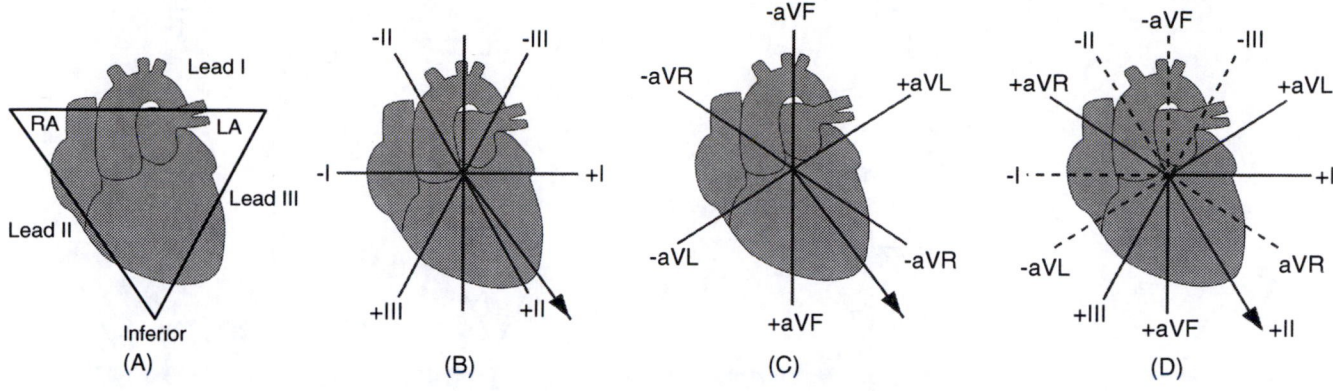

Figure 4-5 In View A, a triangle is formed by leads I, II, and III. View B shows the intersection of the lines of I, II, and III as they form the skeleton of the hexaxial figure. View C incorporates the addition of aVR, aVL, and aVF. View D shows the completed hexaxial system.

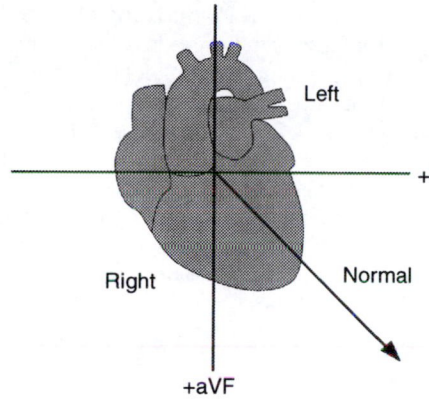

Figure 4-6 The mean flow of current in a heart with normal ventricular conduction. When referencing the mean flow current or the mean vector, a heavy arrow is used to indicate the direction of flow.

2. Identify the lead perpendicular and positive to this lead. (Remember, lead I is at a right angle to aVF, lead II is at a right angle to aVL, and lead III is at a right angle to aVR. The flow of current, or axis, will be parallel to the perpendicular lead.

Figure 4-7 illustrates the two-step method.

Another method used to calculate axis is the quadrant method. This method is useful when there are no equiphasic complexes or when there is more than one lead with equiphasic deflections. The quadrant method is as follows:

1. Look at lead I and determine if the flow of current is to the right or the left; draw an arrow in that direction. Remember that a positive (+) QRS indicates the flow is to the left and a negative (-) QRS indicates the flow is to the right.

2. Look at lead aVF and determine if the flow is superior or inferior; draw an arrow in that direction. Remember that a positive (+) QRS indicates the flow is inferior, toward aVF, and a negative (-) QRS indicates the flow is superior, away from aVF.

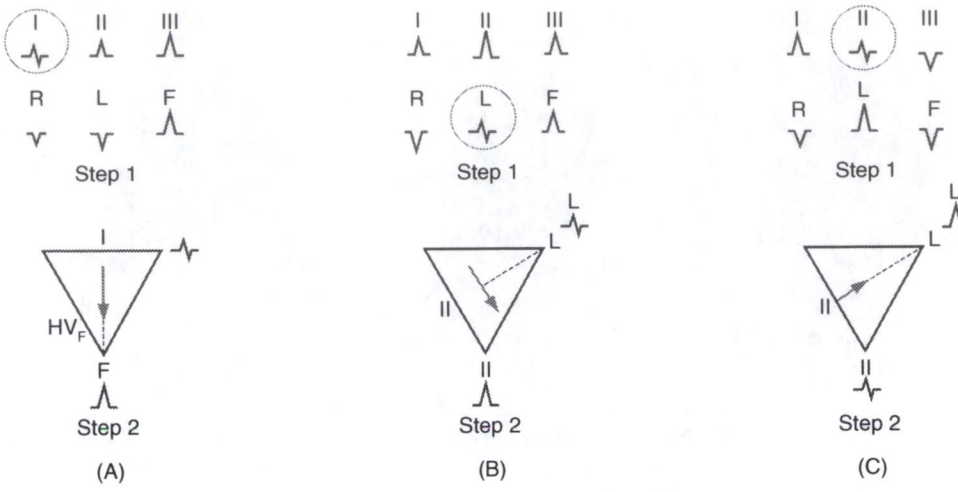

Figure 4-7 In View A, step 1: Look for the equiphasic deflection; in this figure, it is lead I. Step 2: Look for the lead perpendicular (at a right angle) to lead I; in this example, it is lead aVF. Conclusion: The current (axis) is flowing inferior toward the positive electrode of aVF. In View B, step 1: Look for the equiphasic deflection. In this figure, it is lead aVL; therefore, the current flow must be perpendicular to that lead. Step 2: Look at the lead perpendicular to lead aVL; it is lead II. Conclusion: The flow of current is directed inferior toward the positive electrode, lead II. In View C, step 1: Look for the equiphasic deflection. In this figure, it is lead II; therefore, the current flow must be perpendicular to that lead. Step 2: Look at the deflection in the lead perpendicular to lead II; in this example, it is lead aVL. Conclusion: The current is flowing superior toward the positive electrode of aVL. (Adapted with permission from *Understanding Electrocardiography*, 6th Ed., by M. B. Conover, 1992, St. Louis: C. V. Mosby.)

3. This creates a quadrant—look for the most positive lead in that quadrant. This will tell you the direction (axis) of current flow for that patient's QRS.

Figure 4-8 illustrates the step-by-step use of the quadrant method.

It is important to remember that if the QRS in leads I and II are both positive, there is no deviation from normal and no other calculation is necessary. If the QRS in either lead I or II is negative, there is a deviation from normal and further calculation is required.

A flow of current far to the left (superior) is considered a deviation from the normal flow, that is, left axis deviation (LAD). The QRS will be more positive in leads I and aVL than in lead II; leads II and III will be predominantly negative.

A flow of current far to the right (inferior) is considered a deviation from the normal flow, that is, right axis deviation (RAD). The QRS will be more negative in leads I and aVL than in lead II; leads II and III will be predominantly positive, III being most positive.

Another quick method is the Handal-Lewis method, which is as follows:

1. Look at lead I: if the current flow is toward the right, lead I will be the most negative deflection of the three limb leads.

2. Look at lead III: if the current flow is too far right (inferior), lead III will be very positive and the greatest positive deflection of the three limb leads. This is right axis deviation.

or:

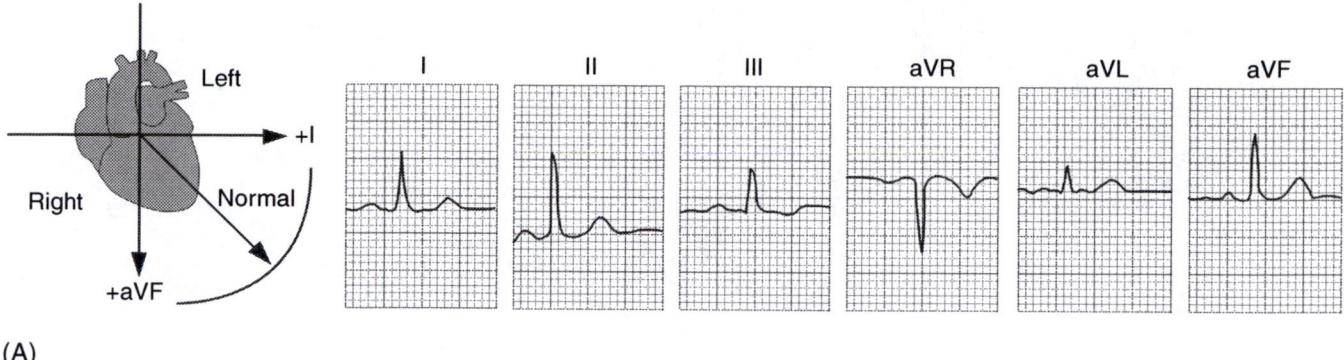

(A)

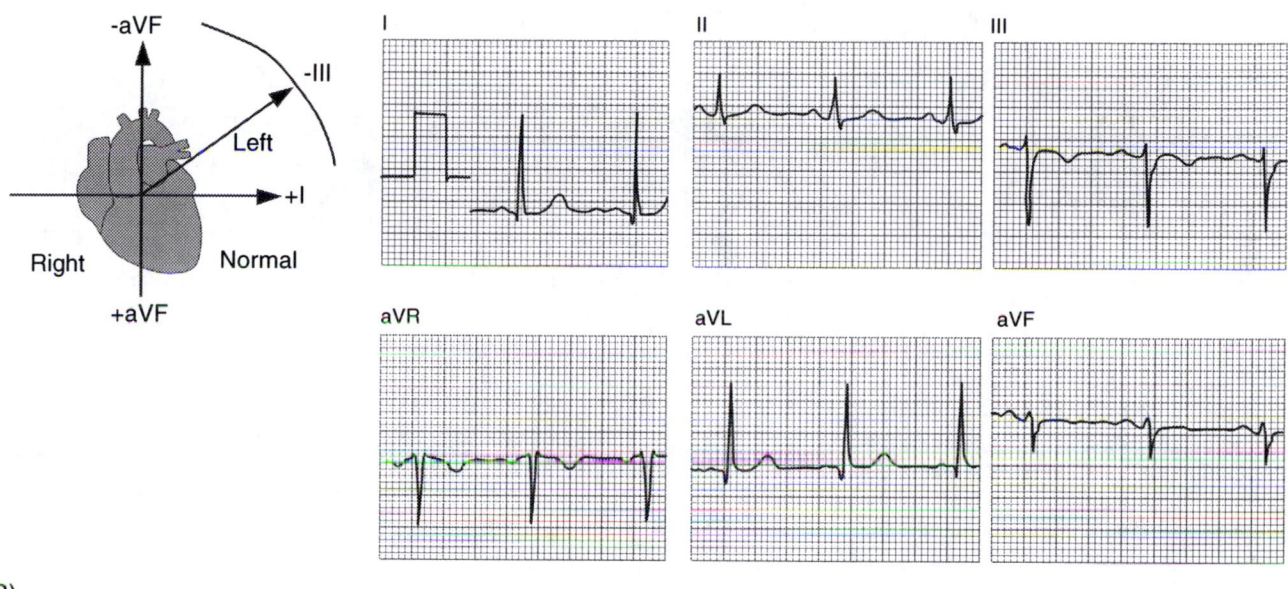

(B)

Figure 4-8 In View A, lead I is positive; the first arrow should be drawn toward the positive electrode in the lead. Next, lead aVF is perpendicular to lead I and the QRS in lead aVF is positive, so, draw an arrow toward aVF. You have now localized the flow of current between leads I and aVF. The QRS in lead II is most positive, so the current of flow is directed inferior and to the left, within the normal limits. In View B, lead I is positive; the first arrow should be drawn toward the positive electrode in that lead,   Next, lead aVF is perpendicular to lead I and the QRS in lead aVF is negative, so, draw an arrow away from the positive electrode in aVF. You have now localized the flow of current between the positive electrode in lead I and the negative electrode in lead aVF. The QRS in lead III is negative, so the current flow is directed superior and to the left, outside the normal limits. This deviation from normal is called left-axis deviation. (Adapted from *Understanding Electrocardiography*, 6th Ed., by M. B. Conover, 1992, St. Louis: C. V. Mosby.)

1. Look at lead I: if the current flow is toward the left, lead I will be the most positive deflection of the three limb leads.

2. Look at lead III: if the current flow is too far left (superior), lead III will be very negative and the greatest negative deflection of the three limb leads. This is left axis deviation.

Figure 4-9 illustrates the application of the Handal-Lewis method, noting the net area in leads I and III as a quick reference to determine axis.

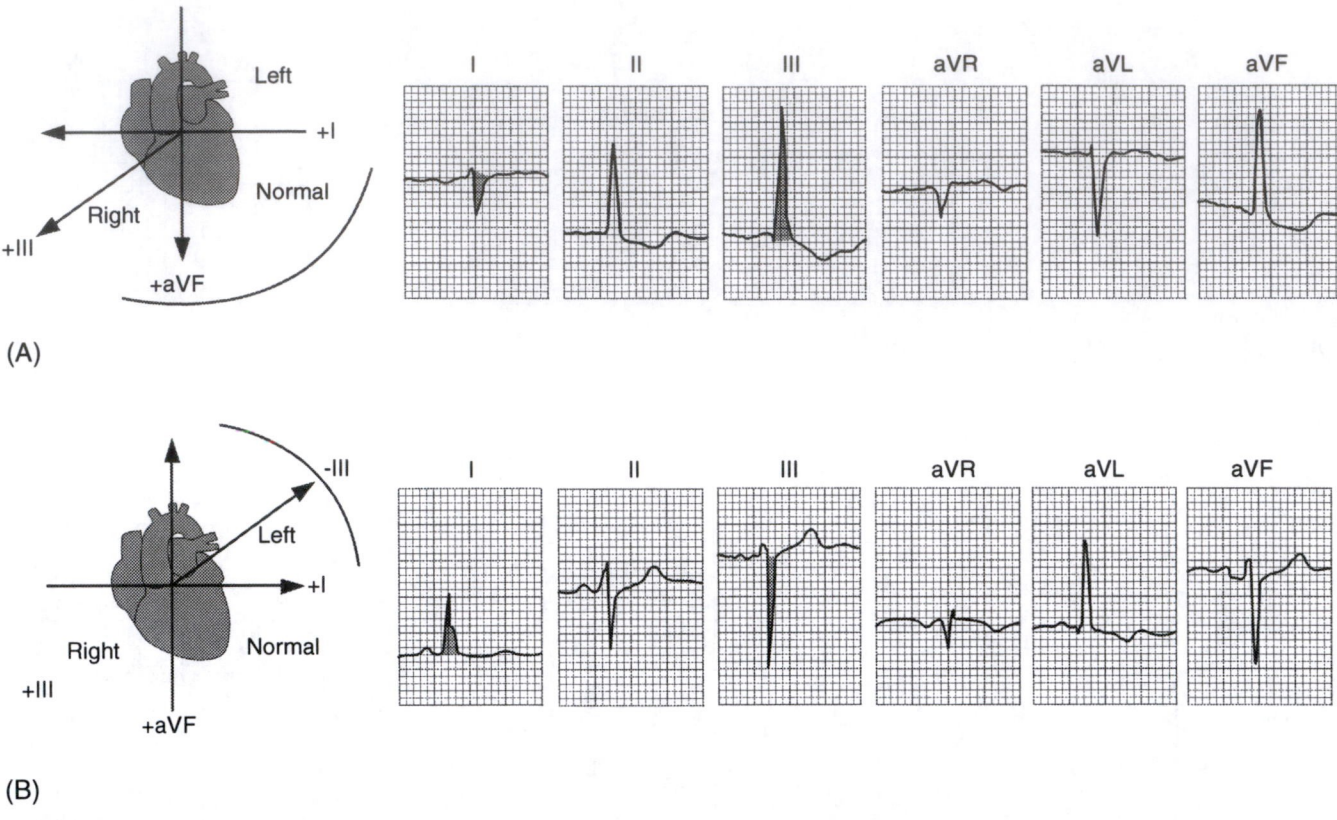

(A)

(B)

Figure 4-9 View A shows an ECG tracing of leads I, II, and III highlighting the net QRS complex in leads I and III. Note that in lead I, the net QRS is negative, and in lead III, the net QRS is positive. Note also that the net QRS in lead III is the most positive net QRS seen in the limb leads. View B shows an ECG tracing of leads I, II, and III highlighting the net QRS complex in leads I and III. Note that in lead I, the net QRS is positive, and in lead III, the net QRS is negative. Note also that the net QRS in lead III is the most negative net QRS seen in the limb leads.

NORMAL AND ABNORMAL VALUES

We have learned that deviation of current to the far left of normal is considered abnormal. This may be caused by a problem with conduction in the left anterior fascicle of the bundle branch system, driving the net current upward and to the left.

Deviation to the far right of normal is also considered abnormal. This may be caused by a problem with conduction in the left posterior fascicle of the bundle branch system, driving the net current to the far right of normal.

Identify the axis by degrees so that each lead has a landmark:

Lead I	=	0 degrees
Lead II	=	+60 degrees
Lead III	=	(+) at +120 degrees (right) or,
		(-) at -60 degrees (left)
Lead aVF	=	(+) at +90 degrees (normal)
		(-) at -90 degrees (superior or far left)

Once calculations are complete, the interpretation would be, for example, "left axis deviation at −60 degrees" or "right axis deviation at +120 degrees."

The Lewis Circle

Another quick reference for calculating axis and the related degrees is the Lewis circle. Figure 4-10 illustrates the heart with the degree values assigned to the limb leads. Note the arrows imposed on the circle to aid in identifying the axis value.

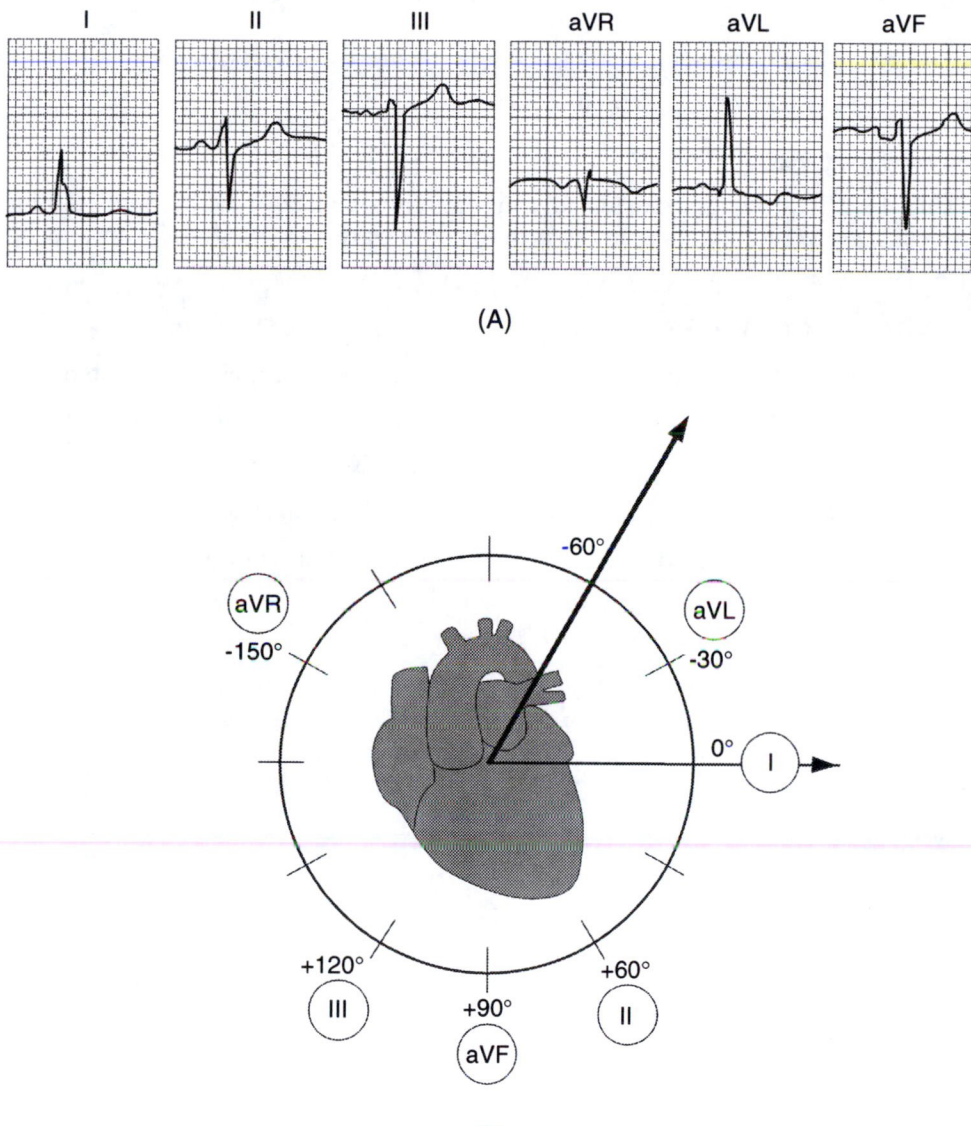

(A)

(B)

Figure 4-10 View A is an ECG tracing showing leads I and II being different in polarity; leads I and aVL are positive; lead III has the greatest negative net area. View B shows the heart with the Lewis circle and degree values assigned to the various leads to provide quick reference and reporting of axis value. Lead I is positive, so an arrow is drawn toward lead I. Lead III is the greatest negative, so an arrow is drawn away from Lead III. Lead aVL is also positive, but lead III has the greater value. Conclusion: Axis deviation superior and to the left at –60 degrees .

Summary

The ECG is a sensitive tool and the limb leads provide valuable information about the intraventricular conduction system. With the evolution of an anteroseptal infarction, there may be development of significant intraventricular conduction defects. Once a QRS complex is reported to be greater than 0.10 second, the clinician should assess the polarity of the QRS to determine if fascicular block is present, and, if possible, to what degree. This involves calculating the QRS axis, for which there are several systems available to the clinician.

Self-Assessment Exercises

● Matching

Match the ECG finding in the left column with the definitions in the right column and compare your answers with those in the back of the book. Definitions may be used more than once.

ECG Finding	Definition
_____ 1. rS greater than 0.10sec in II, III, aVF	A. Left anterior fascicular block
_____ 2. rS greater than 0.10sec in I, aVL	B. Left posterior fascicular block
_____ 3. QRS axis at -60 degrees	C. Normal axis
_____ 4. QRS axis at +30 degrees	D. Right axis deviation
_____ 5. QRS axis at +120 degrees	E. Left axis deviation

● ECG Rhythm Identification Practice

Identify the ECG criterion listed below each ECG tracing. Compare your answers with those in the back of the book.

Figure 4-11

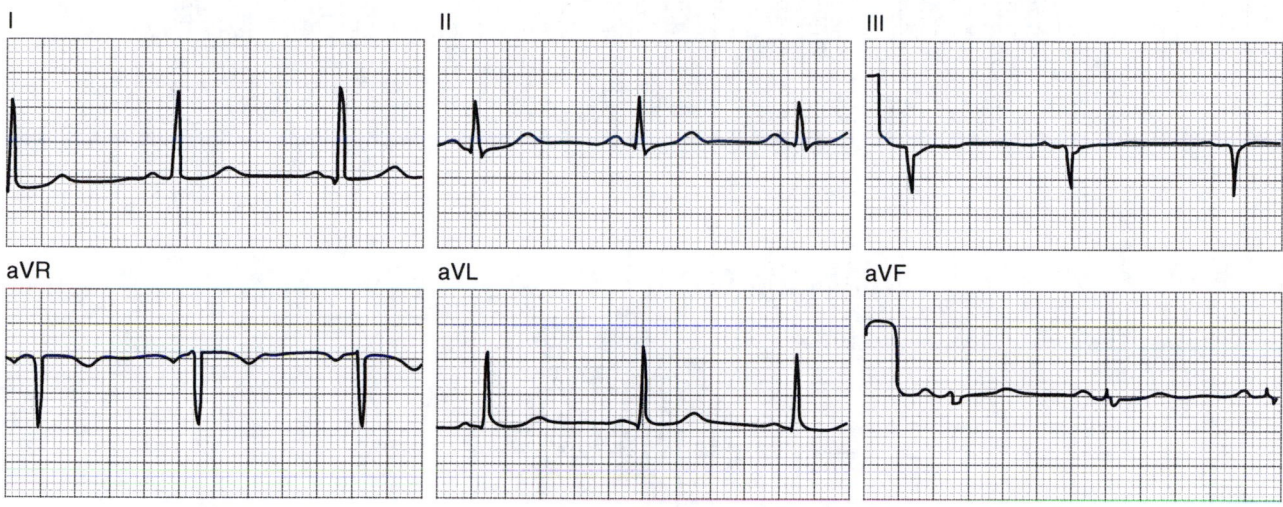

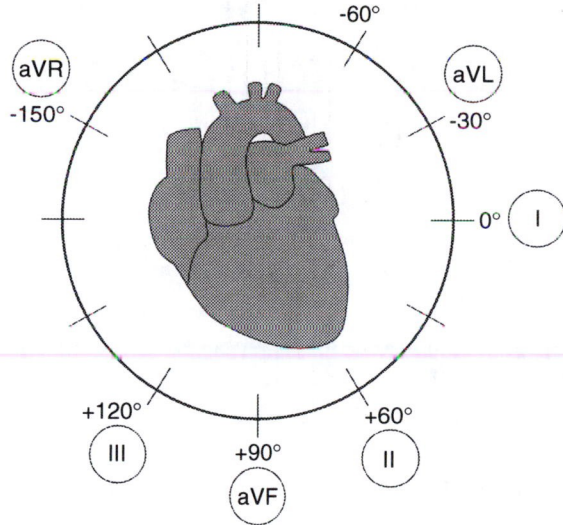

1. What is the underlying rhythm? _____
2. What is the axis? _____
   a. Look at leads I and II; are they positive? _____
   b. Are there equiphasic deflections? _____
   c. Draw the arrows on the Lewis circle to verify your calculations.
3. What is your interpretation? _____

Figure 4-12

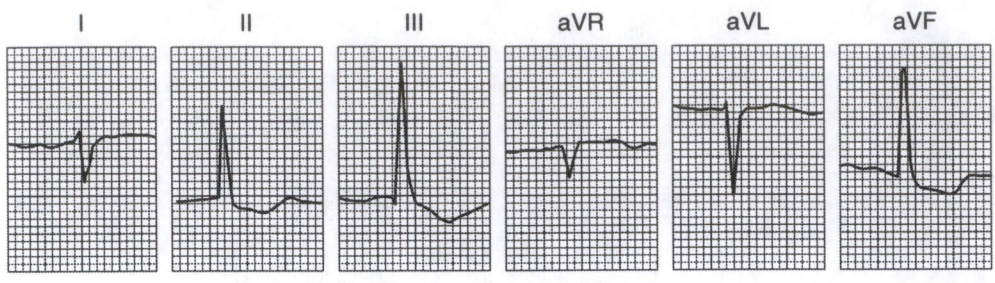

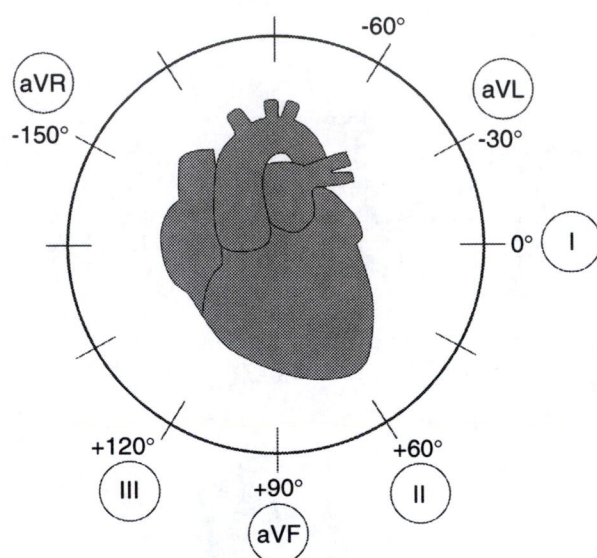

1. What is the underlying rhythm? _____
2. What is the axis? _____
   a. Look at leads I and II; are they positive? _____
   b. Are there equiphasic deflections? _____
   c. Draw the arrows on the Lewis circle to verify your calculations.
3. What is your interpretation? _____
   _____

Figure 4-13

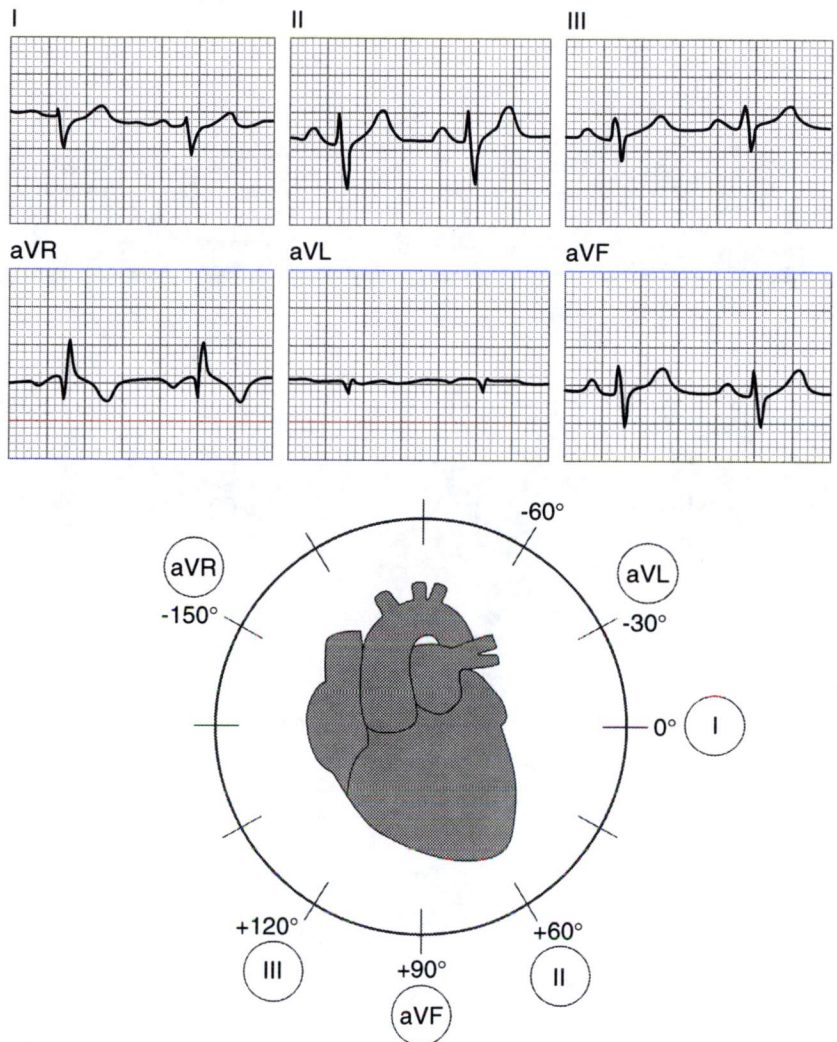

1. What is the underlying rhythm? _____
2. What is the axis? _____
   a. Look at leads I and II; are they positive? _____
   b. Are there equiphasic deflections? _____
   c. Draw the arrows on the Lewis circle to verify your calculations.
3. What is your interpretation? _____
   _____

Figure 4-14

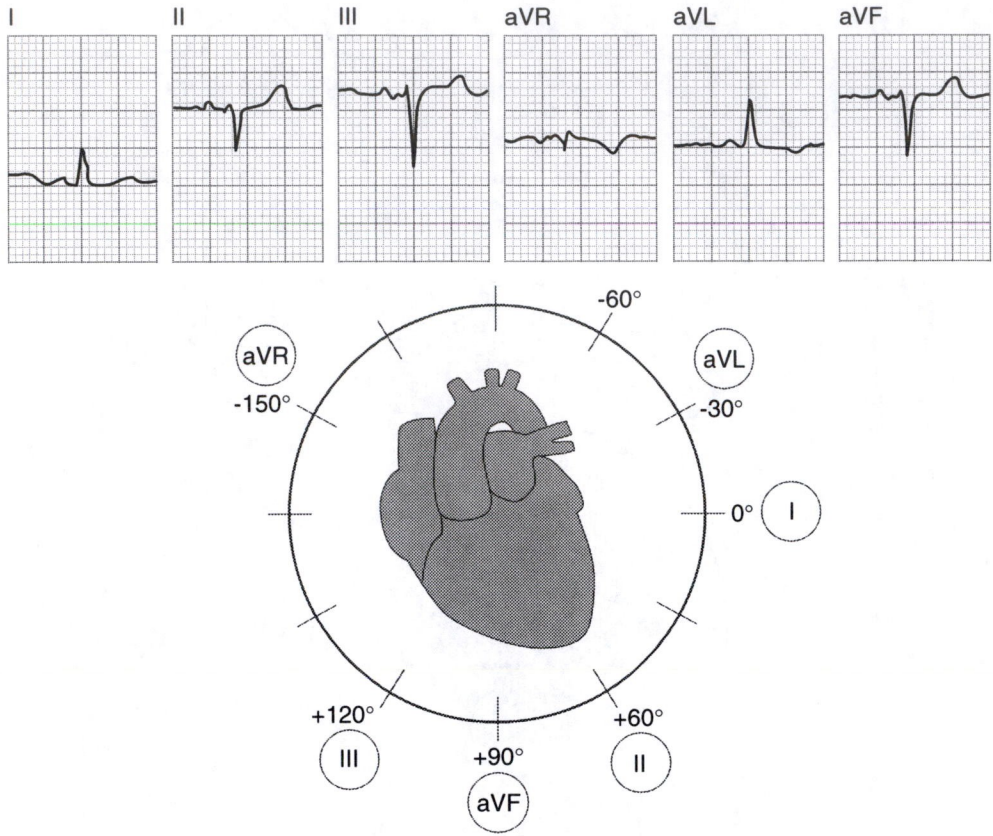

1. What is the underlying rhythm? _____
2. What is the axis? _____
   a. Look at leads I and II; are they positive? _____
   b. Are there equiphasic deflections? _____
   c. Draw the arrows on the Lewis circle to verify your calculations.
3. What is your interpretation? _____
   _____

Figure 4-15

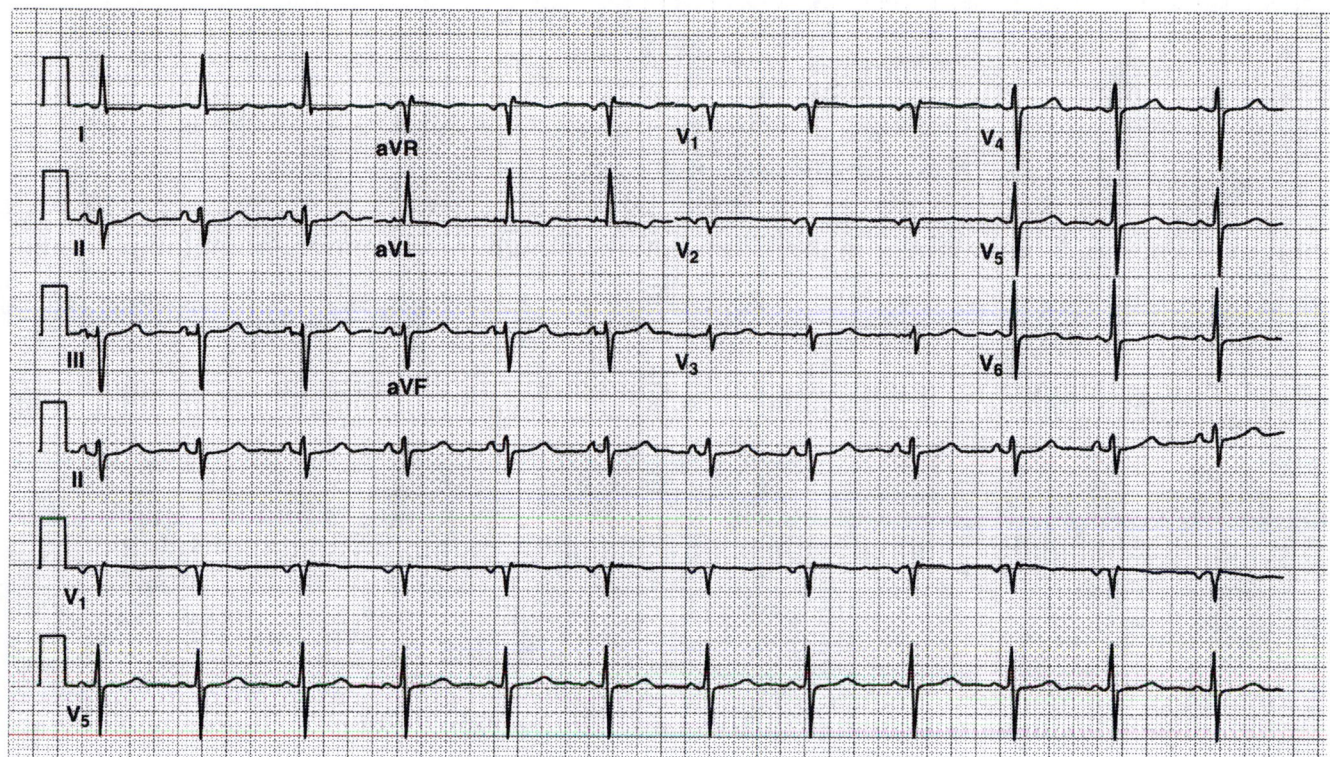

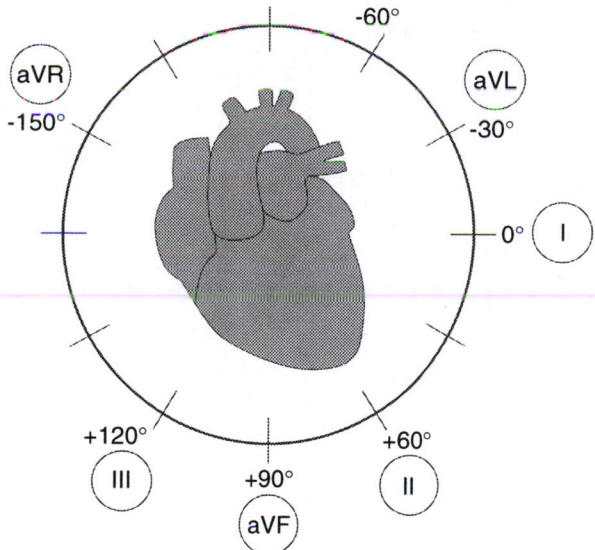

1. What is the underlying rhythm? _____
2. What is the axis? _____
   a. Look at leads I and II; are they positive? _____
   b. Are there equiphasic deflections? _____
   c. Draw the arrows on the Lewis circle to verify your calculations.
3. What is your interpretation? _____
   _____

References

Conover, M. B. (1996). *Understanding electrocardiography: Arrhythmias and the 12-lead ECG.* (7th ed.). St. Louis: Mosby-Year Book.

Conover, M. B. & Wellens, H. J. (1993). *The ECG in emergency decision making.* Philadelphia: W. B. Saunders.

Goldberger, E. (1982). *Textbook of clinical cardiology.* St. Louis: C. V. Mosby.

Marriott, H. J. & Conover, M. B. (1989). *Advanced concepts in arrhythmias.* (2nd ed.). St. Louis: C. V. Mosby.

Topol, E. (1998). *Textbook of clinical cardiology.* Philadelphia: Lippincott-Raven.

Sinus Rhythm and the Arrhythmias

> **Premise** ● Abnormalities of heart rhythm are relatively easy to figure out. Most of the time, the key is to find the P wave.

Objectives

After reading the chapter and completing the Self-Assessment exercises, the student should be able to:

1. Identify sinus mechanisms
2. Identify junctional mechanisms
3. Identify atrial mechanisms
4. Identify ventricular mechanisms
5. Identify ECG signs of aberrant ventricular conduction
6. Identify AV conduction defects
7. Identify arrhythmias caused by accessory pathways
8. Recognize ECG signs of pacemaker function

Key Terms

aberrancy

accessory pathway

arrhythmia

bradycardia

complete AV block

fibrillation

first-degree AV block

fusion beat

junctional rhythm

premature atrial
   complex (PAC)

premature junctional
   complex (PJC)

P prime (P′)

paroxysmal

reentry

SA block

second-degree AV
   block

sinus arrest

supraventricular

tachycardia

Introduction

Normally, the heart depolarizes spontaneously and rhythmically. The rate is controlled by the pacemaker that depolarizes at the highest rate. The sinus node normally has the highest rate of discharge. Subsequent depolarization of atrial tissue will write a P wave on the ECG. If the impulse succeeds in traveling through the

AV junction and activating the ventricles, a normal QRS complex (0.10 second or less) will follow. Variations in cardiac rate and rhythm can occur in hearts without diagnosed pathology, often as a result of drug use, systemic disease, ischemia, or hypoxia. The following is a brief review of the various abnormalities in heart rate and rhythm. We will not dwell on the different definitions of the terms *arrhythmia* and *dysrhythmia*. The derivation of these terms is well-documented, but not always acknowledged. For the purpose of this text, the term arrhythmia will be used because it is correct, practical, and applicable. Its ease and dominant use are respected.

HOW TO LOOK AT AND ANALYZE WAVE FORMS

A clear, organized, and consistent approach is necessary to accurately analyze ECG wave forms. Abnormalities of cardiac rhythms are particularly easy to work out— the key is the P wave.

1. Plot out P waves, calculating rate and rhythm

2. Plot out QRS complexes, calculating rate and rhythm

3. Confirm the association between each P wave and the QRS complex

Labeling the ECG

ECG rhythms are usually labeled with two terms. The first term indicates the energy source, the pacemaker. The second term indicates the effects of the conduction on heart rate or rhythm.

For example, sinus rhythm is interpreted using the sinus node as the pacemaker. The heart rate is between 60 and 100 beats per minute. Junctional tachycardia implies the pacemaker is in the AV junction and the rate is greater than 100 beats per minute. For example:

Sinus	Tachycardia at 110 beats per minute
pacemaker site	rate/rhythm/event

Sinus	Arrhythmia at 75-100 beats per minute
pacemaker site	rate/rhythm/event

Sinus	at 87 with 2° AV block V rate 44
pacemaker site	rate/rhythm/event

Junctional	Rhythm at 56 with frequent PVCs
pacemaker site	rate/rhythm/event

In the case of the back-up pacemakers, the inherent rate range for the AV junction is 40 to 60 beats per minute and the ventricular escape rate range is 20 to 40 beats per minute. When each of these accelerates, but remains less than 100 beats per minute, the term *accelerated* precedes it. Thus, an AV junctional rate of 75 will be termed *accelerated junctional rhythm at 75 beats per minute*; a ventricular pacer at 80 will be termed *accelerated ventricular rhythm at 80 beats per minute*.

It is important to qualify each identification with the specific rate per minute. Coupled with the patient's vital signs, level of consciousness, and overall presentation, this information provides the greatest insight into the arrhythmia and guides interventions.

How to Assess a Monitor Pattern

Atrial activation (P wave) is usually followed by ventricular activation (a QRS complex), and there is normally one P wave for each QRS complex. To assess a monitor pattern, follow the steps outlined here.

1. Determine if the rhythm is supraventricular or ventricular in origin. If the QRS is 0.10 second or less, it is likely supraventricular in origin—from the sinus node, from within the atria, or from the AV junction.

2. Look to the left of the QRS for a P wave for every QRS. If the QRS is 0.10 or less, and the P wave is:

   a. (+), it is probably sinus in origin;

   b. (-) or absent and the QRS is regular, it is probably junctional;

   c. (+) and premature, it is probably atrial in origin.

3. Is the PR interval consistent?

4. Analyze if different complexes are premature (early) or escape (late). Plot out the P waves.

   a. If the P waves plot out regularly, the ectopic is probably ventricular in origin.

   b. If the P waves do not plot out regularly, the ectopic is probably supraventricular in origin; most likely, atrial.

5. Calculate the rate.

   a. Plot P to P and QRS to QRS at the baseline, *not* peak to peak. Some QRS complexes are notched or otherwise altered by artifact and make the peak-to-peak method inaccurate.

   b. If Ps or QRSs are regular, divide the number of large boxes between 2 regularly occurring wave forms and divide into 300. In rapid rates, divide the number of small boxes between 2 regularly occurring wave forms and divide into 1,500.

6. Describe any other deviation.

   a. ST segment elevation or depression

   b. T wave changes such as inversion

   c. Widening of the QRS

   d. Change in rhythm, sudden (paroxysmal), gradual, or sustained

Measuring ventricular rate and rhythm involves plotting wave forms. For example, when plotting ventricular rate, the practitioner will measure from the beginning of the QRS, whatever its configuration, to the next QRS at the baseline. When plotting the measurements, it is important to remain at the baseline.

To accurately identify the rhythm, specific criteria must be evaluated. In each of the mechanisms, the criteria will be addressed in a consistent manner so the reader can develop a consistent pattern of identification.

SINUS MECHANISMS

Normally, the sinus node is the primary pacemaker. As long as the sinus node fires and atrial tissue responds, the process recurs normally at a given rate of speed. The clue is to look to the left of each QRS. If a single, positive P wave is present for each and every normal QRS, that is the sinus mechanism.

To describe the rhythm of the heart as sinus rhythm—the impulse originating in the sinoatrial (SA) node, the normal pacemaker of the heart—without qualifications, certain criteria must be met:

1. P Wave   The P waves are positive (upright) and uniform in lead II. Every P wave is followed by a QRS complex.

2. PR Interval   The PR interval (from the beginning of the P wave to the beginning of the QRS complex) is constant and consistently between 0.12 and 0.20 second.

3. QRS Complex   The QRS complex duration is 0.10 second or less. Every QRS complex is preceded by a single, predictable, positive P wave.

4. QRS Rate   A "normal," predictable heart rate is between 60 and 100 beats per minute in the adult patient.

5. QRS Rhythm   The rhythm is regular. Sinus rhythm is the standard against which most arrhythmias are measured, compared, and analyzed (Figure 5-1).

Sinus Tachycardia

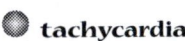

tachycardia

Heart rate greater than 100 beats per minute

Tachycardia means fast (tachy) heart (cardia), that is, a rate greater than 100 beats per minute. Recall that the word *sinus* appearing before the word *tachycardia* indicates that the origin of the rhythm is the SA node, the normal pacemaker of the heart.

If all the criteria for a sinus mechanism have been fulfilled, but the heart rate is greater than 100 beats per minute, the rhythm is called sinus tachycardia. The range for a sinus tachycardia is usually 100 to 180 beats per minute (Figure 5-2). The sinus node rarely exceeds 180 beats per minute, although rates up to 200 beats per minute have been seen with exertion.

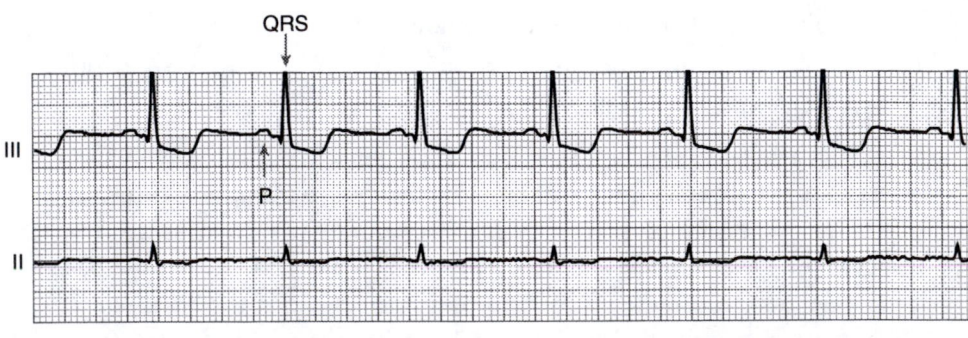

Figure 5-1 An ECG tracing from a patient showing simultaneous leads. Note the difference in the ECG wave forms as depicted in the two leads. Lead III is more clear. This example illustrates that relying on only one lead can be misleading.

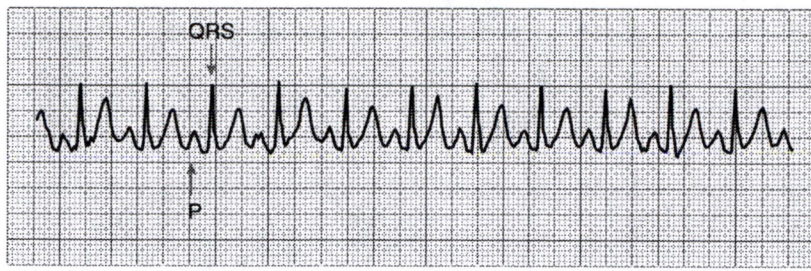

Figure 5-2 An ECG tracing showing one positive P wave to the left of each QRS complex; the PR interval is consistent and the heart rate is greater than 100 beats per minute. Interpretation: sinus tachycardia at 125 beats per minute.

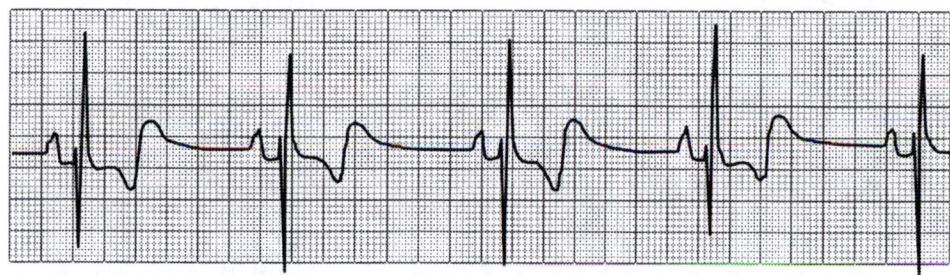

Figure 5-3 An ECG tracing showing one positive P wave to the left of each QRS complex; the PR interval is consistent and the heart rate is 43 beats per minute. Interpretation: sinus bradycardia at 43 beats per minute; 1 mm ST ↓ and ↓ T waves.

Sinus Bradycardia

Bradycardia means slow (brady) heart (cardia). If the heart rate is under 60 beats per minute, but all the criteria for a sinus mechanism have been fulfilled, the rhythm is known as sinus bradycardia (Figure 5-3).

⬤ **bradycardia**
Heart rate less than 60 beats per minute

Sinus Arrhythmia

In sinus arrhythmia, the impulse has its origin in the sinus node and subsequent conduction is normal. In sinus arrythmia, the rhythm of impulse formation, and thus the heart's response, is irregular; *irregular* (ar-) *rhythm* (-rhythmia). The PR intervals are consistent, but the PP and RR intervals are continually changing (Figure 5-4). The heart rate varies from about 86 to 100 beats per minute, about a 10 percent variation.

Sinus Arrest

Sinus arrest is an event caused by a sudden failure of the SA node to initiate a timely impulse. In sinus arrest, multiples of PQRST complexes are missing, sometimes 2, sometimes 3, or sometimes 4. There does not have to be a pattern to the frequency of occurrences. In other words, a patient can have periods of SA arrest, missing 2 or 3 PQRST complexes. This may not recur for several minutes or hours and then an episode of missing several complexes can occur.

⬤ **sinus arrest**
A sudden failure of the SA node to initiate a timely impulse

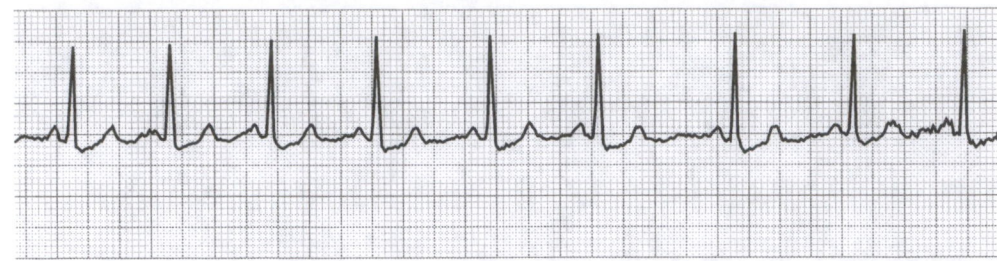

....

Figure 5-4 An ECG tracing showing sinus arrhythmia. Note the gradual increase and decrease of heart rate. There is one positive P wave to the left of each QRS complex; the PR interval is consistent but the heart rate varies. Interpretation: sinus arrhythmia at 66 to 100 beats per minute; 1 mm ST ↓.

If the period of arrest is more than 1 cycle length, physiologically another pacemaker should take over and initiate a new rhythm (Figure 5-5). In most cases, it is the AV junction that takes over as pacemaker.

Sinoatrial (SA) Block

Sinoatrial (SA) block is also called *sinus exit block*. SA block is an event that does not always reflect disease within the sinus node. In SA block, the SA node initiates the impulse, but the propagation over atrial tissue is blocked, so the atria are not depolarized. Therefore, there is no P wave or QRS complex. SA block represents a failure of transmission of the impulse over atrial tissue (Figure 5-6).

SUMMARY OF SINUS MECHANISMS

Normally, the sinus node dominates heart rhythm and does so for a lifetime. An arrhythmia is present when the heart rate is too slow, too fast, or irregular, or when depolarization does not propagate over atrial tissue, and, finally, when the SA node fails to produce a stimulus at all.

In each of the sinus mechanisms, the visible P wave is positive and precedes each and every QRS. Where there is no P wave, there is no atrial depolarization.

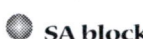 **SA block**

A disorder where the atria are unable to respond to the sinus stimulus, resulting in a missed PQRST complex; sinus cadence is usually undisturbed

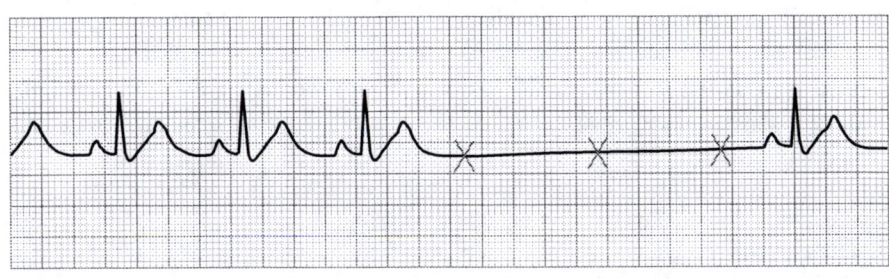

....

Figure 5-5 An ECG tracing showing one positive P wave to the left of each of the first three QRS complexes; the PR interval is consistent and the heart rate is within normal limits prior to the event—the SA arrest. Count the number of large squares between the QRS complexes containing the arrest. Multiply by 0.20 (the value of one large square) for the estimated period of arrest, about 2.76 seconds. Interpretation: sinus rhythm at 75 beats per minute with SA arrest of 2.76 seconds.

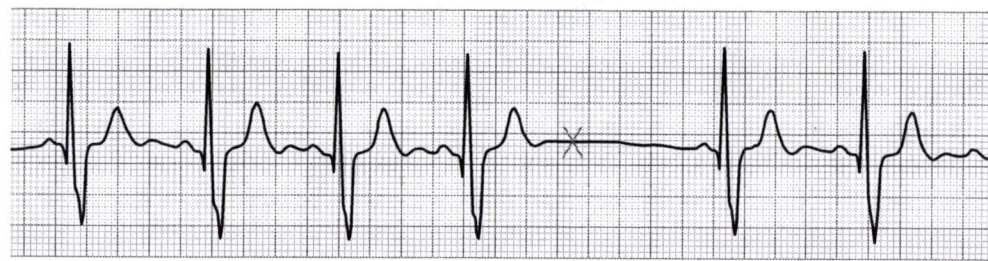

Figure 5-6 An ECG tracing showing a positive P wave to the left of each QRS complex; the PR interval is consistent and the heart rate is within normal limits prior to the event. Plot out the sinus P waves, make an X for the missing P wave. Measure the RR intervals, noting that the RR of the SA block is equal to twice the normal RR interval. Interpretation: sinus rhythm at 75 beats per minute with an episode of SA block. It is necessary to note any other variations, so the final description would include: there are U waves and the QRS complex is 0.16 second with a broad terminal S wave.

Most of the sinus arrhythmias are explainable and patients generally tolerate minor deviations. In most instances, identifying and treating the cause remedies the arrhythmias. When a patient's situation is complicated by persistent bradycardia and accompanying hypotension and hypoperfusion, treating the patient is appropriate.

Table 5-1 is a summary of the sinus mechanisms and the ECG components, to help differentiate the rhythms.

JUNCTIONAL MECHANISMS

When the sinus node fails to function, the next possible pacemaker to respond lies within the AV junction. Conduction into the ventricles usually occurs without problem and the resulting QRS shows little or no difference from a sinus-induced QRS.

The AV junction can function as a back-up or escape pacemaker, generating an impulse at a predictable and satisfactory rate. The AV junction can also function as an ectopic, challenging the sinus node by generating an impulse and taking control of heart rate.

Table 5-1 Summary of the ECG configurations of the sinus mechanisms

Sinus	Rhythm	Bradycardia	Tachycardia	Arrhythmia	SA Block	Sinus Arrest
P waves	(+)/QRS	(+)/QRS	(+)/QRS	(+)/QRS	(+)/QRS	(+)/QRS
PR Interval	0.12–0.20 sec	0.12–0.20 sec	0.12–0.20 sec	0.12–0.20 sec	0.12–0.20 sec	0.12–0.20 sec
QRS duration	≤0.10	≤0.10	≤0.10	≤0.10		
Rate/minute	60–100	<60	>100	60–100		
Rhythm	regular	regular	regular	irregular	regular except for the event	regular except for the event
Event			gradual onset	gradual change	misses one beat; sinus plots through; cadence is regular	misses more than one beat; rhythm after is irregular and slow

An impulse that originates within the nodal-His (NH) region of the bundle of His is conducted through the ventricular bundle branches and results in a narrow QRS complex, not unlike a sinus-induced QRS complex. By convention, the pacing function within AV junctional tissue is referred to as *junctional*. Any P wave that originates from other than the sinus node is referred to as **P prime** (P′). The junction rarely functions in competition with the sinus node because its primary role is that of a back-up pacemaker; it is normally depolarized in sequence with each sinus beat. When the sinus fails, or when the sinus impulse is blocked within the AV node, the bundle of His may reach potential and generate an impulse. This is termed an escape beat. If the bundle of His sustains the role of pacemaker, it is termed a **junctional rhythm**.

An escape beat is one that comes after a delay in the cardiac cycle. There is a pause, as with SA block or SA arrest, and at the conclusion of the delay is a narrow QRS with a retrograde P′ that is seen before, during, or after the QRS; sometimes, the P′ is not visible at all. An escape junctional beat occurs because the sinus failed to maintain control. The junction, not having been stimulated by a sinus-induced wave front, reaches its inherent potential and discharges. If the underlying cause persists, the escape beat can take over the pacemaking function, as in the junctional rhythm described earlier.

The P′ wave may be completely or partially hidden within the preceding T wave or greatly enhance the amplitude and distort the preceding T wave. The P′ waves can be seen before, during, or after the QRS complexes, and are inverted (negative) in leads II, III, and aVF.

The position of the P′ wave depends on whether:

- The atria are depolarized before the ventricles. The P′ wave is inverted in lead II with a short (0.12 second or less) P′R interval.

- The atria and the ventricles may be depolarized simultaneously. The P′ wave is then hidden within the QRS complex and is not visible on the ECG.

- The atria are depolarized after the ventricles. The P′ wave is then inverted in lead II, following the QRS complex.

- When no P′ waves are visible, a 4th possibility exists: the atria are not depolarized because retrograde conduction is blocked. The QRS complex is less than or equal to 0.10 second, with normal ventricular depolarization (Figure 5-7).

Junctional Rhythm

The junction is capable of providing a consistent and predictable heart rate (Figure 5-8). When the junction becomes the dominant pacemaker, the single impulse origination in the junction can travel in 2 directions.

The ventricles are depolarized normally, since the impulse spreads through the bundle of His to the bundle branches and then through to the Purkinje network, leading to ventricular depolarization. The QRS complexes, therefore, are normal in duration, less than or equal to 0.10 second. The atria, however, are depolarized in a manner opposite to that of normal. This is called *retrograde atrial depolarization*, which is reflected on the ECG by a negative (downward, inverted) P′ wave in lead II.

● **P prime (P′) wave**

P wave that is from other than a sinus impulse

● **junctional rhythm**

The role of pacemaker is sustained by the bundle of His

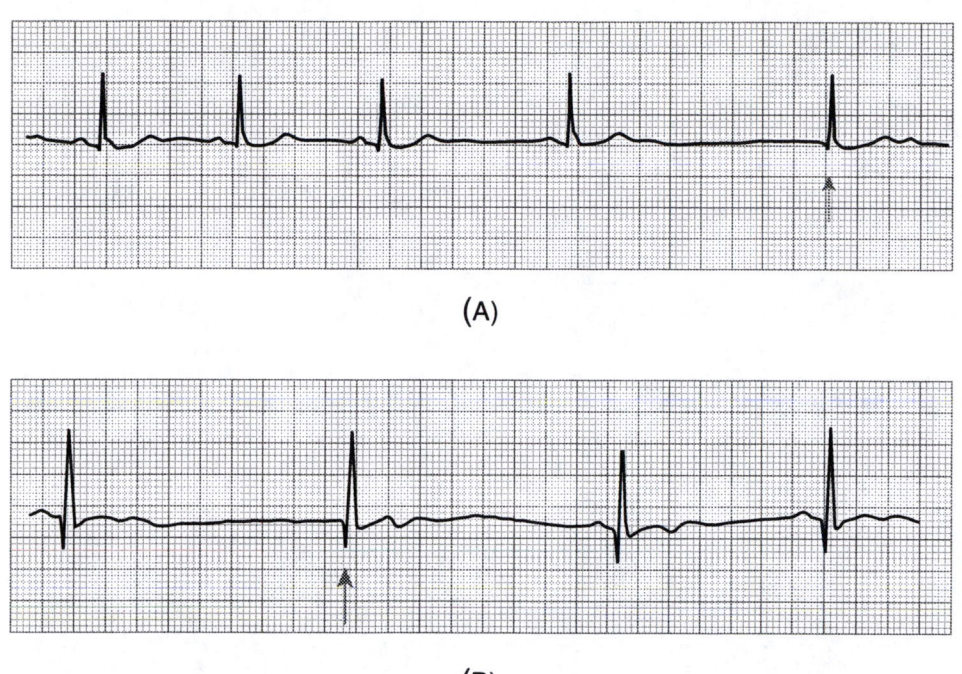

(A)

(B)

Figure 5-7 Two ECG tracings. View A shows one positive P wave to the left of each QRS complex; the PR interval is consistent and the heart rate is within normal limits. The heart rate visibly slows until a long pause of about 1.6 seconds. The next complex is a QRS without the visible sinus P wave to the left. This is the junctional escape beat. View B shows a positive P plus a QRS (a sinus beat), a pause, a QRS with no visible P wave (the junctional escape beat) and a return to a sinus bradycardia. In each example, note the configuration and measurement of the QRS complex does not vary despite the difference in origin.

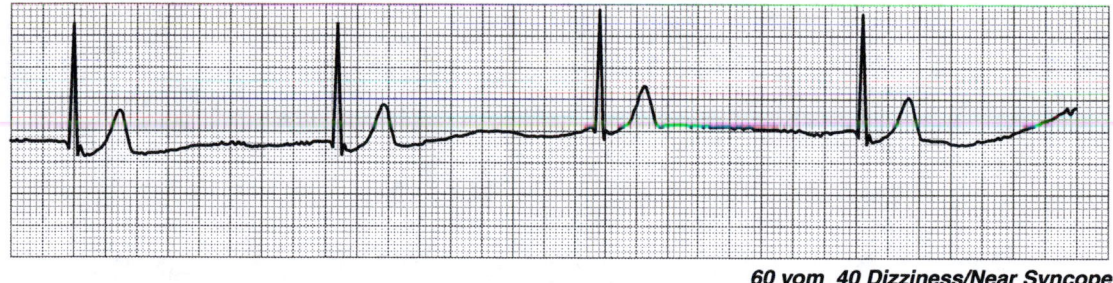

60 yom 40 Dizziness/Near Syncope

Figure 5-8 An ECG tracing showing a narrow QRS complex, but no preceding P wave. This indicates the junctional mechanism. Interpretation: junctional rhythm at 35 beats per minute.

Premature Junctional Complex

In the case of a **premature junctional complex** (PJC), the P′ wave may be completely or partially hidden within the preceding T wave, or it may greatly enhance the amplitude and distort the preceding T wave (Figure 5-9). The P′ waves can be seen before, during, or after the QRS complexes, and are inverted (negative) in leads II, III, and aVF (Figures 5-10 and 5-11).

● **premature junctional complex (PJC)**

A discharge of a junctional ectopic focus that causes earlier than normal retrograde atrial depolarization; represented on the ECG by a negative (-) P′; can occur before, during, or after the QRS complex.

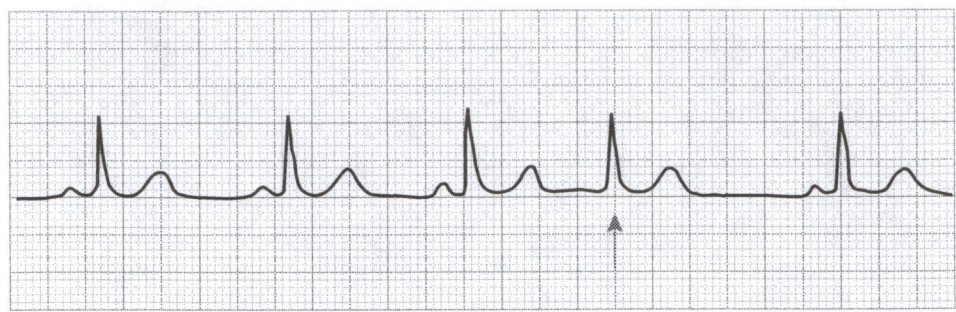

Figure 5-9 An ECG tracing showing one positive P to the left of each of 3 sinus beats. The 4th QRS complex is similar to the sinus QRSs but is clearly early (premature) and has no P wave preceding it. The sinus P waves do not plot through the event. Interpretation: sinus rhythm at 63 beats per minute with a PJC.

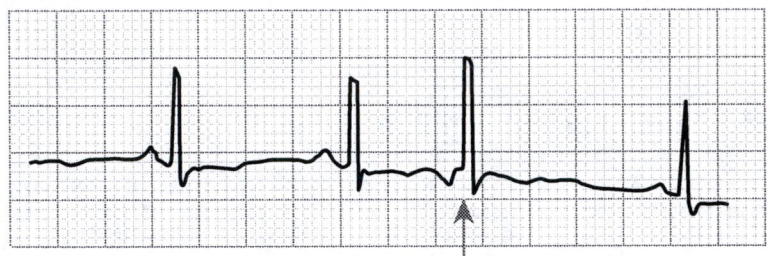

Figure 5-10 An ECG tracing showing one positive P to the left of each of 2 sinus beats. The 3rd QRS complex is similar to the sinus QRSs but is clearly early (premature) and has a negative P' preceding it. The sinus P waves do not plot through the event. Interpretation: sinus rhythm at 77 beats per minute with a PJC.

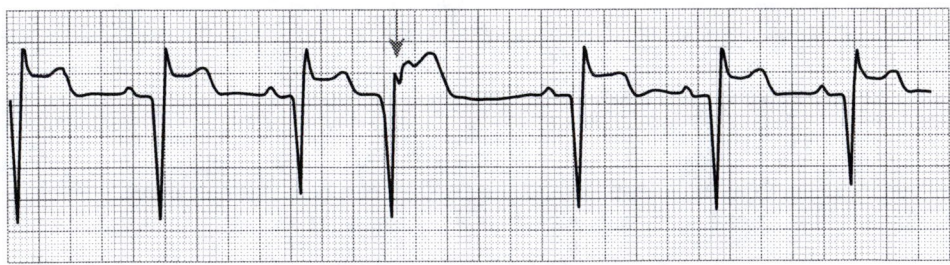

Figure 5-11 An ECG tracing showing a positive P wave for each of 2 clearly visible QRS complexes, indicating a sinus mechanism. The 4th QRS is clearly premature, with no positive P prior to the QRS. There is a negative deflection in the ST segment of the premature complex, which may indicate the retrograde conduction to the atria. The P waves do not plot through the event, but resume cadence afterwards. There is 3 to 4 mm ST segment elevation and deep Q waves (18 mm and 0.06 second). Interpretation: sinus rhythm at 67 beats per minute with one PJC, 3 to 4 mm ST segment elevation, and Q wave at 18 mm.

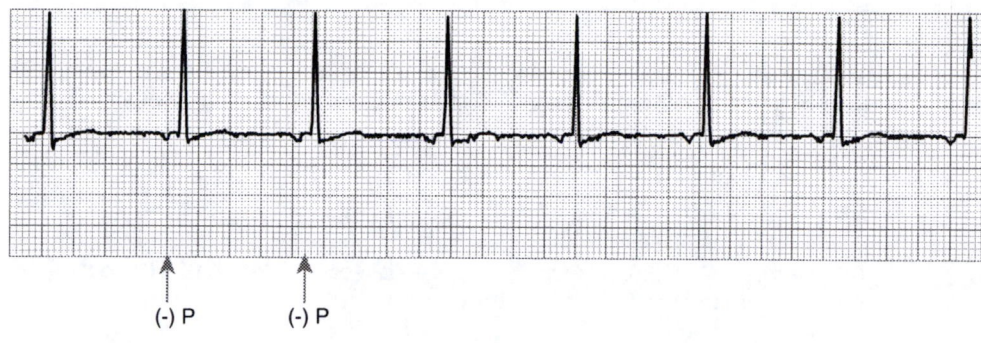

(-) P   (-) P

Figure 5-12 An ECG tracing showing a regular, narrow QRS with a negative P' to the left of each QRS. The QRS rate is 67 beats per minute. Interpretation: accelerated junctional rhythm at 67 beats per minute.

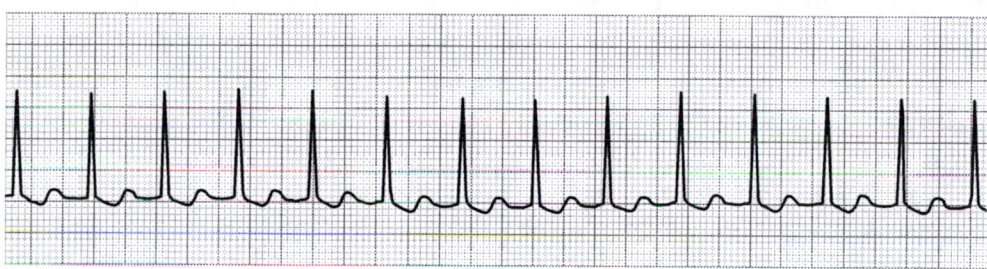

Figure 5-13 An ECG tracing showing narrow QRS with no identifiable P wave to the left of the QRS. The QRS rate is 125 beats per minute. Interpretation: junctional tachycardia at 125 beats per minute.

Accelerated Junctional Rhythm and Junctional Tachycardia

Accelerated junctional rhythm is the term used to describe a junctional rate between 60 and 100 beats per minute (Figure 5-12). The ECG characteristics of junctional tachycardia are similar to those of junctional rhythm and accelerated junctional rhythm, with the exception of rate. In junctional tachycardia, the rate is 100 to 140 beats per minute (Figure 5-13). Table 5-2 is a summary of ECG configurations for the junctional mechanisms.

ATRIAL MECHANISMS

Atrial arrhythmias are usually a manifestation of abnormal electrical activity in the atria. Atrial stretch, hypoxia, drug use, medications, and chemical imbalance are factors that contribute to enhanced or triggered automaticity resulting in atrial ectopy.

Table 5-2 Summary of ECG configurations of junctional mechanisms

	Junctional Escape Beat	Junctional Rhythm	Accelerated Junctional Rhythm	Junctional Tachycardia	Premature Junctional Complex (PJC)
P' waves	(-) or none	(-) or none	(-) or none	(-) or none	(-) or none
P'-R interval	≤0.12 sec	≤0.12 sec	≤0.12 sec	≤0.12 sec	≤0.12 sec
QRS duration	≤0.10	≤0.10	≤0.10	≤0.10	≤0.10
Ventricular rate per minute		40–60	60–100	>100	
Ventricular rhythm		regular	regular	regular	

Premature Atrial Complex

A sinus-induced QRS presents with a single positive predictable P wave preceding each QRS with a consistent PR interval. A junction-induced QRS may present with either a single negative predictable P wave preceding each QRS, or a single negative predictable P wave following each QRS, or no visible P wave at all.

In the case of atrial ectopy, a P' will occur; however, the P' will be positive. The intrinsic sinus rhythm will be disturbed and sinus P waves will not plot through rhythmically, but the QRS complex is usually less than or equal to 0.10 second, since the impulse will be conducted normally.

Premature atrial complexes (PACs) occur when an ectopic atrial focus propagates an impulse before the next normal sinus beat. The ectopic atrial beat is usually easily identified. The morphology of the QRS complex will be narrow and relatively unchanged. The preceding P' will be early (premature) and may vary in size and configuration from the sinus P waves.

Finally, PACs disrupt the regularity and rhythm of the sinus rhythm. The sinus P waves will not plot through the premature event, since the premature depolarization will affect sinus activity (Figure 5-14). When the sinus node regains control, the rhythm and regularity will be restored.

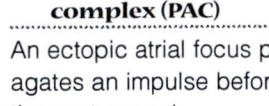
premature atrial complex (PAC)

An ectopic atrial focus propagates an impulse before the next normal sinus beat

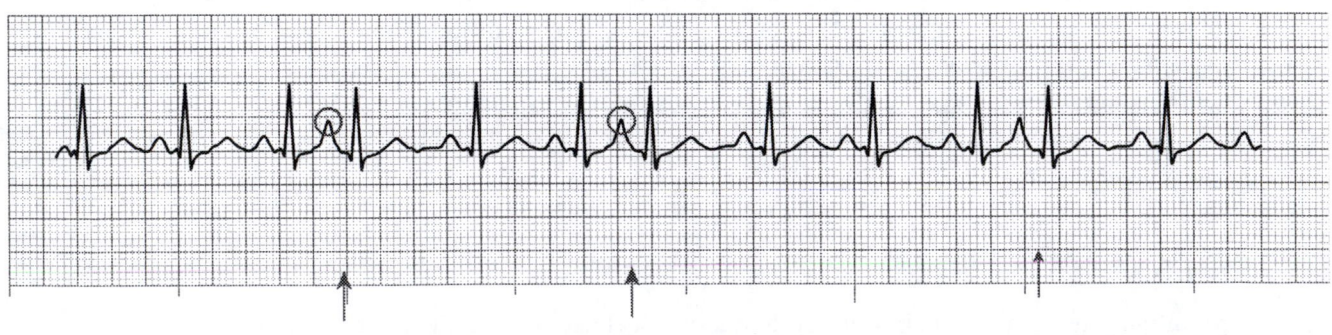

Figure 5-14 An ECG tracing showing one positive P wave to the left of each of the first 3 sinus beats, a sinus rhythm at 96 beats per minute. The next QRS complex is similar to the sinus QRSs but is early (premature) and has a positive P' superimposed on the previous T wave. The sinus P waves do not plot through the event. The PACs recur (arrow) each time disturbing the sinus rhythm. Interpretation: sinus rhythm at 96 beats per minute with frequent PACs.

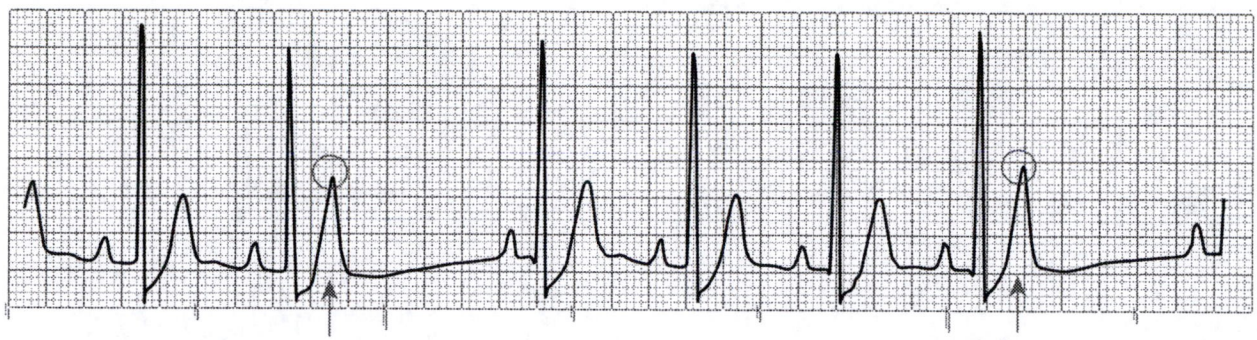

Figure 5-15 An ECG tracing showing one positive P wave to the left of each of the first 2 sinus beats, a sinus rhythm. There is a sudden pause in the cadence of the sinus mechanism. Look back at the last T wave and note the increased amplitude. The height of the T wave is a combination of P and T wave amplitudes. The sinus P waves do not plot through the event, and the cadence of the sinus rhythm resumes at about 75 beats per minute. Interpretation: sinus rhythm at 75 beats per minute with frequent, nonconducted PACs.

An atrial ectopic may not successfully conduct into the ventricles. Ability to conduct is a matter of timing and opportunity. For instance, if the PAC finds the AV node or the bundle branches completely refractory, the impulse will not conduct into the ventricles. This is called a *blocked*, or *nonconducted*, PAC. The position of the atrial P′ may be hidden within the ST segment or T wave and can usually be recognized when there is an alteration of T wave morphology. For example, when the amplitude of the T wave changes suddenly, or appears notched, the cause is a premature P′ superimposed on that T wave.

Figure 5-15 is an ECG tracing of a sinus rhythm with two nonconducted PACs. Note the increased amplitude of the T waves just prior to the pause in the rhythm. The P′ generated an additive influence on these T waves. The P′ did not conduct into the ventricles; therefore, there was no QRS, and this absence of conduction created the pause seen in the tracing.

Figure 5-16 is an ECG tracing of a sinus rhythm with a nonconducted PAC, causing a sudden pause in the cadence of the sinus rhythm. The pause is followed

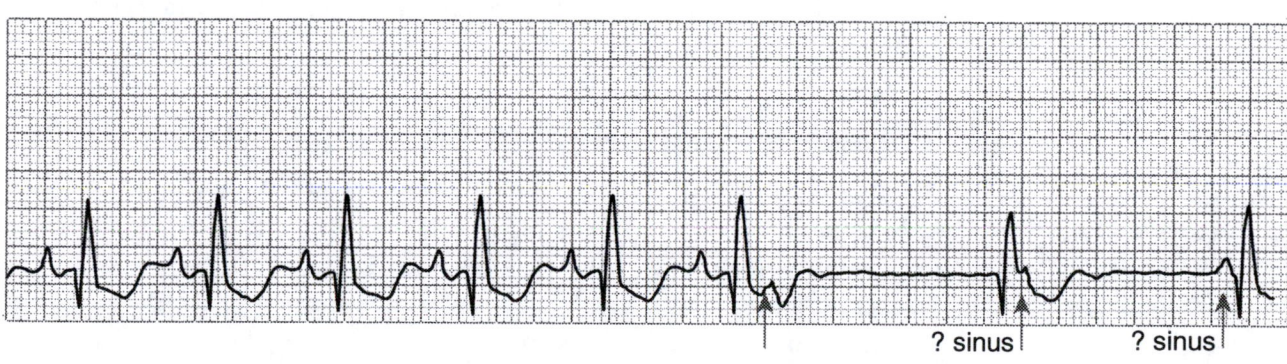

Figure 5-16 An ECG tracing showing one positive P wave to the left of each of the first 6 sinus beats, a sinus rhythm. There is a sudden pause in the cadence of the sinus mechanism. Look back at the ST segment and note the appearance of the P′. The sinus P waves do not plot through the event. An escape junctional rhythm is the source of the last 2 QRSs. The emerging sinus is seen as sinus P waves (arrows). The sinus rate has not yet overcome the junction, thus the fusion of sorts is on the last complex. Interpretation: sinus rhythm at 86 beats per minute with a nonconducted PAC, followed by a junctional escape rhythm at 50 beats per minute.

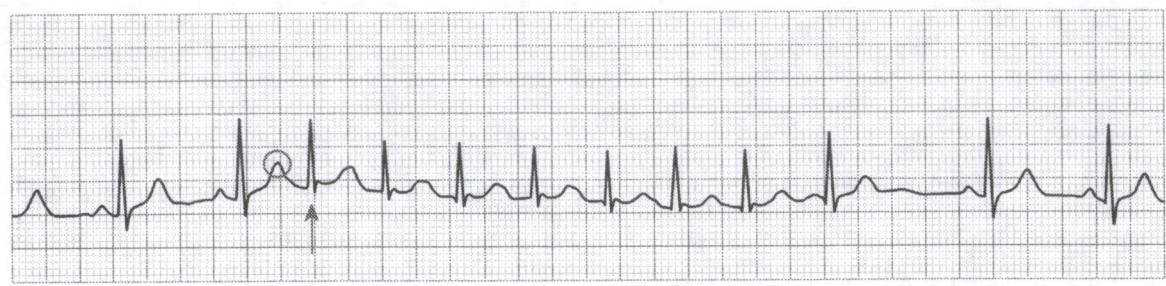

Figure 5-17 An ECG tracing showing a narrow QRS complex of similar configuration throughout. Plotting out the P waves, the atrial rate is 86 beats per minute for the first 2 complexes. The rate changes suddenly. Note the PAC (arrow) at the beginning of the tachycardia. The rate here is 136 beats per minute, T waves are distorted and "lumpy" indicating the atrial ectopics. The rate changes again, beginning with a pause, and reverting back to a sinus rhythm. The visible sudden onset and sudden end of the tachycardia is the paroxysm. Interpretation: sinus at 86 beats per minute → paroxysmal atrial tachycardia (PAT) at 136 beats per minute → sinus at 86. The sinus P waves do not plot through this event.

by junctional escape beats. In this tracing, the P′ is visible in the ST segment. The PAC did not conduct into the ventricles and this created the pause visible in the tracing. There is a junctional escape mechanism for 2 beats, which is not uncommon following atrial ectopics. Sinus P waves seem to be surfacing, and perhaps as the sinus accelerates, it will capture and conduct as it did earlier in the tracing.

Atrial Tachycardia

In atrial tachycardia, an atrial ectopic discharges a stimulus at a rate of 130 to 250 beats per minute. Fortunately, the AV node protectively blocks many of the impulses and the resulting ventricular rate is usually slower. The ventricular rhythm can be regular or irregular. Figure 5-17 is an example of atrial tachycardia. Note the rate of the (+) P′ waves, so the atria are tachycardic at 136 beats per minute. An atrial ectopic focus may develop a rapid rate of depolarization, thus creating a tachycardia. When this arrhythmia is seen to appear and disappear suddenly, it is referred to as **paroxysmal** atrial tachycardia. If the AV node supports the rhythm, every atrial impulse will be conducted through to the ventricles. Figure 5-17 and Figure 5-18 are examples of atrial tachycardias.

● **paroxysm**
An abrupt start or stop

Supraventricular Tachycardia

● **supraventricular**
A site above the ventricles, that is, the SA node, atria, or AV junction

The term **supraventricular** has several connotations. First is the category of rhythm; the origin is from above (supra) the ventricles (ventricular). Hence, the term *supraventricular* (SVT) also denotes when an atrial ectopic has taken pacemaker control over the atria, and the AV node unwittingly supports the tachycardia. The 3 most common mechanisms are:

1. AV Nodal Reentry: a retrograde P wave coincidental with abnormal, narrow QRS (most common).

2. Concealed Bypass Tract: no evidence of heart disease, a younger "healthy" patient, but QRSs are wide, with no clinical evidence of preexisting bundle branch block.

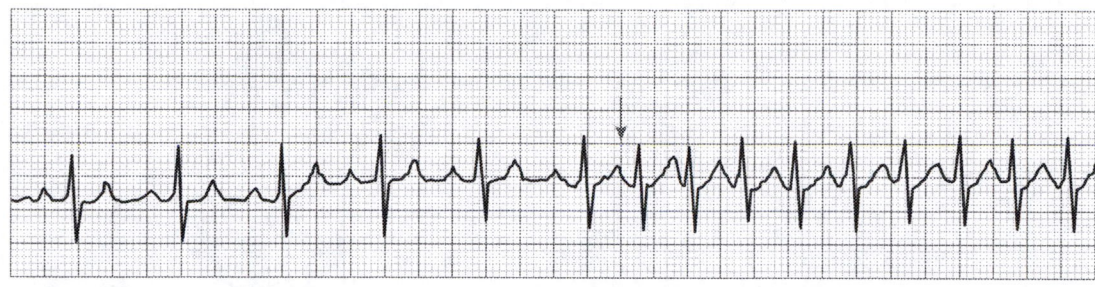

Figure 5-18 An ECG tracing showing sinus rhythm at 100 beats per minute. A PAC (arrow) begins the sudden change in rate at 188 beats per minute.

3. SA Nodal/Atrial Reentry: presence of P' waves before the narrow QRS in the presence of organic disease.

Reentry is the ability of an impulse to reexcite some region of the heart through which it has already passed. Reentry usually occurs when an impulse deviates into a circular conduction pathway, forming a loop.

Like atrial tachycardia, SVT with reentry begins abruptly. At the onset, the tachycardia is preceded by a prolonged P'R interval. This mechanism establishes the reentry circuit. The P' waves may distort the QRS; however, there should be no alteration of the QRS amplitude.

Two AV nodal reentrant tachycardias can result: one accessing the fast path downward and the slow path in a retrograde fashion (fast-slow), which is often seen in children; and the other accessing the slow path downward and the rapid path in a retrograde fashion (slow-fast). Since it uses the slow pathway for return to the atria, the RP' is longer than the P'R interval. The slow-fast is almost always triggered by a PAC associated with a prolonged P'R interval preceding it. Sometimes, the P' is lost or blended into the narrow QRS and is impossible to see.

Many small potential circuits—microcircuits—normally exist within the conduction system, such as the AV node, atrial, and ventricular tissue where the terminal Purkinje fibers attach to cardiac muscle. Macrocircuits, or larger circular pathways, may also form. These circuits are at least partially composed of cardiac conduction tissue. An example of this phenomenon would be a circuit formed by a congenital accessory pathway, or by AV node microcircuits functionally grouped together into 2 major pathways. Figure 5-19 is composed of three sketches. The first is the AV node exhibiting normal conduction, the second shows an atrial ectopic with AV nodal reentry, and the third shows the Kent bundle as a potential pathway for conduction.

Reentry circuits can exist in normal cardiac tissue. In reentry, the impulse travels through the conduction fibers in an even and synchronous manner. The impulse collides with itself in these circuits. Conditions of ischemia, systemic disease, and some medications can affect selected portions of these conduction fibers, altering their speed of conduction. These cells recover slowly from previous impulses and may not conduct new approaching impulses. When the block occurs, there is an abrupt stop to the tachycardia. This is not to be confused with aberrant conduction pathways.

● **reentry**

Ability of an impulse to reexcite some region of the atria through which it has already passed

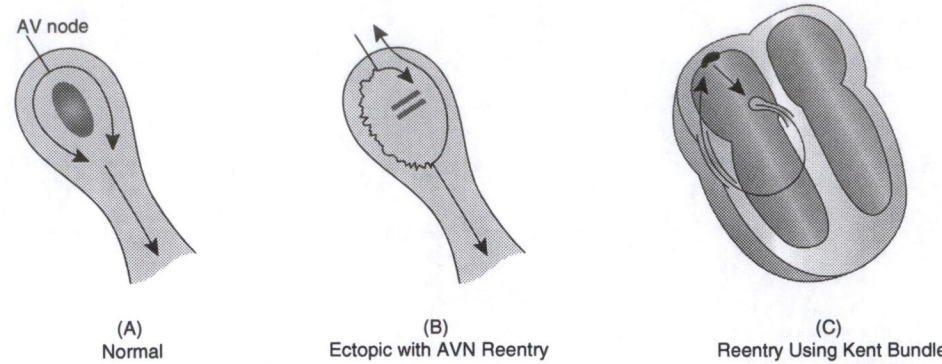

(A)
Normal

(B)
Ectopic with AVN Reentry

(C)
Reentry Using Kent Bundle

Figure 5-19 Three examples of AV conduction: normal AV conduction (A); a PAC and AV nodal reentry (B); and a reentry circuit using the accessory Kent bundle (C).

An altered circuit may be partially or totally refractory. If the circuit is partially refractory in only 1 direction, the impulse will be blocked from transmitting in that direction.

When the impulse is blocked in 1 direction through a pathway, it is called a *unidirectional block*. When an impulse encounters refractory tissue, the impulse detours away from the blocked area and deviates around the conduction pathway, forming a loop. Impulse transmission then becomes asynchronous.

The impulse enters the ischemic area in a retrograde direction and is conducted through ischemic tissue slowly. Remember, ischemic cells are slow cells that have prolonged refractory periods. If tissue surrounding the previously blocked area has recovered sufficiently to be excitable, the emerging impulse will reenter the adjacent tissue. As a result, an original impulse will now reexcite or depolarize the area through which it has just passed. Figure 5-20 illustrates the concept of unidirectional block and subsequent reentry.

If the reentrant impulse exits early in repolarization, when the disparity in recovery is still pronounced, the impulse may recycle within the circuit, producing a chain-reaction response. This response often disintegrates into chaotic activity.

Atrial Flutter

One consequence of PACs is the occurrence of atrial flutter. A common mechanism is a reentry circuit within the right atrium. Atrial depolarization will be seen as sharp deflections at a rate of 200 to 300 beats per minute. The atrial P' waves are referred to as *flutter* waves. In atrial flutter, the rapid atrial rate may take on a sawtooth appearance (Figure 5-21), but this is not critical. The ventricular rate and rhythm are a direct reflection of the AV node's ability to slow down the impulses coming to it. Remember, the physiological function of the AV node is to therapeutically delay conduction and protect ventricular response.

When atrial flutter is new to the patient, it often presents with a ventricular rate of about 150 beats per minute. In other words, every other atrial impulse is conducted through to the ventricles. The arrhythmia is often termed *atrial flutter with two-to-one conduction*. The atrial flutter waves will plot through regularly.

Atrial flutter with 2:1 block can be misdiagnosed as sinus tachycardia. However, in sinus tachycardia, the P and T waves are usually distinctly different from

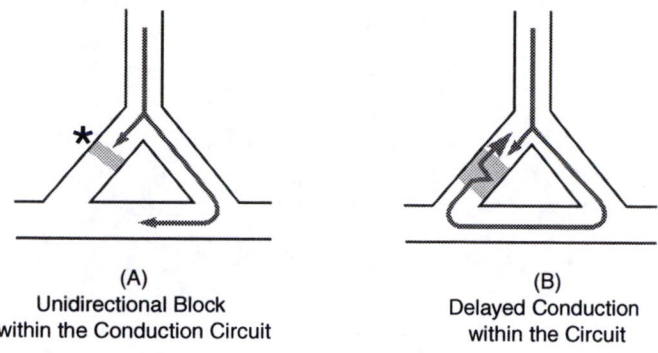

(A)
**Unidirectional Block
within the Conduction Circuit**

(B)
**Delayed Conduction
within the Circuit**

Figure 5-20 Reentry with unidirectional block (A) and delayed conduction of the reentry circuit (B).

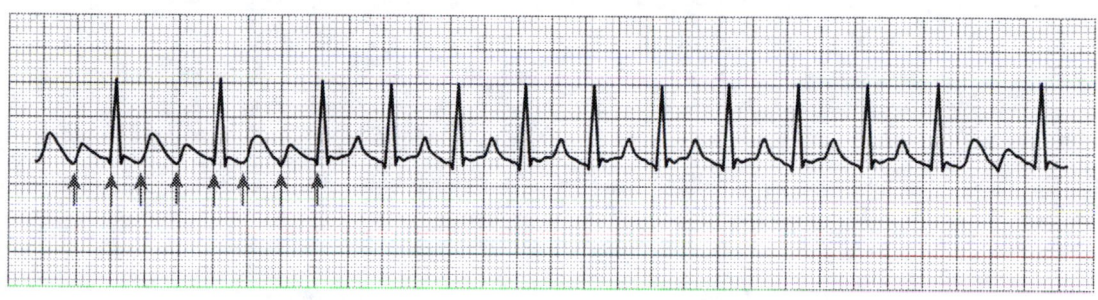

Figure 5-21 An ECG tracing showing a narrow QRS-complex tachycardia with varying ventricular rate. Note the illustration of the flutter waves as they are plotted out across the tracing. The flutter waves cause occasional distortions in the QRS complex.

each other. In other words, Ps plot with Ps and Ts plot with Ts, but the T-P-T is not rhythmic and regular. Also, looking at the negative deflections, one can plot out the flutter waves more easily.

Another clue to differentiating sinus tachycardia at 150 beats per minute from atrial flutter with 2:1 AV block is finding the P' midway between the QRS complexes. One should suspect there is an additional P' within the QRS complex, and in fact be able to detect distortion of the P'. Distortion of the QRS by suspected P' is called *Ta distortion*.

Finally, the patient with atrial flutter may complain of a sudden onset of the rapid heart rate, along with feelings of weakness and dread (Figure 5-22). These symptoms are less likely to occur with sinus tachycardia.

Atrial Fibrillation

Another consequence of PACs is the occurrence of atrial **fibrillation**, a chaotic and erratic depolarization state within the atria. In contrast to atrial flutter, atrial fibrillation is one of the most commonly seen arrhythmias. The rate of atrial depolarization cannot be measured, as it often exceeds 300 to 600 beats per minute, producing results in a chaotic baseline. The atrial P' waves are sometimes referred to as *fib* waves. Atrial kick is lost, as the atria are quivering and there is no organized atrial contraction. Mural thrombi are a common consequence of long-term atrial fibrillation.

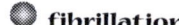 **fibrillation**

Chaotic activity due to multiple ectopic foci

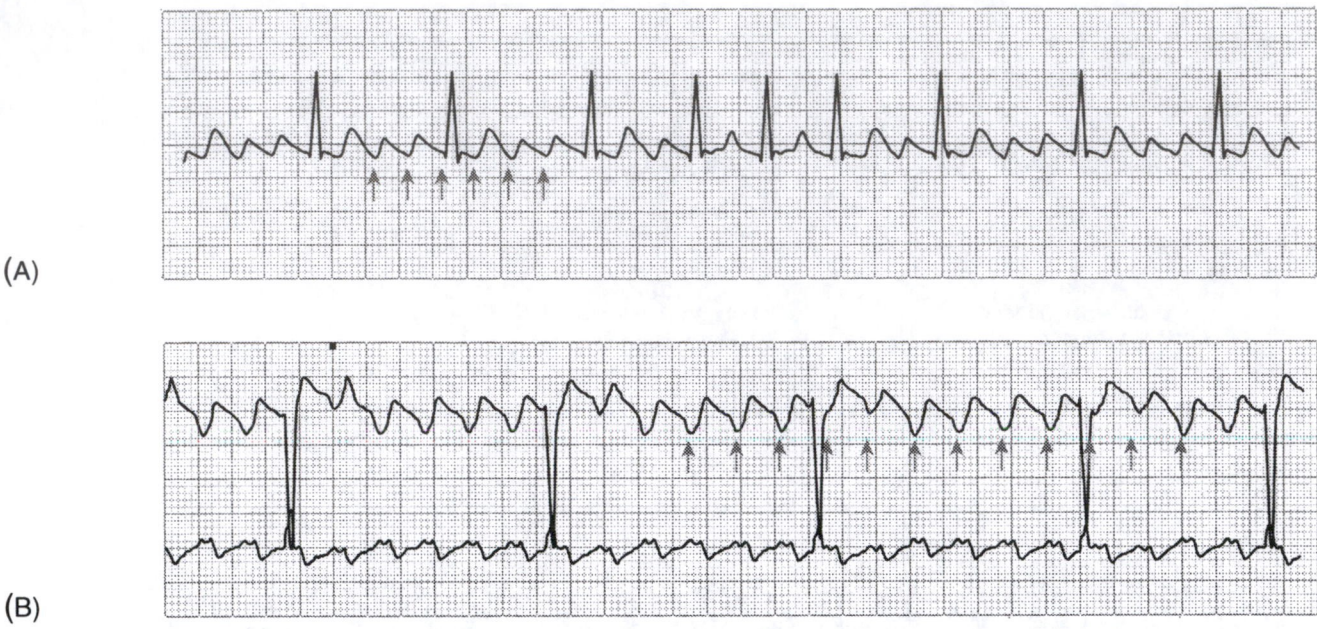

(A)

(B)

Figure 5-22 ECG showing new-onset atrial flutter in a patient (A) and a continuous ECG tracing from a patient with recurrent atrial flutter (B). The patient was taking Lanoxin 0.25 mg daily, for 37 days.

The irregular fibrillatory waves are usually easy to recognize and may be referred to as *coarse* atrial fibrillation (Figure 5-23A). In other cases, the fibrillation is of such low amplitude, it is occasionally referred to as *fine* atrial fibrillation (Figure 5-23B).

Assessing the tracings to determine the arrhythmia will help the practitioner with that identification. For example, in Figure 5-23, the QRS complexes are narrow, indicating a supraventricular origin. However, there are no identifiable P waves with consistent PR intervals, so the rhythm is not sinus in origin.

Next, the QRS rhythm in both examples is irregular, so it cannot be identified as junctional in origin. The only other option for the origin of the narrow QRS is atrial. There are no flutter waves so, by the process of elimination, the rhythms are identified as atrial fibrillation. The ventricular rate range should be reported, to provide an indication of the protective blocking ability of the AV node. The coarse or fine appearance of the fibrillatory waves has no clinical relevance.

In atrial fibrillation, the AV node is bombarded by hundreds of atrial ectopics, at varying rates and amplitudes. The AV node therapeutically and randomly conducts impulses at a varying rate of speed, so the ventricular response is irregular. When a patient first experiences atrial fibrillation, the atrial rates are immeasurable and the ventricular rhythm is irregular and very rapid (Figure 5-23B). A rapid ventricular rate may compromise the patient. It is important to note the ventricular rate when reporting this arrhythmia, as well as the patient's medication and medical history.

SUMMARY OF THE ATRIAL MECHANISMS

When arrhythmias are said to be supraventricular in origin, this means they come from above the ventricles, but, more specifically, are probably caused by atrial

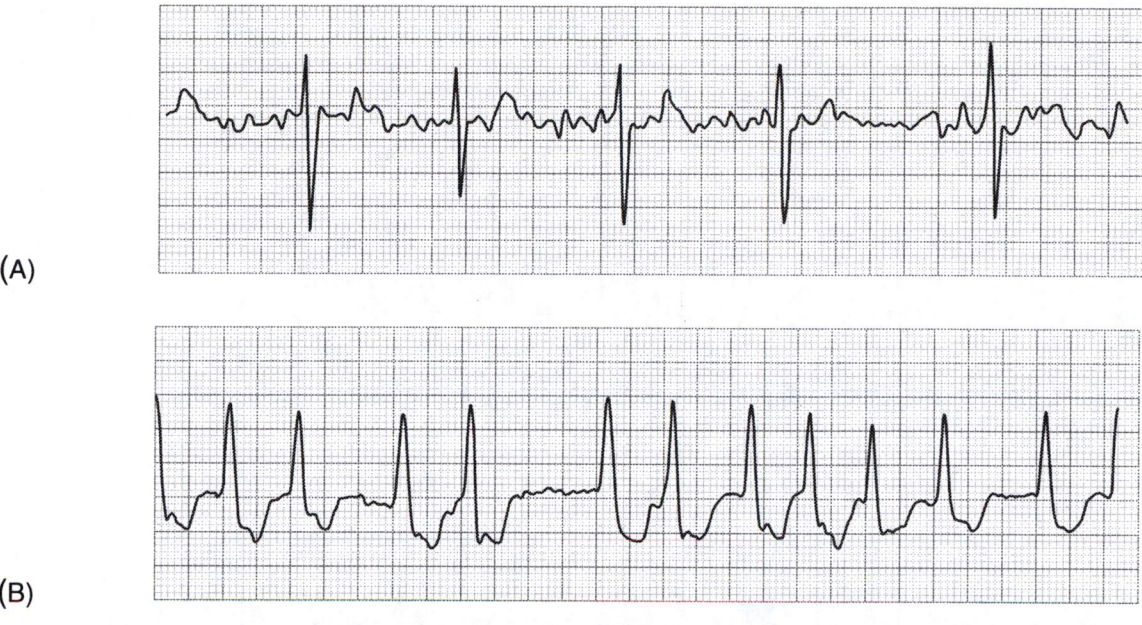

(A)

(B)

Figure 5-23 (A) is an ECG tracing showing narrow QRS complex with an irregular rhythm at 48–88 per minute. The chaotic pattern between the QRS complexes is the atrial fibrillation. This coarse pattern is easily seen. (B) is an ECG tracing from a patient with narrow QRS complex with an irregular rhythm. Similar to (A), there are no identifiable P waves or a consistent PR interval. The baseline between QRS complexes is finely distorted. This is referred to as atrial fibrillation. Ventricular rate is 75–166 per minute, with 5 to 6 mm ST segment ↓.

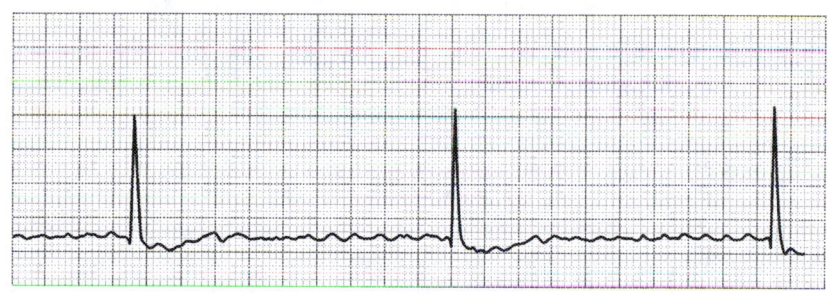

Figure 5-24 An ECG tracing from a patient in atrial fibrillation with an escape junctional rhythm. Note the regularity of the narrow-QRS complex. Identification: atrial fibrillation with an escape junctional rhythm at 36 beats per minute.

Table 5-3 Differentiation of the source of the narrow QRS by assessing P waves

Look at the P waves:	
Sinus:	One (+) P for each QRS
Junctional:	A (-) P′ in front of or behind each QRS, or no P at all
Atrial:	A different (+) P′ in front of the QRS

ectopics.   Differentiation among the various sources of supraventricular tachycardia is based largely on the rate and how it starts off. Table 5-3 provides a simple tool for differentiating the source of the narrow QRS arrhythmia by assessing the P waves. Table 5-4 is a summary of atrial mechanisms.

Table 5-4 ECG characteristics of the various atrial mechanisms

	PAC	Flutter	Fibrillation	Tachycardia	SVT with AVN Reentry	SVT with Aberrancy
P' waves	(+)/QRS (+)no/QRS	usually sawtooth >250/min	unable to identify	sometimes 1:1 with the QRS; sometimes independent RP>PR rate <250	within the QRS; distorts the QRS at its beginning or at its end	(+) with a PAC at the beginning of the tach
P'R interval	different					0.12–0.20 second
QRS duration	≤ 0.10	≤ 0.10	≤ 0.10	≤ 0.10	≤ 0.10	confused with a PVC >0.10
Ventricular rate/minute		60–100 usually	60–100 when controlled with medication	>100	>150/minute often >180/minute	>100/min
Ventricular rhythm		regular or irregular	irregular; beware if regular or slow	regular starts suddenly	regular	regular

VENTRICULAR MECHANISMS

Previous sections have dealt with *supra*ventricular arrhythmias, those rhythm disturbances that arise either in the sinus node, the atria, or the AV junction with normal ventricular depolarization. In this section, we will deal with ectopics and arrhythmias that have their origin in ventricular tissue and cause abnormal ventricular depolarization.

Characteristics of a Ventricular Ectopic

An impulse whose origin is within ventricular tissue, and outside the normal ventricular conduction system, creates a QRS different from any supraventricular QRS (Figure 5-25). The QRS often has an increased amplitude with a T wave of opposite polarity to the QRS. For instance, a positive QRS is followed by a negative T wave. Similarly, a negative QRS is followed by a positive T wave.

The QRS morphology of the PVC is usually, but not always, greater in amplitude and wider than the dominant QRS. Ventricular activation that begins at a site of the ectopic ventricular focus travels across ventricular muscle mass instead of using the His-Purkinje system. Depolarization then takes longer, resulting in a broad QRS complex (greater than 0.10 second). Remember, the P in PVC means "premature," so by definition, a PVC will be seen to occur earlier than the normally conducted beats.

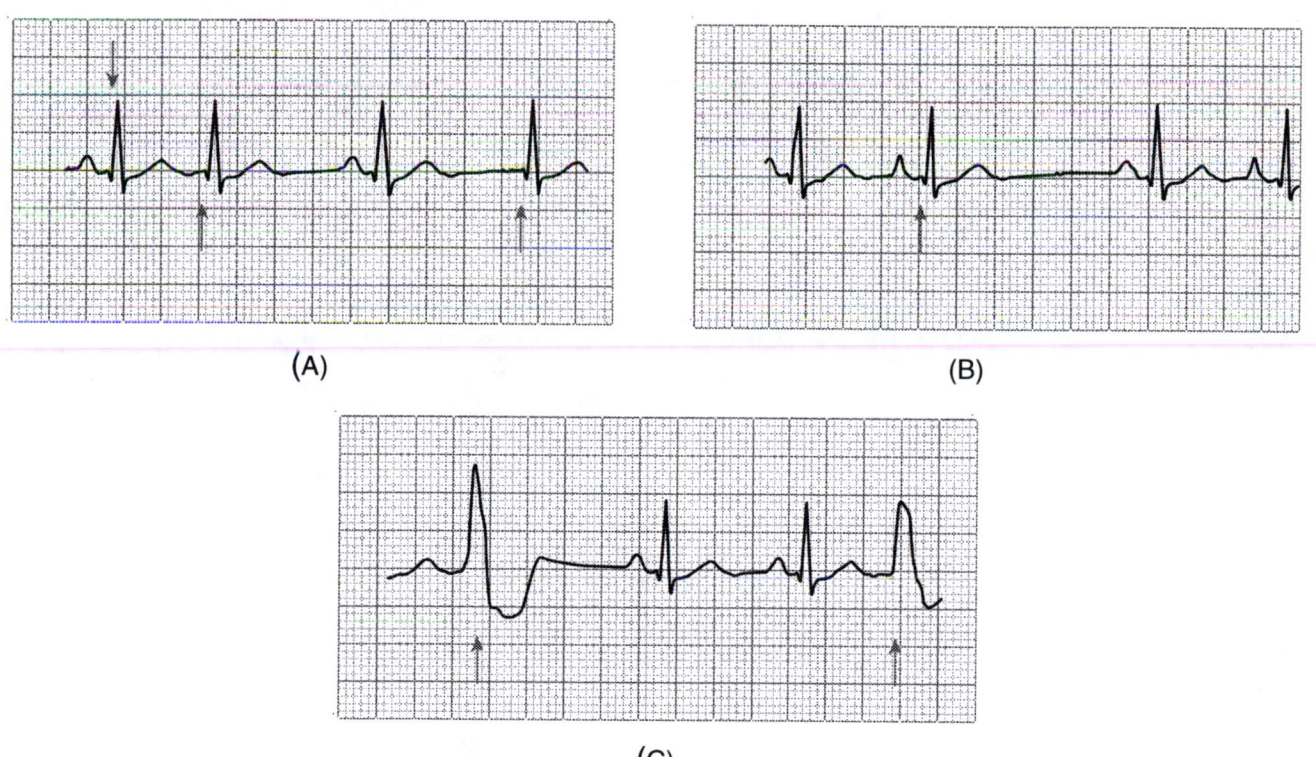

(A)   (B)

(C)

Figure 5-25 ECG tracings showing a sinus-induced QRS followed by a PJC → sinus followed by a junctional escape beat (A); sinus with PACs (B); and sinus with PVCs (C). In A and B, all the QRS complexes are similar as each uses the bundle branch system normally. In C, the QRS complex of the PVC is different and that QRS is opposite in direction from its T wave. The PVC occurs within the ventricular musculature, outside the bundle branch conduction system, causing an abnormal configuration.

Narrow Complex PVCs

PVCs originating within the intraventricular conduction system are narrower than PVCs that occur outside the bundle branch system. This is because the bundle branch system supports the conduction in a different but relatively normal fashion. For a fascicular PVC, the initial wave form and the direction of the QRS vary depending on which fascicle is the origin.

For example, an anterior fascicular PVC has an inferior, rightward direction, appearing positive in lead II and negative in lead I. A posterior fascicular PVC has a superior leftward direction, appearing negative in lead II and positive in lead I.

In either instance, the fascicular PVC has an rSR′ configuration in precordial lead V₁, since the impulse originates within the left ventricular fascicles and the right bundle branch is the last to be activated. Figure 5-26A is a graphic of the ECG and ventricular conduction system, showing the formation of the PVC in the left anterior fascicle (LAF) of the left bundle branch and the resulting wave forms in leads I and II. Figure 5-26B is a graphic of the ECG and ventricular conduction system, showing the formation of the PVC in the left posterior fascicle (LPF) of the left bundle branch and the resulting wave forms in leads I and II. Figure 5-26C is an ECG

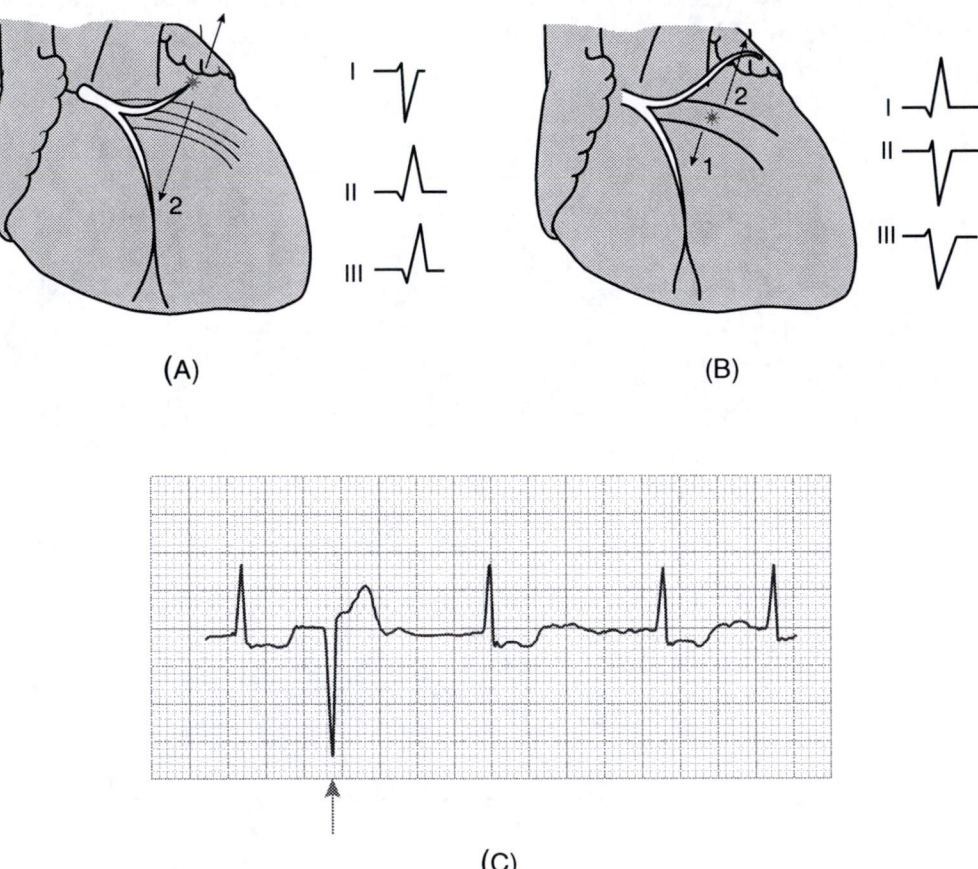

(A)

(B)

(C)

Figure 5-26 View A shows the origin of a left anterior fascicular PVC and how it appears on ECG limb leads, I, II, and III. View B is another example of the direction of current flow of a PVC whose origin is in the area of the left posterior fascicle. In View C, the ECG interpretation is atrial fibrillation, 67 to 100 beats per minute, 2 mm ST segment depression, with a narrow-complex PVC. This is confirmed on a 12-lead ECG.

tracing of atrial fibrillation and a narrow-complex, fascicular PVC, confirmed on 12-lead ECG.

Variations in PVCs

There are several variations of PVCs. By and large, they are named for where they occur within the cardiac cycle:

- End-Diastolic: a PVC at the end of or just after a sinus P wave (Figure 5-27).

- Interpolated: a PVC between two consecutive sinus beats (Figure 5-28).

- Uniform: PVCs similar to each other in polarity and configuration (Figure 5-29).

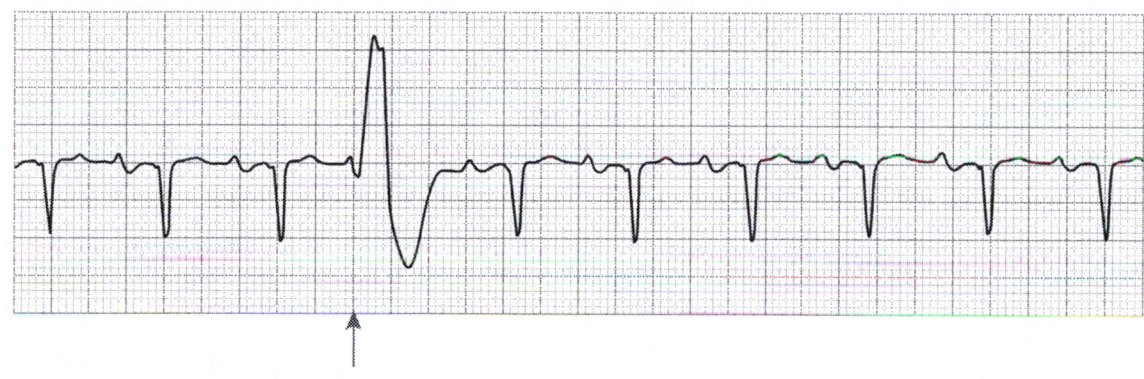

Figure 5-27 An ECG tracing showing sinus at 100 beats per minute with an end-diastolic PVC. Note the presence of the PVC just after the sinus P wave. The PR interval is 0.24 second indicating AV node delay. 9–10 mm Q waves are present.

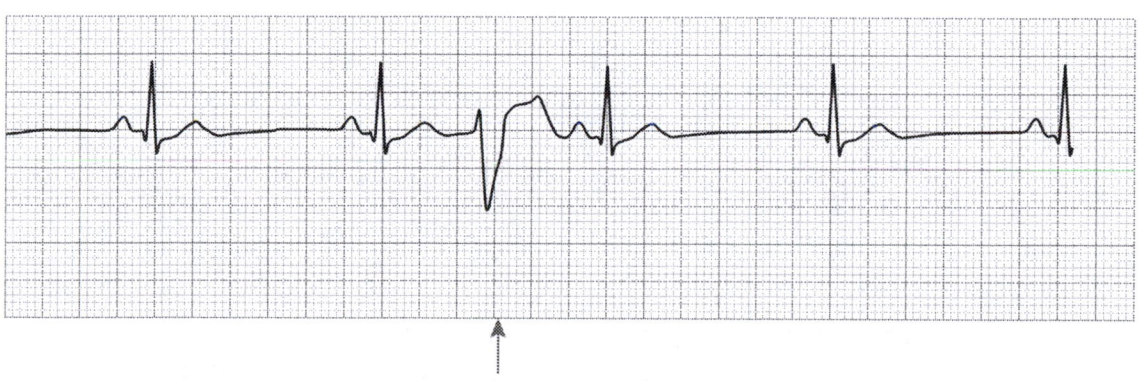

Figure 5-28 An ECG tracing showing sinus bradycardia with an interpolated PVC. Note that the sinus P waves plot through undisturbed. The ECG interpretation would be sinus bradycardia at 50 beats per minute, with 1 to 2 mm ST segment ↓ and an interpolated PVC.

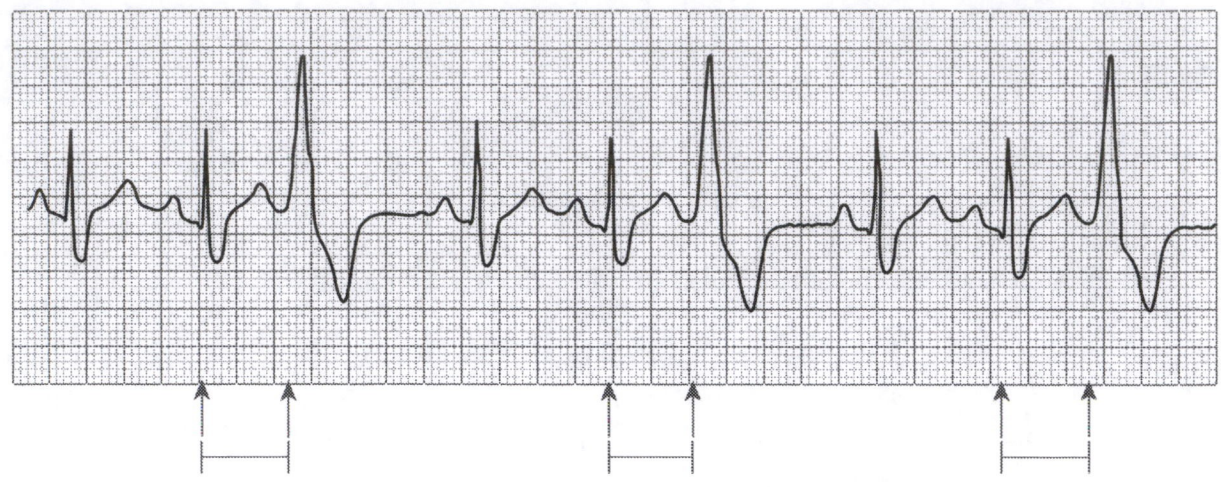

Figure 5-29 An ECG tracing showing sinus rhythm at 86 beats per minute with frequent, uniform PVCs. Notice that the distance (arrow) between the normal QRS to the PVC is similar in each instance. In this tracing, every 3rd beat is a PVC: this is called ventricular trigeminy.

- **Multiform:** PVCs different from each other in polarity and configuration (Figure 5-30).

- **Paired or Couplet:** 2 PVCs in succession with uniform appearance (Figure 5-31).

- **Bigeminy:** every other beat is a PVC (Figure 5-32A).

- **Trigeminy:** every 3rd beat is a PVC (Figure 5-32B). In ventricular bigeminy or trigeminy, the underlying rhythm can be sinus, atrial, or junctional in origin.

- **R-on-T:** a PVC superimposed onto the T wave of the preceding beat (Figure 5-33).

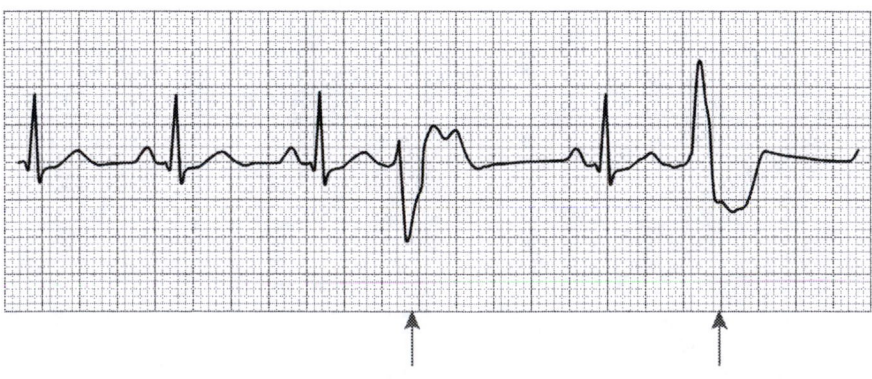

Figure 5-30 Note the difference between the PVCs. Interpretation: sinus rhythm about 78 beats per minute with frequent multiformed PVCs.

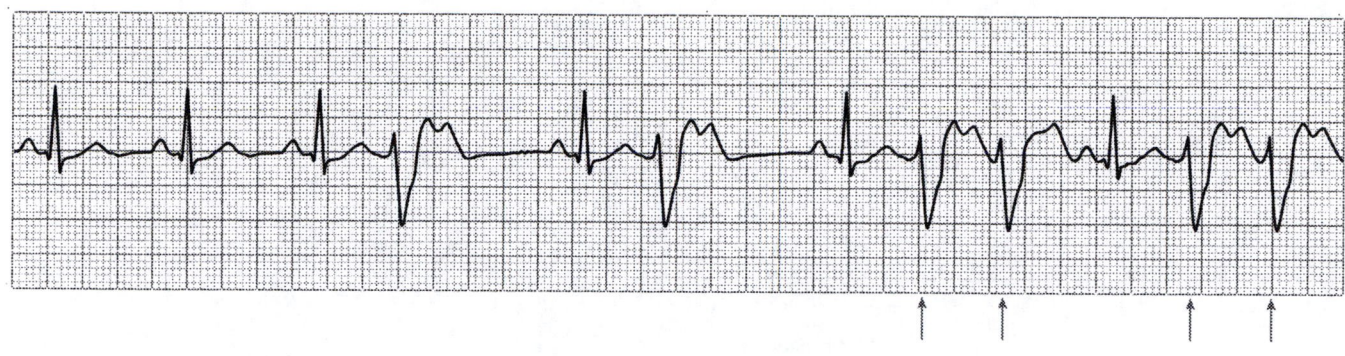

Figure 5-31 An ECG tracing showing sinus rhythm with frequent uniform PVCs and 2 examples of paired PVCs or couplets (arrows). Couplets indicate the beginning of reentry and are regarded as dangerous to the patient.

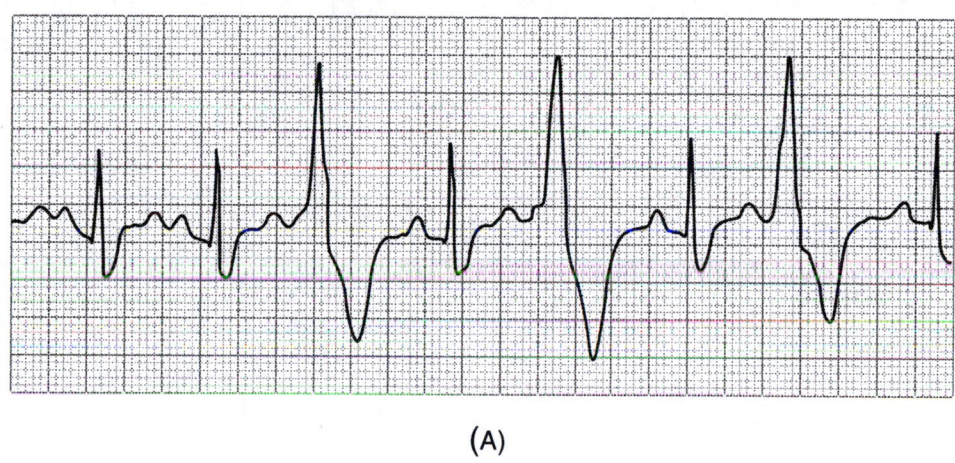

(A)

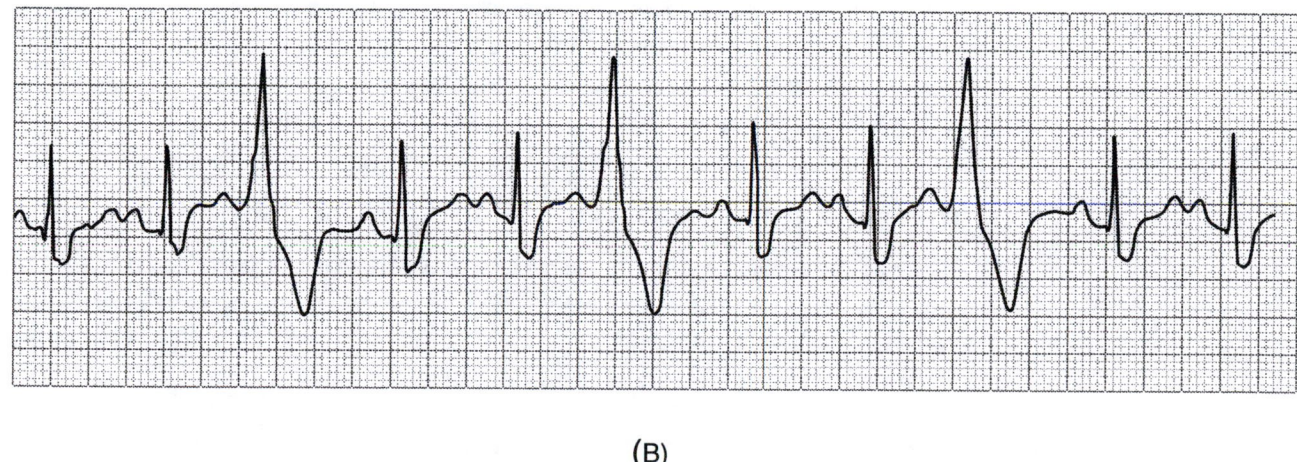

(B)

Figure 5-32 Continuous ECG tracing from a patient illustrating ventricular bigeminy, where every other complex is a PVC (A); and trigeminy, where every third complex is a PVC (B). The QRS is 0.16 second with a broad S wave of 0.08 second.

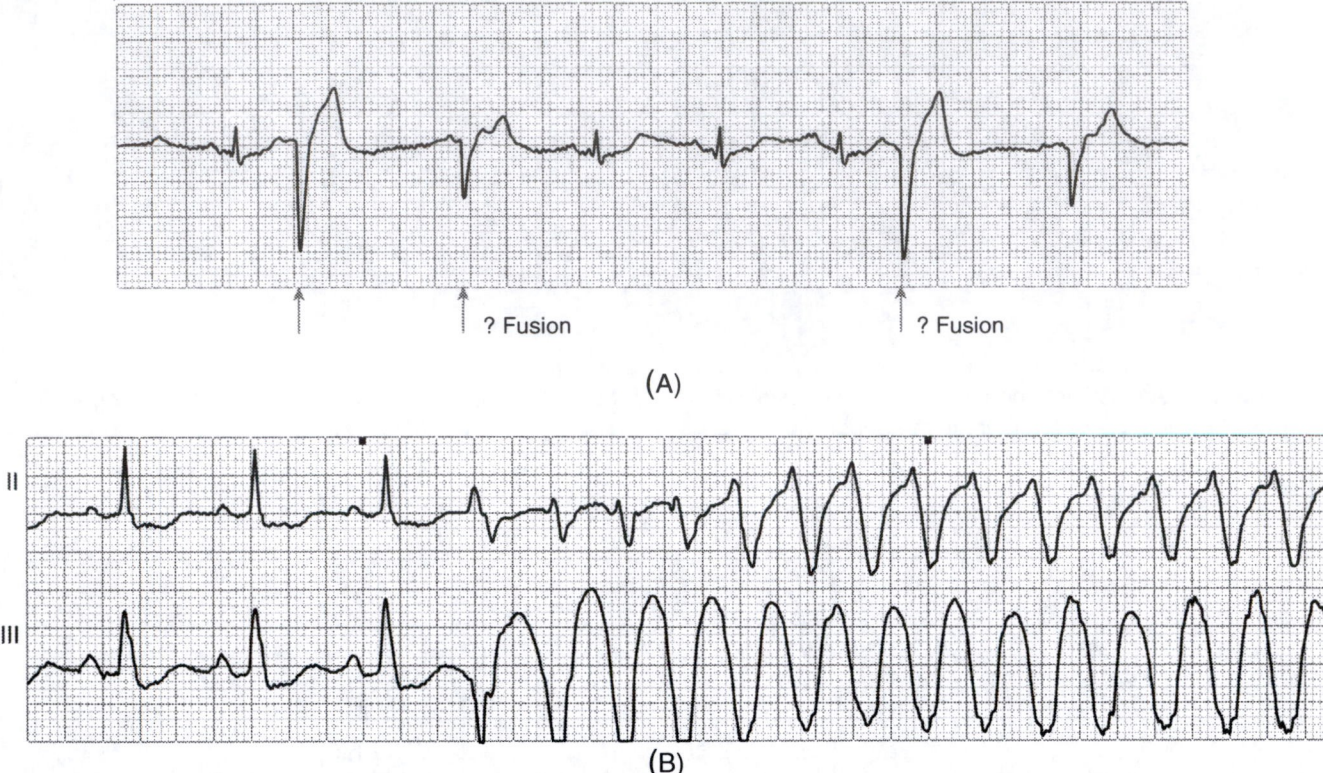

? Fusion   ? Fusion

(A)

II

III

(B)

Figure 5-33 Two examples of R-on-T PVCs. (A) an ECG tracing showing sinus rhythm with frequent R-on-T PVCs in a 61-year-old male with chest pain. Note that the PVCs are narrow, perhaps fascicular in origin. The complex to the right of the PVC is a **fusion beat**. The patient later developed ventricular fibrillation. (B) an ECG tracing from a 55-year-old patient who developed ventricular tachycardia. The patient responded to antiarrhythmic medication and was reportedly successfully reperfused.

● **fusion beat**

An abnormal QRS complex that occurs when the ventricles are activated partly by sinus, atrial, or junctional impulse and partly by the PVC

Ventricular Tachycardia

When 3 or more PVCs occur in a row, and their rates exceed 100 beats per minute, the arrhythmia is labeled ventricular tachycardia. *Ventricular tachycardia* may break through in spite of adequate sinus rate and often occurs suddenly. It is usually initiated by a distinctly premature PVC, but can occur without any warning. When the ECG shows only ventricular tachycardia, it is described as sustained ventricular tachycardia, or sustained V-tach (Figure 5-34).

Intermittent Ventricular Tachycardia

During sinus, atrial, or junctional rhythms, there may be a "run" or "salvo" of 3 PVCs in a row. For instance, one may see 3 PVCs in a row, that is, a burst of ventricular tachycardia, then 2 more sinus beats, followed by more PVCs. Figure 5-35 is an illustration of 2 rhythms, each with episodes or runs of ventricular tachycardia.

Polymorphic Ventricular Tachycardia

Polymorphic ventricular tachycardia has a changing polarity of the QRS pattern. Many polymorphic ventricular tachycardias terminate spontaneously; others

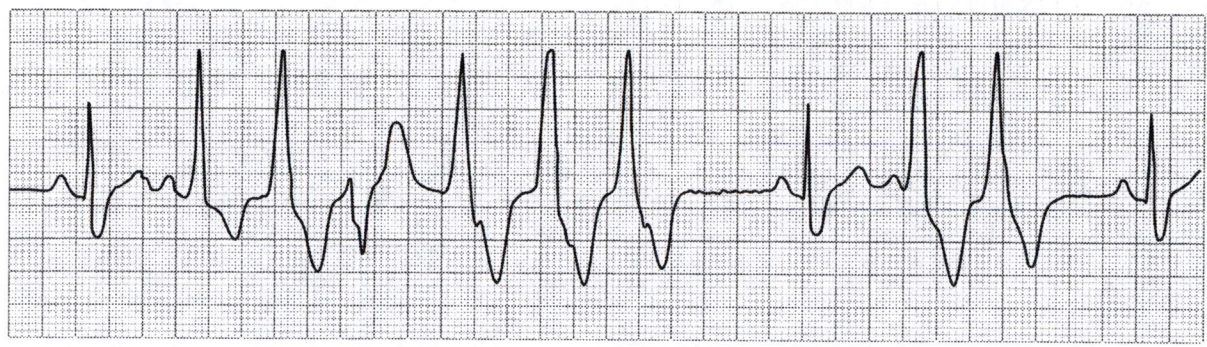

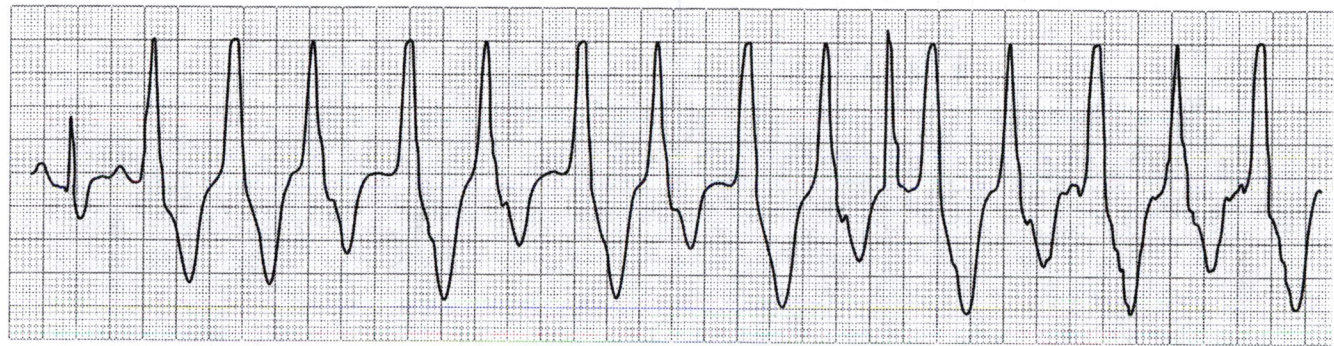

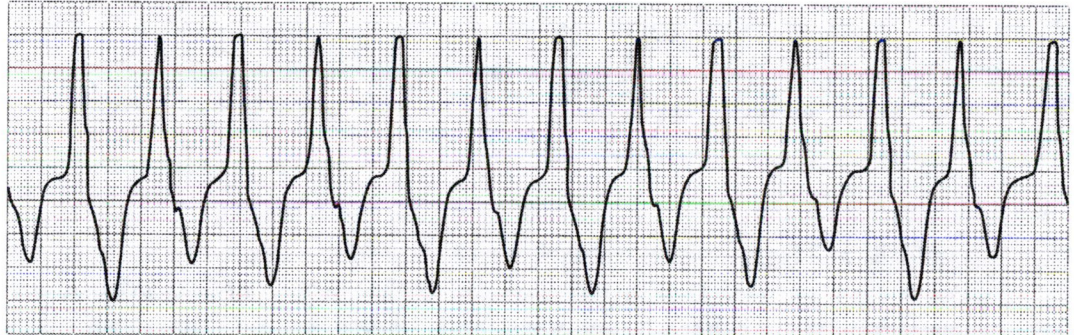

Figure 5-34 Continuous ECG tracing from a patient with sinus rhythm, frequent paired PVCs, and episodes of ventricular tachycardia; finally, the ventricular tachycardia sustains itself. Sinus P waves are sometimes visible and can be plotted out. Sinus cadence is independent of the ventricular tachycardia. As the tachycardia rate increases, the P waves become indistinct.

become sustained at very rapid rates and deteriorate into ventricular fibrillation. Polymorphic ventricular tachycardia can occur as a result of a congenital long QT interval, or it can be acquired as a result of medications, drug use, or disease. Polymorphic ventricular tachycardia that occurs despite normal QT intervals is simply called polymorphic ventricular tachycardia.

Torsade de Pointes (TdP) is the term given to polymorphic ventricular tachycardia that has a distinctive spindle-like pattern on the ECG. For example, there will be QRS complexes of one polarity, followed by beats of the opposite polarity, separated by beats of an intermediate form. The alteration in polarity usually occurs

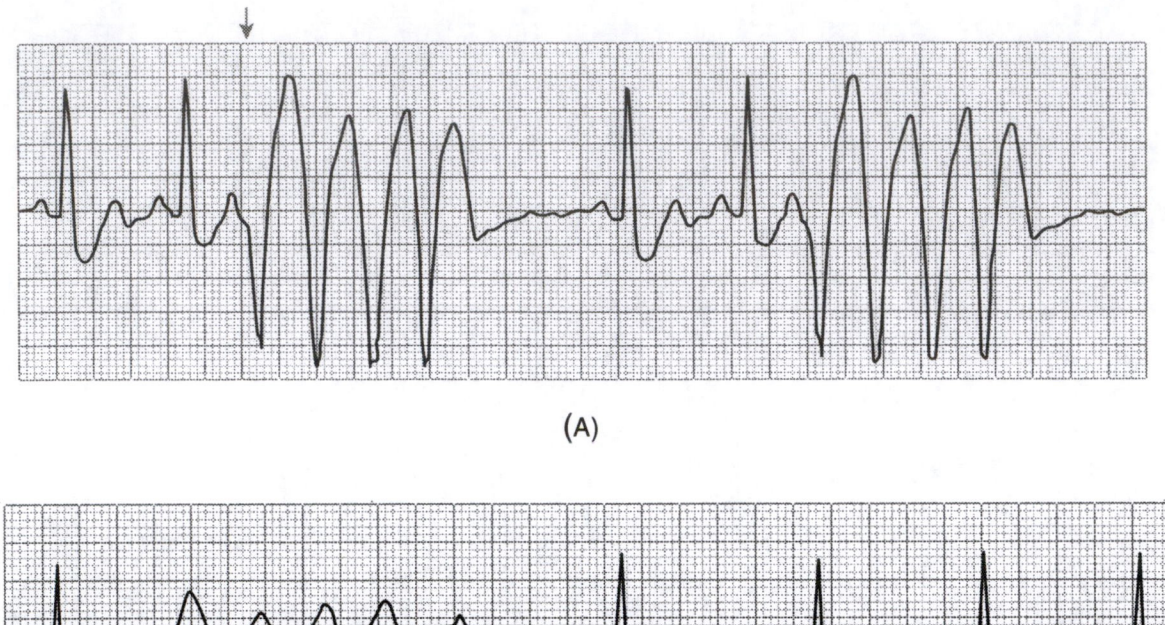

(A)

(B)

Figure 5-35 Two ECG tracings each showing sinus mechanisms with runs of ventricular tachycardia each beginning with R-on-T PVCs.

gradually and is repeated several times in succession. The singular form, Torsade de Pointes, is used to refer to a single episode, while the plural form—*Torsades*—is used when there is more than one episode or an episode of sustained duration. TdP is frequently initiated by a PVC occurring on a prolonged T or TU wave. The rate range of the tachycardia is usually 250 to 350 beats per minute. Figure 5-36 presents two examples of Torsade de Pointes.

Ventricular Fibrillation

Multiple, disorganized complexes characterize ventricular fibrillation and cause cardiac arrest. Ventricular fibrillation may be of sudden onset or may follow PVCs, ventricular tachycardia, or ventricular flutter, or it may occur without any warning ectopic.

Ventricular fibrillation is a terminal rhythm, meaning that there is no natural conversion to a normal rhythm. There is no condition that involves intermittent episodes of ventricular fibrillation.

Clinically, there is no pulse and no cardiac output with ventricular fibrillation. Occasionally, there are erratic movements in the extremities, or agonal breath sounds that accompany this rhythm. The practitioner should not presume that

QT 0.54 sec

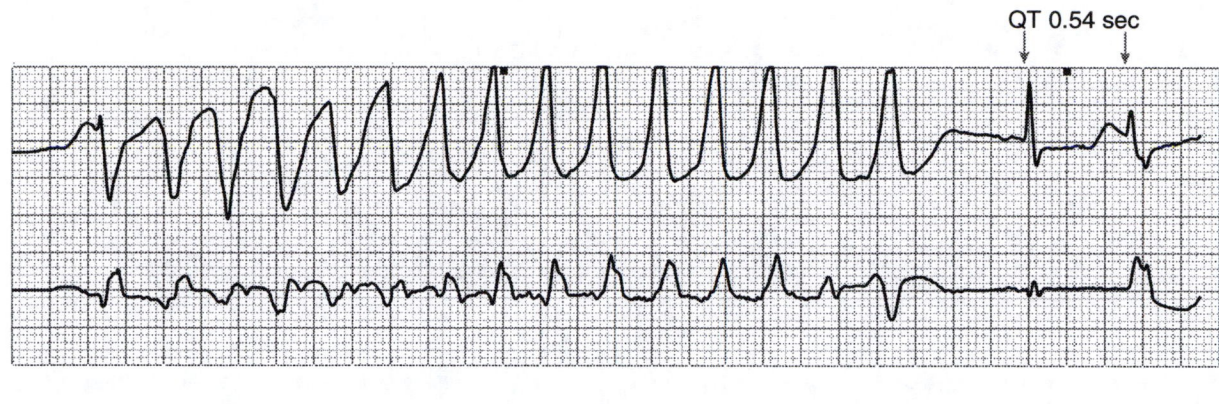

(A)

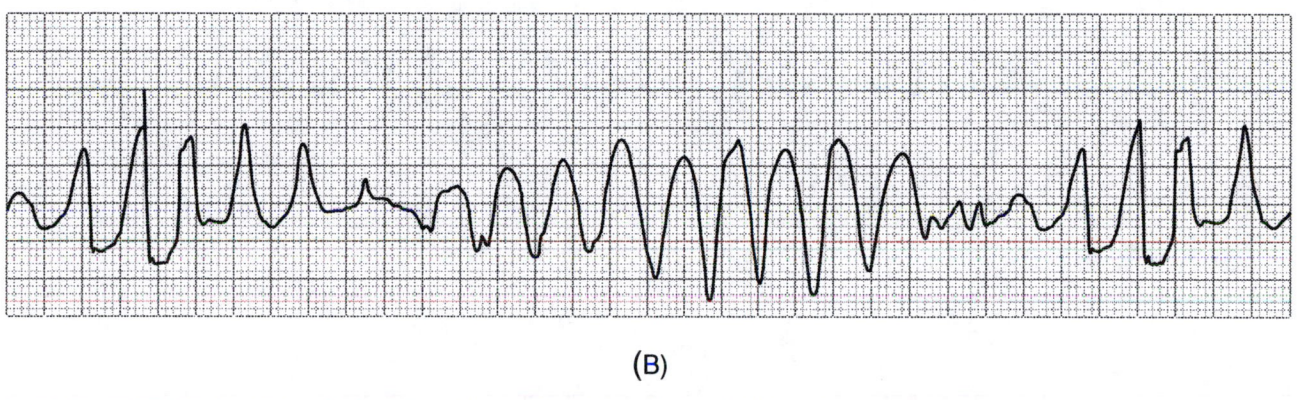

(B)

Figure 5-36 Two ECG tracings showing Torsade de Pointes. In View A, the rhythm spontaneously converted after being managed with intravenous (IV) magnesium. The patient was reportedly taking amiodarone. In View B, the patient was defibrillated. This patient had alleged tricylic overdose.

because these movements occur, the rhythm is probably not ventricular fibrillation. These movements are explained as terminal events that may accompany the myocardial fibrillation.

Ventricular fibrillation may be confused with artifact, for example, when the patient is unresponsive and cannot be roused, or is in a seizure state or shivering. The clinician should assess and confirm pulses and responsiveness. Figure 5-37 shows three examples of ventricular fibrillation.

Despite the chaos, ventricular fibrillation has a direction to the flow of current. It is easily recognized in a lead parallel to that flow of current and is often referred to as *coarse*. If the flow is off in another direction, the amplitude may be diminished. If the fibrillation is of low amplitude, frequently called *fine v-fib*, it may be confused with asystole. The clinician should switch to lead I and lead III to differentiate between ventricular fibrillation and asystole.

Once ventricular fibrillation is confirmed, immediate defibrillation is the treatment of choice. There is no clinical difference between fine and coarse ventricular defibrillation. The term *coarse* ventricular fibrillation does not imply a more easily

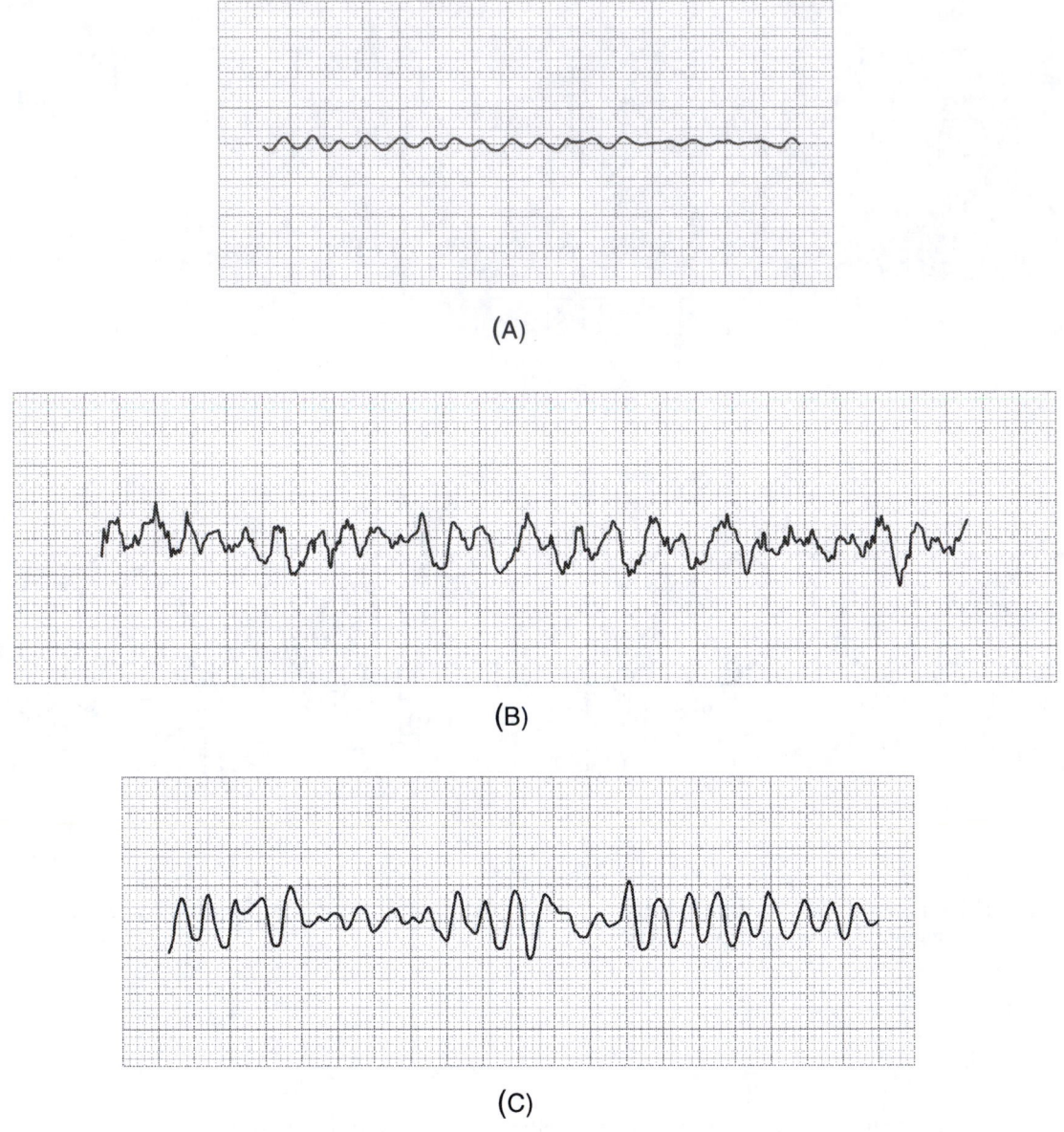

(A)

(B)

(C)

Figure 5-37 ECG tracings from 3 patients with ventricular fibrillation.

converted rhythm; nor does the term *fine* ventricular fibrillation imply a more lethal situation. Figure 5-38 provides illustrations of ventricular fibrillation of varying amplitudes as recorded in different leads.

Ventricular Escape: Idioventricular Rhythm

The ventricular pacemaker is not as efficient as supraventricular pacemakers. Idioventricular rhythm is lowest of the series of pacemakers, and may become dominant when the higher pacemakers have failed. It may function as an "escape" or "safety" rhythm and, as such, should never be suppressed.

Idioventricular rhythm (IVR) appears in the presence of depressed conduction, when the ventricles assume control of the rhythm. The ventricles have the abil-

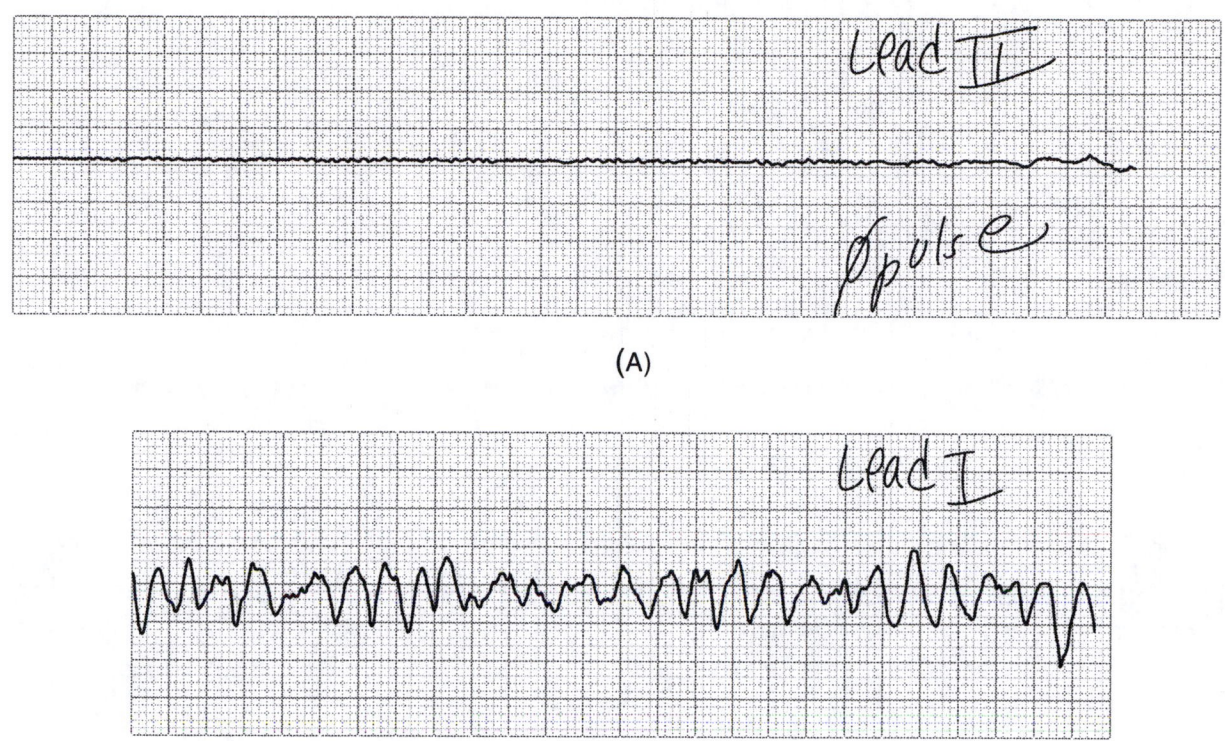

Figure 5-38 ECG tracings from the same patient. View A shows an apparent asystole or fine ventricular fibrillation, while View B shows ventricular fibrillation was confirmed on lead I.

ity to initiate impulses at 20 to 40 beats per minute. The rhythm is usually regular. IVR is clinically significant because it is slow, and usually may not provide effective perfusion. IVR may accelerate or progress to ventricular tachycardia or fibrillation. Figure 5-39 provides examples of IVR.

Accelerated Idioventricular Rhythm

Accelerated idioventricular rhythm (AIVR) refers to three or more ventricular complexes in succession, with a rate of between 40 and 100 beats per minute. AIVR often begins with a long coupling interval and terminates as the sinus rate emerges when it can conduct through to the ventricles. Figure 5-40 is an example of atrial fibrillation with an episode of AIVR. Figure 5-41 shows the two fusion beats commonly seen with AIVR.

Aberrant Ventricular Conduction

Not every wide-complex QRS is ventricular in origin. Abnormal ventricular activation will occur if 1 or more of the bundle branches are partially refractory at the time of the next electrical stimulation. This may occur when there is a transient AV conduction defect, right bundle branch block, or any intraventricular conduction defect.

Some PACs deviate from the normal conduction pathways and produce changing QRS complexes that appear ventricular in origin. Therefore, it is important for

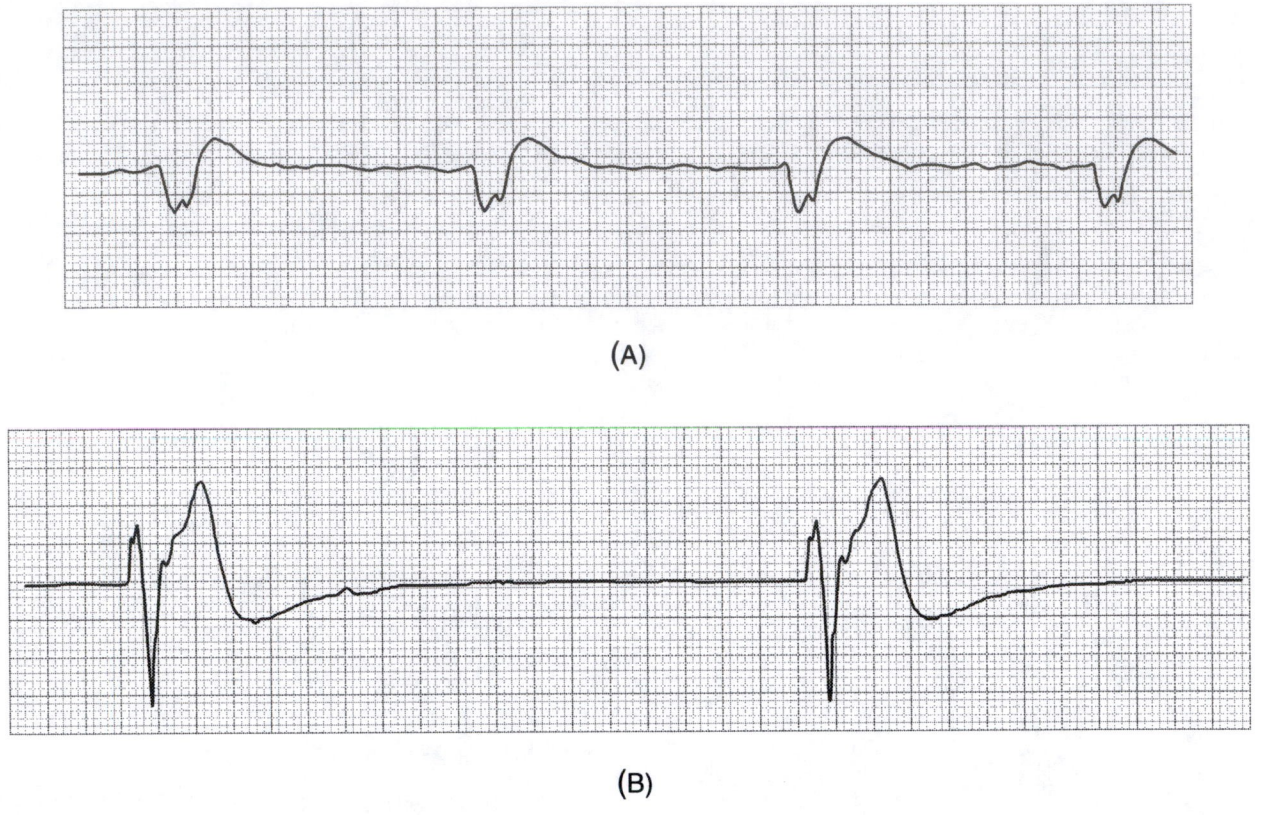

(A)

(B)

Figure 5-39 ECG tracings showing idioventricular rhythm (IVR) at 37 beats per minute (A); and an IVR at 16 beats per minute (B). Neither patient had a pulse nor responded to epinephrine, atropine, or to transcutaneous pacing.

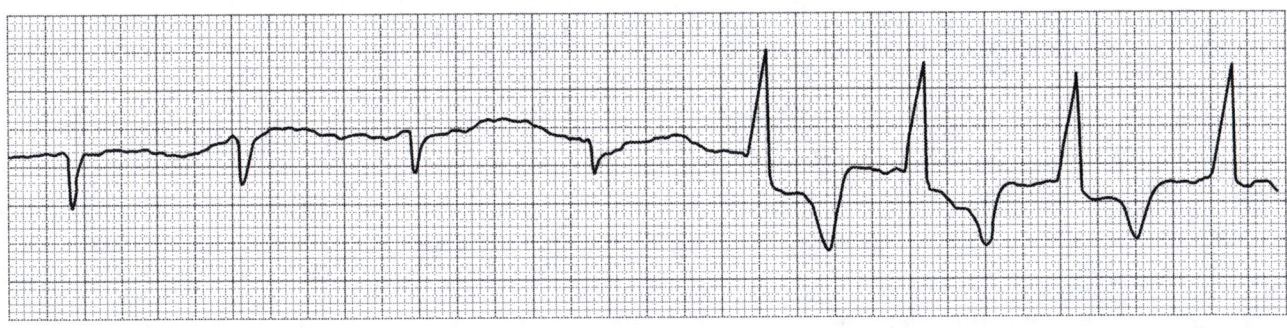

Figure 5-40 An ECG tracing showing atrial fibrillation with an accelerated junctional rhythm of 67 beats per minute progressing to an accelerated idioventricular rhythm (AIVR) at 75 beats per minute.

the clinician to look for the premature P′ that may be hidden in the previous ST segment or T wave.

Another way to recognize the PAC with aberrant ventricular conduction is to carefully plot out the sinus-conducted P waves. Remember, in a regularly occurring sinus rhythm, the sinus P's will plot through, usually undisturbed by a PVC, but be reset by the PAC.

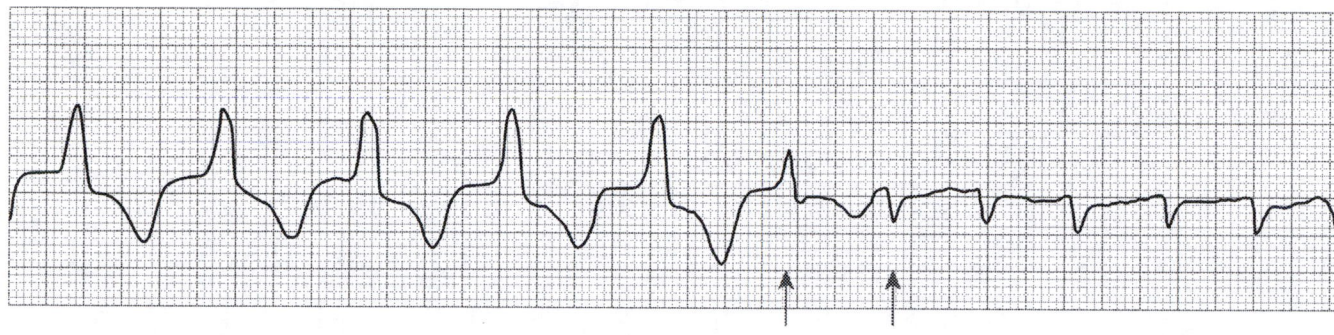

Figure 5-41 An ECG tracing showing AIVR R 84 beats per minute progressing to atrial fibrillation. Note the 2 fusion beats commonly seen with AIVR.

Remember, too, that PVCs are different from sinus-conducted beats; the QRS is usually opposite from the T wave and PVCs are usually greater than 0.12 second in duration. However, there are PVCs that are fascicular in origin and while they are "different," they are not broad and bizarre and may be interpreted as PACs. Again, the clinician should plot out the sinus P waves—they should march through any PVC event without disturbing the cadence of the sinus rhythm.

In most hearts, the right bundle branch has the longest refractory period. Therefore, aberrantly conducted PACs usually find the right bundle branch still refractory and conduct with a right bundle branch block pattern, that is, rSR'. The PAC with aberrant ventricular conduction may present with its T wave in the same direction. Again, the clinician should plot out the sinus P waves—they should march through any PVC, but be altered if the abnormal beat is atrial in origin.

Although PACs are the source of most aberrantly conducted beats, PJCs can conduct abnormally. These complexes are difficult to differentiate from PVCs. Once again, if these abnormal QRSs occur in a sinus rhythm, the sinus rate is not disturbed provided there is no retrograde conduction from the bundle of His to the atria. This hint is not applicable if the underlying rhythm is sinus arrhythmia. QRS complexes that are different from the underlying rhythm should be considered ventricular in origin, until confirmed by 12-lead ECG. Figure 5-42 provides examples of sinus with PACs and aberrant ventricular conduction. Figure 5-43 summarizes the differences between PVC and PAC with **aberrancy**.

Asystole

Cardiac asystole is the absence of electrical and mechanical cardiac activity. Ventricular asystole occurs when there are no ventricular complexes, indicating the ventricles are inactive. In some instances, the atria continue to beat in their own time. Asystole must be confirmed in at least 2 leads. The treatment for asystole and ventricular fibrillation is very different; inappropriate treatment could lead to the patient's demise.

Recall that ventricular fibrillation is the result of chaotic activity within the ventricular system. Many fibers are depolarizing and there is no effective perfusion. When the flow of current is largely parallel to the monitoring lead, the fibrillation is

⬤ **aberrancy**

QRS distortion that occurs with abnormal impulse transmission; often used when referring to a PAC or SVT with abnormal ventricular conduction; the QRS complex, instead of being narrow, is wide and distorted.

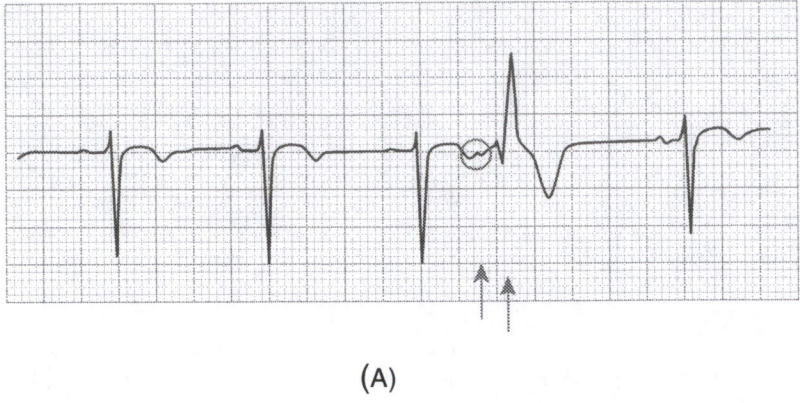

(A)

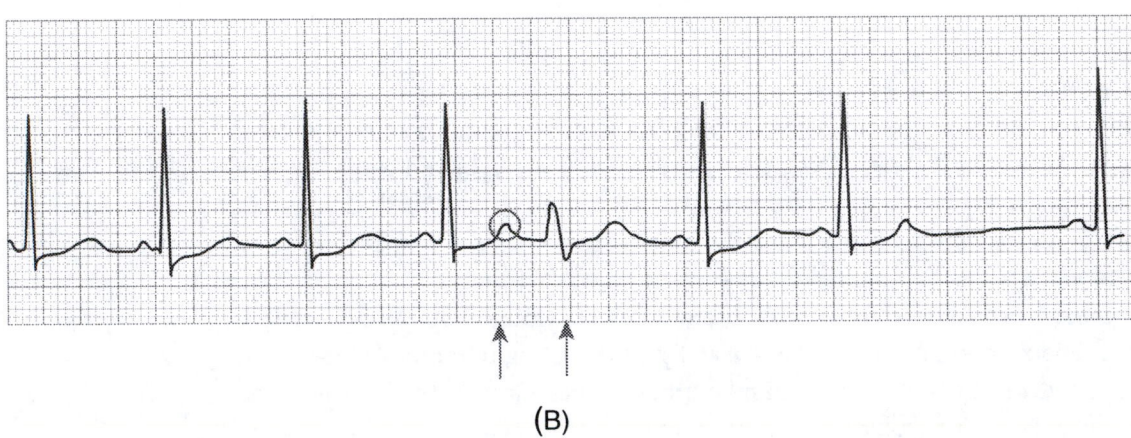

(B)

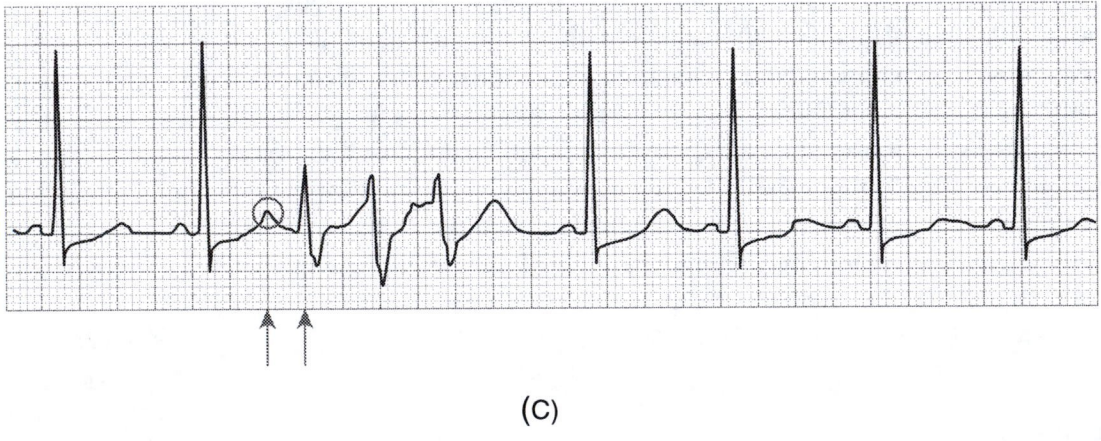

(C)

Figure 5-42 Three ECG tracings illustrating aberrant ventricular conduction. Note in View A that there is a PAC in the previous ST segment. Interpretation: sinus at 75 beats per minute with a PAC and aberrant ventricular conduction. The sinus P waves do not plot through the event. In Views B and C, the T wave amplitude prior to the aberrant QRSs is increased. The increased amplitude of the T wave is additive; that is, the combined amplitude of the P' superimposed on the previous T wave. View B interpretation: sinus at 75 beats per minute with a PAC with aberrant ventricular conduction and a nonconducted PAC. Here too, the sinus P waves do not plot through. View C interpretation: sinus at 75 beats per minute, 1 to 2 mm ST segment depression, a PAC with aberrant conduction → 3 per beat run of tachycardia. The sinus P waves do not plot through the event. Note that the T wave just prior to the tachycardia is increased in amplitude. That amplitude is additive and measures as the total of the T wave plus the P wave of complexes prior to the event. PACs that occur that early in the cardiac cycle often find the tissue partially refractory and thus the impulse conducts abnormally, or aberrantly.

Differentiation of PVC and PAC with Aberrancy

● Look for the sinus P waves and plot them through the event. Sinus-conducted P waves usually plot out independently of the event. The chance of the event being a PVC is better than 12:1 (Conover 1996; Wellens and Conover 1992).

● If the sinus-conducted P waves are disturbed in their cadence, and the rhythm is not sinus arrhythmia, look to the left of the event for a P' in the preceding ST segment or T wave.

● Look for other PACs and PVCs in the same patient. If you see conducted or blocked PACs, the chance of the event being a PAC with aberrant ventricular conduction is now better than 14:1 (Conover 1996; Wellens and Conover 1992).

● If you are dealing with a tachycardia, look at its onset. A PAC will begin the PSVT and a PVC will begin the tach or fib. Also, you will be able to see the previous QRSs before the event started.

Figure 5-43 Summary of the differences between PVC and PAC with aberrancy.

---

easily recognized. However, when the flow of current is at right angles to the monitoring lead, the ECG may look like asystole. Switch to leads I and III to differentiate asystole from ventricular fibrillation. Figure 5-44 presents ECGs showing asystole in lead II confirmed in lead I and asystole in lead II confirmed as v fib in lead I.

Table 5-5 is a summary of the ECG characteristics of ventricular mechanisms.

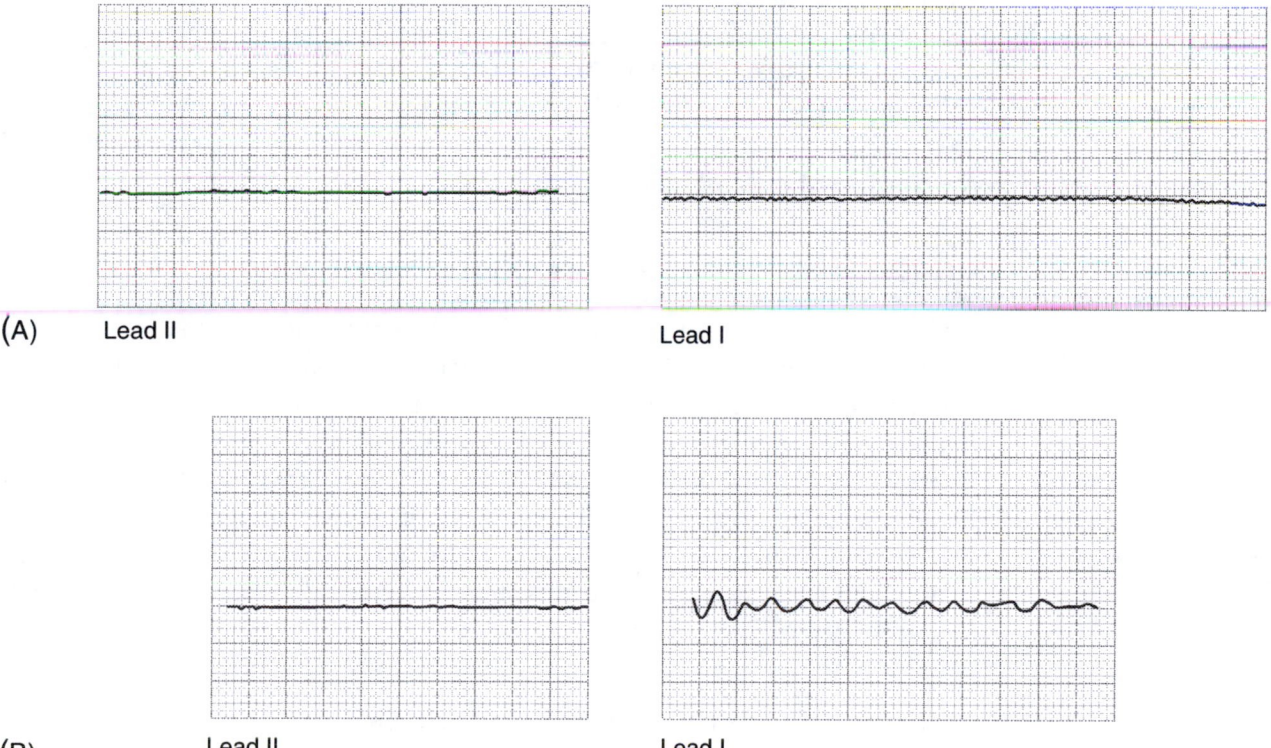

(A)   Lead II   Lead I

(B)   Lead II   Lead I

Figure 5-44 In View A, a patient's ECG shows two leads that confirm the asystole. In View B (another patient), the asystole was, in reality, ventricular fibrillation as confirmed in the second lead.

Table 5-5 Guide to ECG analysis of ventricular mechanisms

	PVC	Idioventricular Rhythm	Accelerated	Tachycardia	Fibrillation	Asystole
P waves	independent or none	independent or none	independent or none	independent or none	unable to see or none	independent or none
PR Interval						
QRS duration	≥ 0.10 QRS opposite the T wave	≥ 0.10 QRS opposite the T wave	≥ 0.10 QRS opposite the T wave	≥ 0.10 QRS opposite the T wave	≥ 0.10 QRS opposite the T wave	
Rate/minute		20–40	40–100	>100		
Rhythm		regular	regular	regular	irregular	

AV CONDUCTION DEFECTS

Recall that electrical activation normally begins with the SA node, and the wave of depolarization spreads outward through the atrial muscle to the AV junction. In the AV junction, there is a natural delay in the AV node, and then the impulse travels down the bundle of His and its branches into the ventricles. This is especially helpful in atrial flutter and fibrillation. In these arrhythmias, the AV node functions in a protective manner, so the resulting ventricular rate is usually slower.

In AV conduction defects, the conduction of the normal wave front can be delayed or blocked at any point after atrial depolarization. This can occur within the AV node, below the bundle of His, or infranodally, or involve 1, 2, or all of the bundle branches. Analysis of the ECG must be correlated to patient presentation and the clinical setting in which it occurs.

Sinus Rhythm with First-Degree AV Block

The time taken by the spread of depolarization from the SA node to the ventricular muscle is seen on the ECG by the PR interval and is not more than 0.20 second. Interference with the conduction process within the AV node results in a lengthening of the PR segment and thus the PR interval. When this lengthening of the PR interval is consistently greater than 0.20 second, it is referred to as **first-degree AV block**. Table 5-6 shows the difference in the ECG configurations between sinus rhythm and first-degree AV block. Note the only difference is the PR interval. Figure 5-45 is an example of a consistently prolonged PR interval reflecting first-degree AV block.

Sinus with Second-Degree AV Block: The Intermittent Conduction Defects

In **second-degree AV block**, one or more sinus impulses fail to reach the ventricles. Most sinus beats are conducted and the PR may be normal or prolonged, but is always constant. The hallmark of second-degree block is that there is a predictable

⬤ **first-degree AV block**

A delay in AV conduction reflected in a consistently prolonged PR interval greater than 0.20 second

⬤ **second-degree AV block**

One or more sinus impulses are blocked and are unable to stimulate the ventricles. There is a fixed PR interval after the missing QRS.

Table 5-6 Comparison in ECG configurations between sinus rhythm and first-degree AV block.

	Sinus	**First-Degree AV Block**
P waves	1 (+) per QRS	1 (+) per QRS
PR interval	0.12–0.20 second	>0.20 second and consistent
QRS duration	≤ 0.10	≤ 0.10
Rate/minute	60–100	60–100
Rhythm	regular	regular

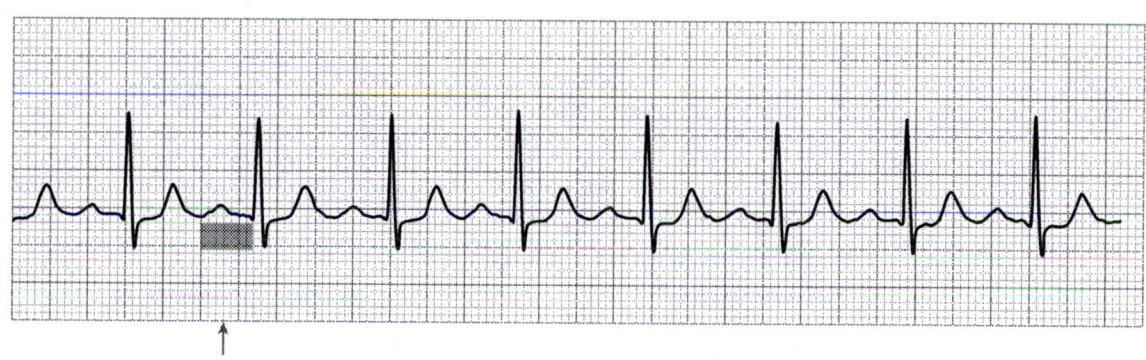

Figure 5-45 An ECG tracing illustrating a sinus rhythm at 60 beats per minute, with a consistently prolonged PR interval that is greater than 0.20 second. Note the PR segment is consistently greater than 0.12 second. Interpretation: sinus at 60 beats per minute with first-degree (1°) AV block.

P wave and an occasional absent QRS complex. There are several variations of second-degree AV block.

It is critical to plot out the cadence of the P waves to differentiate between a nonconducted PAC and an AV block. In the AV conduction defects, sinus P waves will plot through. Certainly it is possible to have a sinus arrhythmia with AV block, but the gradual increase and decrease in sinus rate is easy to plot out. Figure 5-46 is an example of a "missed QRS."

Second-Degree AV Block: The Wenckebach Phenomenon (aka Type I AV Block)

The Wenckebach phenomenon occurs when there is a progressive delay in conducting an atrial impulse, until finally there is no conduction into the ventricles. This phenomenon in conduction delay can occur with sinus rhythm, atrial flutter, or fibrillation. The Wenckebach phenomenon can also occur between sinus depolarization and atrial activation.

In a sinus rhythm, where disease affects the AV node, there is a progressive lengthening of the PR segment until there is no conduction, resulting in the missed

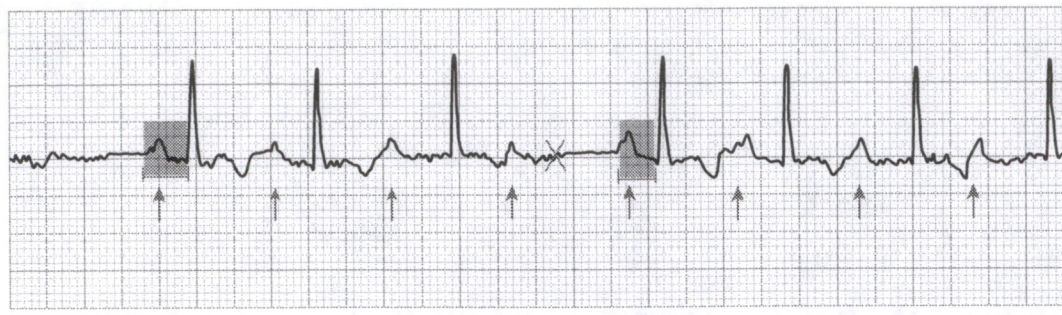

Figure 5-46 An ECG tracing showing sinus rhythm with second-degree (2°) AV block. The sinus P waves (arrows) plot through and there is a positive P wave to the left of each QRS complex. Note the missing QRS (X). Also, note that the PR after the missed QRS complex is consistent. The QRS duration is within normal limits. There is progressive prolongation of the PR segments of the PR intervals, indicating the Wenckebach phenomenon. Interpretation: sinus rhythm at 86 beats per minute, with second-degree AV block, probably type I (QRS = 0.06-0.08sec) with Wenckebach.

QRS complex. The next sinus beat occurs right on time. The PR interval following the missed QRS is the same as the first PR of each group (Figure 5-46).

The cycle may repeat itself, with variations in the numbers of conducted beats. The progressively prolonged PR segment of the PR interval is a warning of progressive conduction problems.

To summarize, the Wenckebach phenomenon is characterized by:

- Group beating
- The group begins and ends with a P wave
- There is one more P wave than QRSs in the group
- The PR after the missed QRS is the same regardless of the number of PQRST complexes in the group
- The greatest PR interval prolongation occurs within the second PR interval of the group
- Irregular or decreasing RR intervals

Figure 5-47 is an ECG tracing showing a sinus mechanism with occasional missed QRS complexes. First, plot out the P waves to confirm or rule out that the

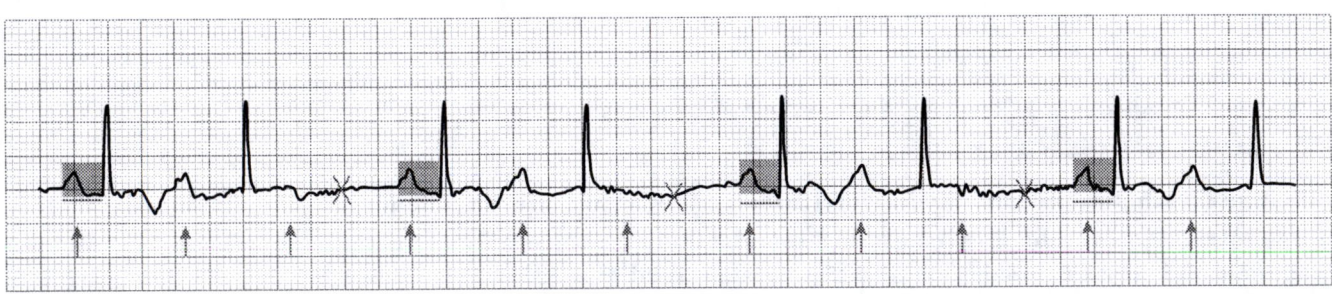

Figure 5-47 An ECG tracing showing progressive prolongation of the PR interval until the sinus P does not conduct into the ventricles. There is no ventricular depolarization, hence the missed QRS. The PR after the dropped beat (shaded) is consistent in each instance. Interpretation: sinus at 86 beats per minute, with second-degree (2°) AV block, Wenckebach, probably type I (QRS = 0.04-0.06 sec) inverted T waves, ventricular rate 57 to 75 beats per minute.

missed QRS is due to a nonconducted PAC. In this example, the P waves plot through regularly. Where there is a missed QRS complex, the PR after the missed beat is constant. The succeeding PR intervals warn of the difficulty in AV conduction by the progressive prolongation of the PR intervals, until finally there is no conduction.

In second-degree AV block, the second PR interval in the group usually demonstrates the greatest amount of prolongation. Its PR segment is usually dramatically greater than the first in the group. After that, there are a series of prolonged PRs. While the PRs do get longer, the amount of increase is less each time. The last event in the group is a P wave without a subsequent QRS.

Second-Degree AV Block with Wide QRS Complex (Type II)

Conduction defects that occur below the bundle of His and within one or more of the bundle branch fascicles may be associated with left coronary artery disease. The left coronary artery supplies most of the right bundle branch as well as the left anterior fascicle, and, partially, the left posterior fascicle. Left coronary artery occlusion produces anterior wall myocardial infarction (AWMI). When intraventricular conduction defects occur, the QRS duration is prolonged and takes on specific morphology reflecting the affected fascicle.

Second-degree AV block Type II may occur as a result of chronic lesions within the conduction system and also may occur in acute myocardial infarction. Second-degree AV block Type II is diagnosed when a dropped QRS complex is not preceded by progressive prolongation of the PR interval. The PR interval may be normal or prolonged, but remains fixed and constant.

The QRS duration and morphology are critical in describing second-degree AV block Type II. This will alert the clinician to assess for evidence of bundle branch pathology. Figure 5-47 is an ECG tracing showing second-degree AV block and the Wenckebach phenomenon. The QRS complex is 0.08 second; the PR after the missed QRS is constant. Figure 5-48, in contrast, shows the Wenckebach phenomenon with QRS that is an rS configuration and 0.12 second. The QRS in this patient on 12-lead ECG confirmed left anterior fascicular block, that is, the disease affected the penetrating portions of the bundle branch system (see Chapter 6).

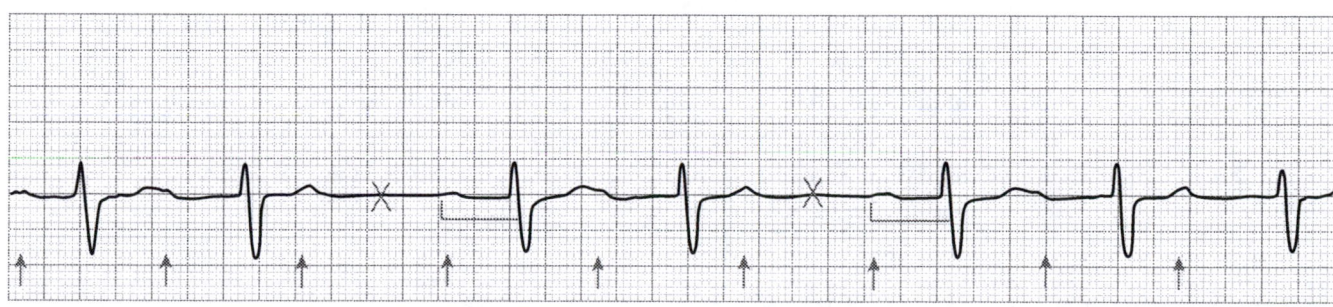

Figure 5-48 An ECG tracing showing second-degree AV block. The P waves plot through and the PR lengthens progressively but the PR is constant after a missed beat. The QRS is broader than normal at 0.12 second and is an rS configuration, which may indicate an intraventricular conduction defect. Interpretation: sinus at 75 beats per minute with second degree AV block, probably Type II, (QRS = 0.12 in an rS configuration), ventricular rate is 37 to 67 beats per minute, with Wenckebach.

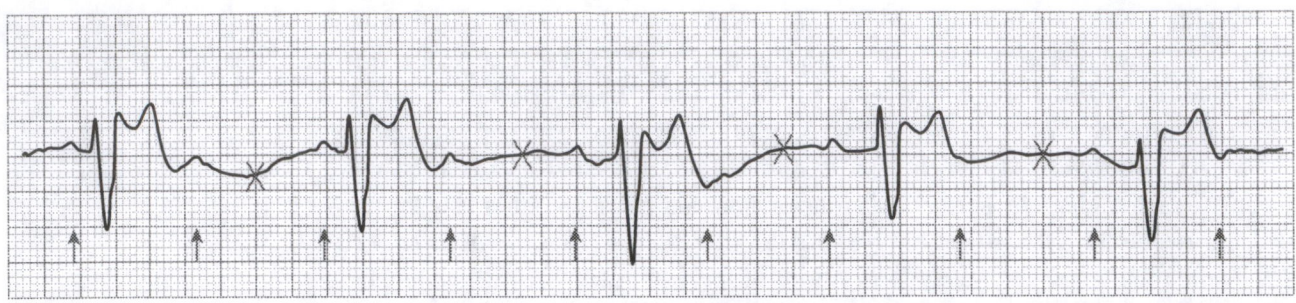

Figure 5-49 An ECG tracing from a patient with confirmed anteroseptal wall myocardial infarction. Plot out each of the P waves as they occur within the ST segment and T waves. The PR interval is constant after the missed QRS and the QRS is 0.16 second and an rS configuration. Every other sinus P does not conduct. The ventricular rhythm is regular. This is an example of AV block with 2:1 conduction. Interpretation: sinus at 86 beats per minute, second-degree AV block, probably type II (QRS = 0.12 in an rS configuration), ventricular rate is 43 beats per minute.

Figure 5-49 is an ECG tracing from a patient who had a confirmed myocardial infarction. Note the difference between atrial and ventricular rates, the fixed PR interval, and the QRS that is 0.16 second in duration.

Second-Degree AV Block: AV Block with 2:1 Conduction (aka Fixed-Rate Second-Degree AV Block)

Second-degree AV block may be an end result of AV nodal or intraventricular conduction defects and may be associated with coronary artery disease. In second-degree AV block that occurs as a result of AV nodal delay, the QRS complexes are narrow—0.10 second or less. In fixed-rate second-degree AV block, that may occur as a result of pathology in the ventricular conduction system, the QRS complexes may be prolonged, and the duration will be greater than the normal 0.10 second, often 0.12 to 0.16 second. Table 5-7 summarizes the differences in pathology, ECG characteristics, and interventions in Types I and II second-degree AV block.

Sinus with High-Grade (Advanced) AV Block

High-grade second-degree AV block can be identified when the atrial rate is reasonable and two or more consecutive atrial impulses are not conducted, but the conducted beats have consistent PR intervals. There is no competition from a subsidiary pacer, as with accelerated junctional rhythm. The ratio of atrial to ventricular conducted beats may vary from 3:1, 4:1, etc. Figure 5-50 is an ECG tracing of high-grade second-degree A-V block.

⬤ **complete AV block**

Independent beating of the atria and ventricles due to complete refractoriness in the AV junction, usually the AV node.

Sinus with Complete AV Block

Pathology involved in AV block can progress in severity until all the sinus impulses are completely blocked, resulting in **complete AV block**. Regardless of the lesion site, there is no conduction through to the ventricles. When complete AV block occurs at the level of the AV node, the bundle of His will control the ventricular

Table 5-7 Summary of differences in pathology, ECG characteristics, and interventions in Types I and II second-degree AV block

Type I, QRS 0.10 or less, with or without Wenckebach Phenomenon	Type II QRS greater than 0.10
AV lesion: above the bundle of His	Lesion in the bundle branch system
Associated with IWMI, digitalis, chronic AV lesions	Associated with AWMI or chronic lesions within the bundle branch system
Nature: ischemic, reversible, transient	Lesion is usually chronic in nature
ECG: Ps plot through; PR interval may prolong prior to missing QRS; PR after the dropped QRS is consistent	P waves plot through; dropped QRS preceded by a fixed PR interval
Ventricular rhythm can be regular or irregular	Ventricular rhythm can be regular or irregular
In the presence of sinus bradycardia, usually responds well to pharmacologic intervention	Usually does not respond well to pharmacologic intervention
Rarely requires electronic pacing	Usually requires electronic pacing

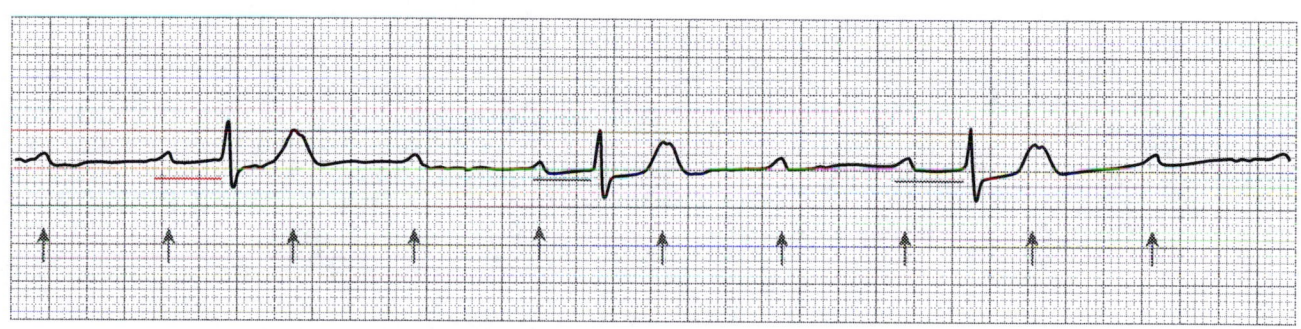

Figure 5-50 An ECG tracing illustrating high-grade, second-degree, (advanced) AV block. Note the atrial rate is 93 beats per minute, the ventricular rate is 30 beats per minute. Also note that the conducted beats have consistent PR intervals. Interpretation: sinus at 93 beats per minute with advanced second-degree AV block, ventricular rate is 30 beats per minute.

rhythm at 40 to 60 beats per minute. The ventricular rhythm will be regular. Figure 5-51 is an example of complete AV block. The QRS rhythm is regular, at 37 beats per minute. The atrial rate is faster, at about 60 beats per minute. The QRS and P waves are independent of each other.

When complete AV block occurs below the bundle of His, the ventricular rhythm is controlled by a ventricular escape mechanism of between 20 to 40 beats per minute. The ventricular rhythm will be regular. Figure 5-52 is another example of complete AV block. The atrial and ventricular rates are independent and regular. The QRS is 0.18 to 0.20 second.

In complete AV block, the atrial rate is faster and independent of the ventricular rate. There is no relationship between P and QRS; thus, there is no PR interval,

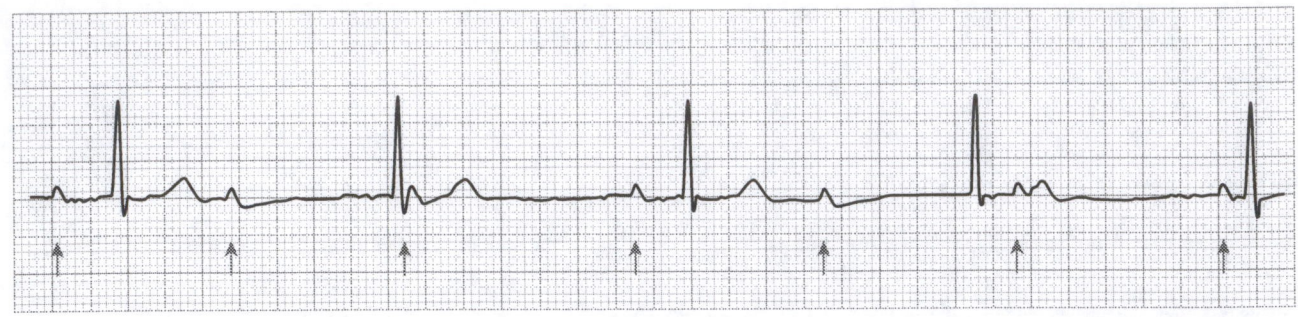

Figure 5-51 An ECG illustrating complete AV block, probably at the level of the AV node since the QRS is 0.06 second. The atrial rate is faster than the QRS rate and the P waves and QRS complexes are independent of each other. There are no consistent PR intervals. Interpretation: sinus at 50 beats per minute with complete AV block, a junctional rhythm with a ventricular rate at 40 beats per minute.

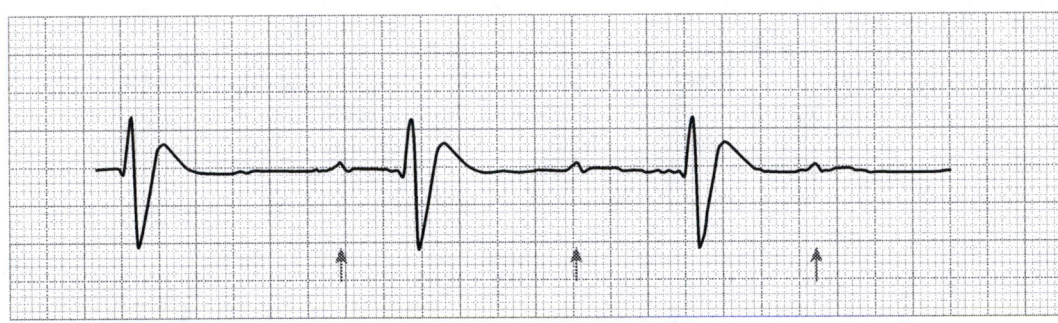

Figure 5-52 An ECG illustrating complete AV block that is probably infranodal, since the QRS is 0.18 to 0.20 second. The sinus rate is faster than the QRS rate and the P waves and QRS complexes are independent of each other. There are no consistent PR intervals. Interpretation: sinus at 50 beats per minute with complete AV block, possibly an idioventricular rhythm (or a QRS showing bundle branch conduction defect) and a ventricular rate at 40 beats per minute.

because, in complete AV block, there is no communication between the atria and the ventricles. They function independently of each other. The atria, remaining under the control of the SA node, or in atrial flutter or fibrillation, are beating at their own intrinsic rate and are completely dissociated from the ventricles. Table 5-8 summarizes the ECG characteristics of the AV conduction defects.

ARRHYTHMIAS DUE TO ABNORMAL CONDUCTION PATHWAYS

Depolarization from the sinus node travels through atrial tissue and terminates at the crest of the AV node. The PR interval comprises the time taken for atrial depolarization; the formation of the P wave; the time taken for depolarization of the AV node, bundle of His, and both bundle branches; and the PR segment. Slow conduction through the AV node accounts for most of the PR segment. If the wave of depolarization can bypass the AV node, then the normal delay that would have been encountered is circumvented, and the PR segment (and thus the PR interval) will be shortened.

Table 5-8 Summary of ECG configurations of first, second, and complete AV blocks

	First-Degree	Second-Degree Wenckebach	Second-Degree 2:1 Type I	Second-Degree 2:1 Type II	Complete
	every P has a QRS	*misses a QRS *PR after dropped QRS is consistent	misses a QRS *PR after dropped QRS is consistent	misses a QRS *PR after dropped QRS is consistent	AV dissociation
P waves	(+)/QRS	independent and regular	independent and regular	independent and regular	independent and regular
PR Interval	>0.20 but consistent	progressively longer, but the PR associated with the missed QRS is the same	can be < or >0.20 second; the PR after the missed beat is the same	can be < or >0.20 second; the PR after the missed beat is the same	there is no PR interval
QRS duration	<0.10	<0.10	<0.10 probably Type I *may present as 2:1 conduction	>0.10 rS, broad S wave, Or (+) notched QRS probably Type II; may present as 2:1 conduction	<0.10 if from a junctional pacer >0.10 and slow if from a ventricular pacing site
Rate/minute	60–100	varies	atrial rate is twice ventricular	atrial rate is twice ventricular	atrial rate is faster than the ventricular
Rhythm	regular	varies	regular	regular	regular

Many patients with accessory pathways (AP) are not diagnosed until adulthood. Males are affected more often than females. There is evidence to support a genetic predisposition to AP and resulting tachycardias.

Preexcitation is a term that describes early ventricular depolarization, using an *accessory* pathway rather than the normal AV conduction system. An **accessory pathway** is an extra bundle composed of ventricular tissue that exists outside the normal, specialized conduction tissue. This bundle forms a connection between the atria and ventricles. *Preexcitation syndrome* is used to describe clinical situations in which preexcitation causes tachycardias.

Several AP connect the atria to the ventricles:

● Kent bundles are accessory AV pathways that connect the atrium to the ventricles. Accessory AV pathways are a common type of preexcitation.

● The James bundle is an AP that connects atrial fibers to the upper part of the AV node. This is also called an *intranodal bypass tract.*

● Mahaim's fibers are an AP that connect the AV node and the ventricle (*nodoventricular*), or those that connect the bundle of His and the bundle branch (*nodofascicular*), or from the bundle branch to the ventricles (*fascicular ventricular*).

● Atriofascicular bypass tracts are fibers that connect the atrium to the bundle of His.

ECG Wave Forms Affected by Preexcitation

The ECG pattern of preexcitation consists primarily of a short PR interval because the descending impulse bypasses the normal AV conduction delay. Often, this is the source of AV nodal reentrant tachycardias. During these tachycardias, the QRS can be narrow, wide, or aberrant. If atrial fibrillation occurs with an AP, the ventricular response is usually very rapid and irregular, with aberrant ventricular conduction.

In addition, the early depolarization of the ventricles will cause a widened QRS complex with characteristic slurring in the initial wave forms of the QRS, called a **delta wave.** The delta wave is caused by slow intramyocardial conduction, rather than normal intraventricular conduction pathways. Also, the widened QRS is a result of the asynchronous depolarization of the ventricles.

The polarity of the delta wave may be positive or negative, depending on the direction of conduction as viewed by a particular lead. If the forces of excitation are toward the positive electrode in a lead, the polarity of the delta wave will be positive. Similarly, if the forces of excitation are away from the positive electrode in a lead, the polarity of the delta wave will be negative and produce an abnormal Q wave in leads III and V_1. Finally, if the forces of excitation are perpendicular to the positive electrode in a lead, the polarity will be isoelectric.

The amplitude of the delta wave depends on several factors, primarily on how quickly the AP conducts the current ahead of the normal wave of depolarization. If normal and accessory wave fronts arrive simultaneously, there may be no delta wave, and the PR interval is unchanged. However, because there are sources depolarizing the ventricles, the resulting QRS is a fusion of both wave fronts.

To summarize, the width of the QRS depends on several factors:

● **accessory pathway**

An extra bundle composed of ventricular tissue that exits outside the normal specialized conduction tissue

● **delta wave**

Initial slurring of the QRS complex; a premature upstroke to the QRS complex due to an atrial ventricular bypass tract as in WPW syndrome

- the length of time it takes to conduct through the AP;
- the location of the AP; and
- the conduction time between the sinus and AV nodes.

Since ventricular depolarization does not follow the normal conduction pathway, repolarization will be out of sequence. The extent of ST segment and T wave abnormalities that occur with altered ventricular repolarization depends on the source and degree of preexcitation.

Degrees of Preexcitation

There are four degrees of preexcitation:

1. *None.* The patient has a latent accessory pathway, and the PR interval and QRS duration are normal. The anatomical source of the pathway is on the lateral side of the left ventricle. This pathway may become active with atrial fibrillation and is capable of antegrade conduction, resulting in a life-threatening arrhythmia.

2. *Minimal.* The size of the delta wave is very small and not seen in all leads.

3. *Less than maximum.* The impulse arrives in the ventricle, first using the AP (short PR interval) and then using the AV node, causing a fusion beat. The resulting QRS may not have the classic delta wave, but may exhibit an abnormal Q wave, distortion of the ascending arm of the R wave, or increased QRS voltage. In less-than-maximum preexcitation, it is difficult to differentiate among ventricular hypertrophy, bundle branch block, and acute myocardial infarction. Clinical presentation, serial ECGs, and enzyme studies will facilitate diagnosis.

4. *Maximum preexcitation.* The term used when both ventricles are activated by the AP. There is almost no PR interval and the fusing of P to the QRS complex results in the widened QRS.

When preexcitation is suspected, the clinician must assess the PR interval and a delta wave in all leads. The PR may not be obviously shortened and a delta wave may not be visible in all leads taken simultaneously. Hints of the existence of an AP may be seen in a resting ECG. Whenever possible, a 12-lead ECG should be taken during the tachycardia episode and compared with the resting or normal ECG to rule out or confirm preexcitation. Figure 5-53 is a diagram with a corresponding ECG tracing for the 4 degrees of preexcitation.

Arrhythmias with Preexcitation

Reciprocating tachycardia occurs when a premature atrial focus conducts down the normal AV conduction system, but uses the AP to reenter the atria. This is also known as circus-movement or reentry tachycardia or orthodromic (narrow QRS) reciprocating tachycardia.

The P′ polarity may be negative or positive in lead I, and may be visible after the QRS complex. There is a short RP interval and QRS alternans may be seen. *QRS alternans* is a term used to describe alteration of the amplitude of the QRS complex's R and S waves. The ECG tracing in Figure 5-54 depicts QRS alternans.

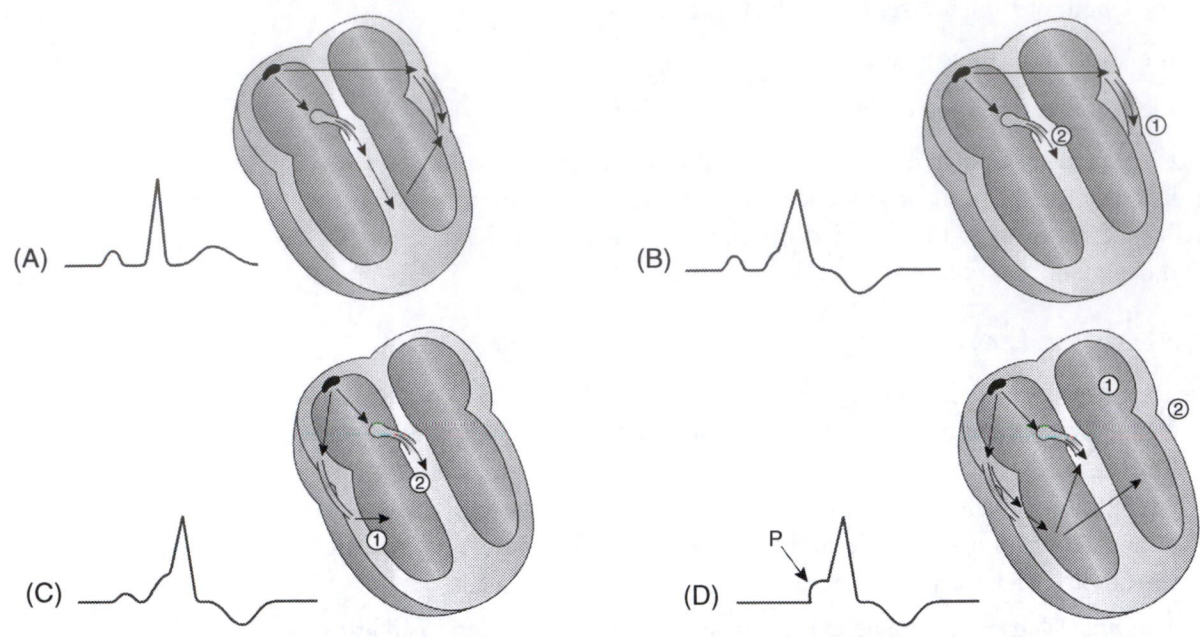

Figure 5-53 Normal activation: QRS complex showing no visible delta wave, no visible change in the QRS to identify the presence of an accessory pathway (A); minimal activation: QRS complex showing positive wave on the ascending arm of the QRS (B); and less than maximal activation: QRS complex showing positive delta wave in ascending arm of the QRS. Note the short PR interval. Diagram shows the fusion of normal and early forces arriving in the ventricle. The QRS will be a fusion of early and normal depolarizing forces (C); and maximum activation: the PR interval is so minimal as to be nonexistent. The delta wave is quite obvious as it fuses into the ascending arm of the QRS (D). (Adapted from *Understanding Electrocardiography: Arrhythmias and the 12-lead ECG,* 7th ed., by M. B. Conover, 1996, St. Louis: Mosby-Year Book, Inc.)

Figure 5-54 QRS alternans. Note the alternating amplitude of the QRS complex in several of the ECG leads in a patient with circus movement tachycardia. Note: alternans is not always visible in all the ECG leads. (From *Advanced Concepts of Arrhythmias,* by Marriott and Conover, 1989, St. Louis: C. V. Mosby.)

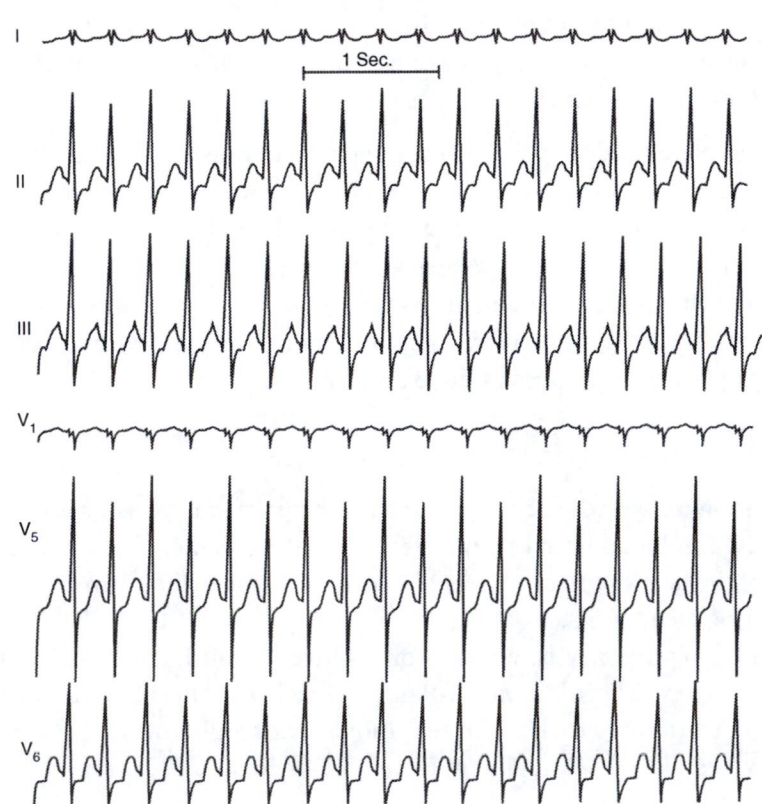

A PVC can cause a tachycardia by accessing the atria via the AP and subsequently traveling down the AV node, bundle of His, and into the ventricles. This will result in a narrow QRS tachycardia. During sinus tachycardia, when a critical rate is reached, the AP is blocked in an antegrade fashion. The impulse may well conduct normally, and reenter the atria using the AP in a retrograde fashion, thus establishing the reentry circuit. Orthodromic tachycardia can occur using a slower conducting AP. The reentry circuit uses the AV node in an antegrade direction and a slower-conducting AP in the retrograde direction. The slower conduction time from ventricle to atria over the slow AP will produce a long RP interval. In fact, the P' will be closer to the QRS that follows it, rather than the one that precedes it. The rhythm appears as a junctional tachycardia, but the ventricular rate is 130 to 200 beats per minute. Figure 5-55 is a 12-lead ECG tracing from a patient with orthodromic reciprocating tachycardia. The QRS complexes are narrow, and delta waves are present in leads III, aVF, and V_2.

Antidromic (wide QRS) tachycardia is a reentry tachycardia that uses the AP in an antegrade fashion and the AV node in a retrograde direction. The resulting QRS will be wide and the ventricular rhythm may be irregular, because retrograde conduction through the ventricular pathways may differ. In some cases, a P' occurs

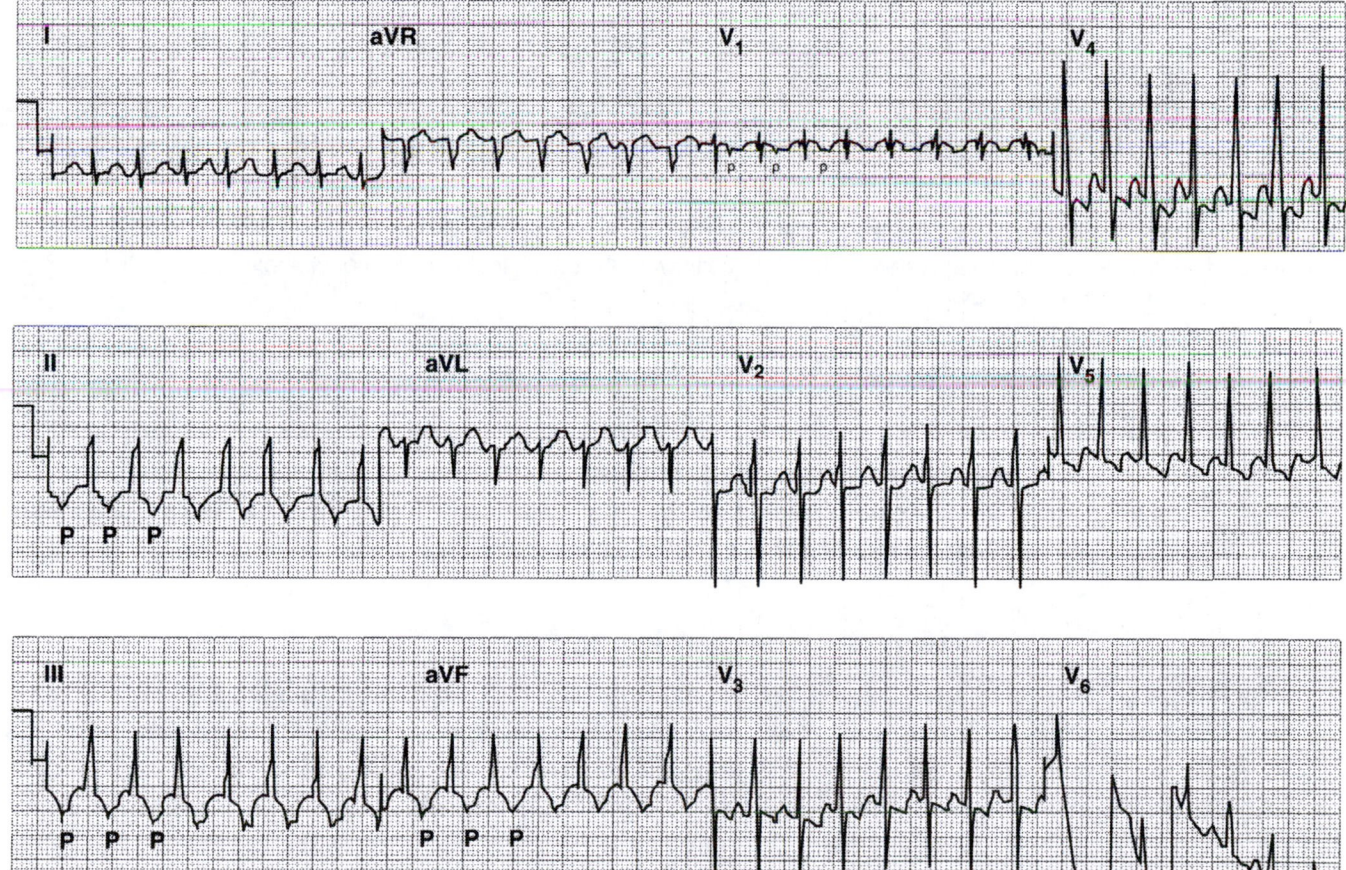

Figure 5-55 A 12-lead ECG of a patient with orthodromic reciprocating tachycardia. Note that the QRS complexes are narrow, PR intervals are short, and delta waves are present in leads III, aVF, and V_2.

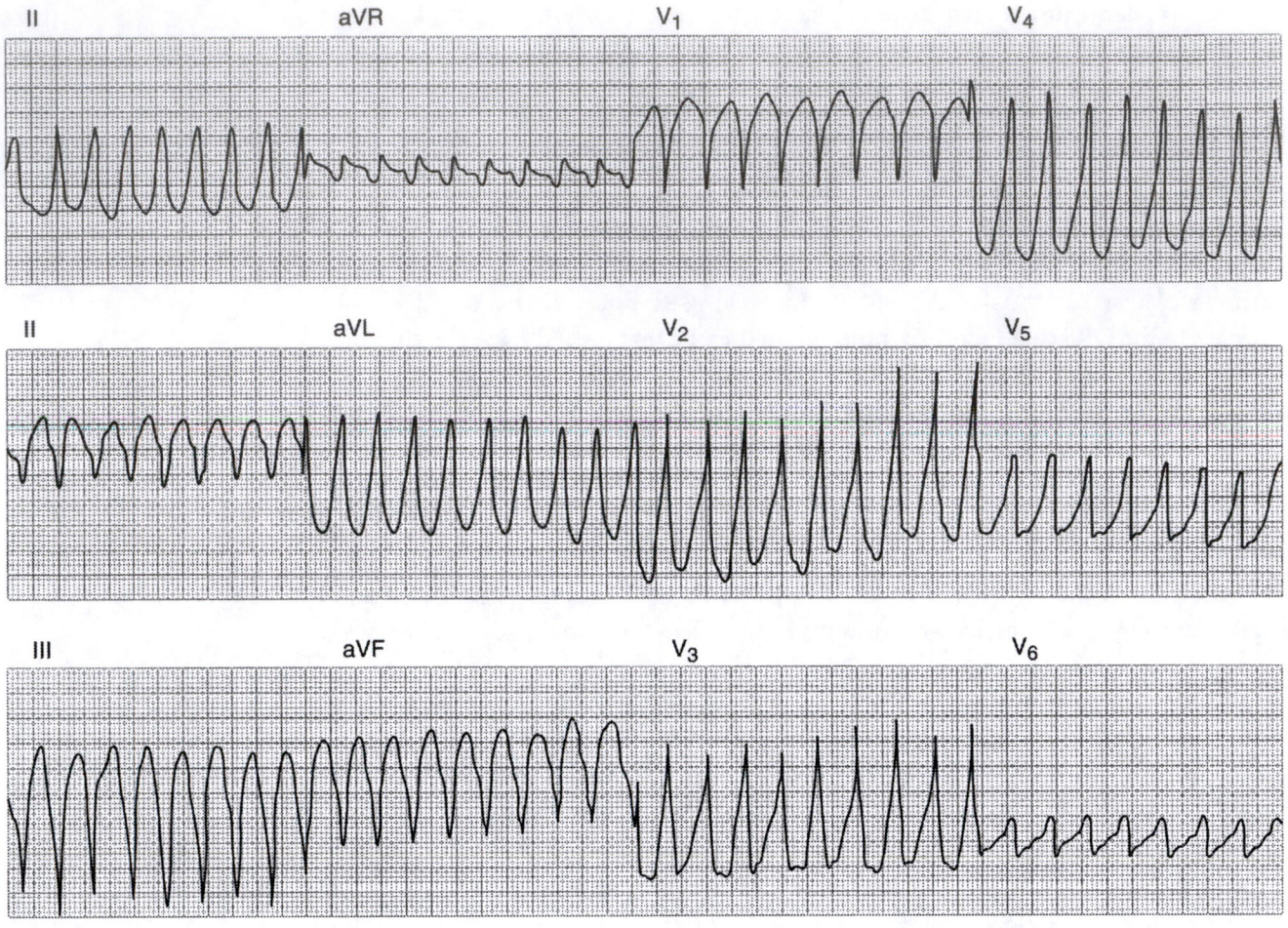

Figure 5-56 A 12-lead ECG of a patient with antidromic reciprocating tachycardia. Note the broad QRS with opposite T wave polarity, similar to ventricular tachycardia. The delta waves on the ascending and descending arms of the QRS have broadened the QRS complex.

because of the retrograde stimulation of the atria. This P′ may be seen after the QRS, but not in all leads, since the QRS is so broad. Figure 5-56 is a 12-lead ECG showing a patient with antidromic reciprocating tachycardia.

Lown-Ganong-Levine Syndrome

Lown-Ganong-Levine syndrome (LGL), also known as intranodal bypass tract syndrome, was initially described as a combination of a short PR interval, normal QRS configuration, and recurrent supraventricular tachycardias. It was subsequently shown that in patients who exhibit LGL, intranodal fibers bypass the crest of the AV node and one of the intranodal fibers terminates near the bundle of His (James' fibers). The major conduction delay in the AV node is thus circumvented and a short PR interval of less than 0.12 second is recorded. Ventricular depolarization takes place via the normal His-Purkinje system, thus generating a normal QRS complex.

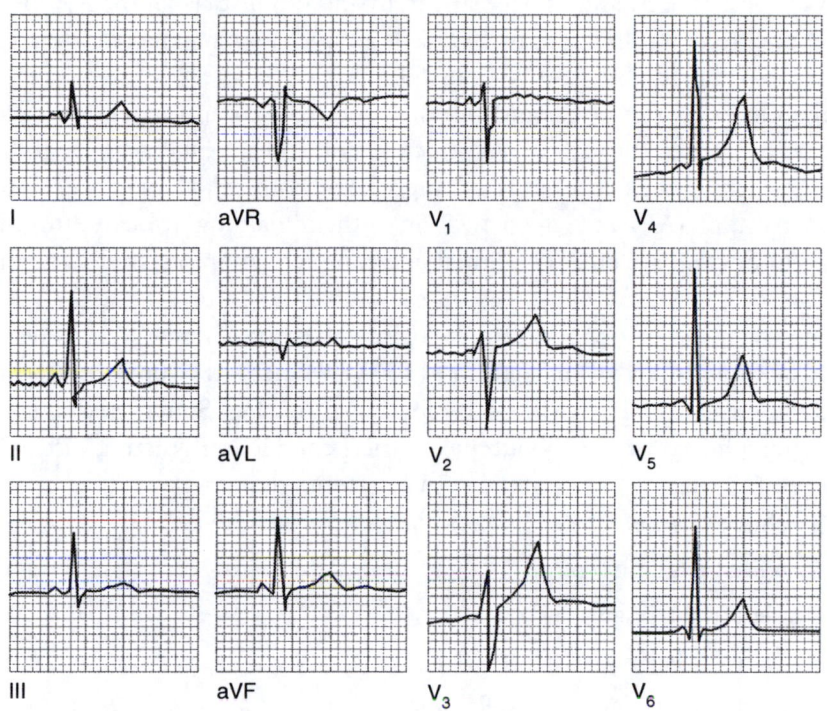

Figure 5-57 A 12-lead ECG showing a short PR interval and a narrow QRS complex in a patient with confirmed Lown-Ganong-Levine syndrome.

Many patients whose ECGs display a short PR interval and a normal QRS complex (Figure 5-57) may or may not be aware of a clinical history of tachycardia. Such tracings probably indicate bypass of the AV node by an intranodal fiber, and should be interpreted as consistent with, but not diagnostic of, Lown-Ganong-Levine presentation.

The three criteria for diagnosing Lown-Ganong-Levine syndrome are:

1. short PR interval (0.12 second or less);
2. normal QRS configuration; and
3. recurrent paroxysmal tachycardia.

Wolff-Parkinson-White Syndrome

Wolff-Parkinson-White (WPW) syndrome is characterized by preexcitation that occurs using accessory AV pathways (Kent bundles) with tachycardia. WPW that occurs without tachycardia is called *WPW pattern*. WPW can occur in healthy hearts. The anatomical presence of the AP may not manifest itself until later in life, or with myocardial infarction or atrial fibrillation.

In WPW, as atrial tissue is depolarized and forms the P wave on the ECG, the depolarizing wave front arrives simultaneously at the crest of the AV node at the AP's atrial end. Conduction through the AV node is normally delayed, but the AP is capable of very rapid depolarization. Thus, ventricular tissue is depolarized before the AV node has permitted normal conduction to continue through the bundle of His.

If all ventricular tissue is depolarized by the impulse using the AP, the resulting QRS is different from the sinus-induced QRS. The resulting widened QRS complex can be confused with bundle branch block or PVCs. However, as the wave of depolarization slowly spreads out from the prematurely depolarized ventricle, conduction is completed through the AV junction and spreads quickly through the His-Purkinje system. The net result is a composite of both initial, premature ventricular depolarization (AP) and later activation of the remaining myocardium using the normal conduction system. The initial aberrant activation generates a slurring of the QRS.

The changes that occur with myocardial infarction, bundle branch block, and ventricular hypertrophy will be masked by the WPW pattern. Confident diagnosis of an AP's existence may be made by electrophysiologic testing. Simply assessing the QRS to draw any other conclusion about the electrical conduction system is discouraged.

The ECG characteristics of the WPW pattern are:

1. short PR interval (0.12 second or less);

2. wide QRS complex;

3. delta wave (Figure 5-58);

4. tachycardias with normal QRS;

5. tachycardias with wide QRS; and

6. normal conduction pattern in which the Kent bundles are not activated and normal pathways of depolarization are followed.

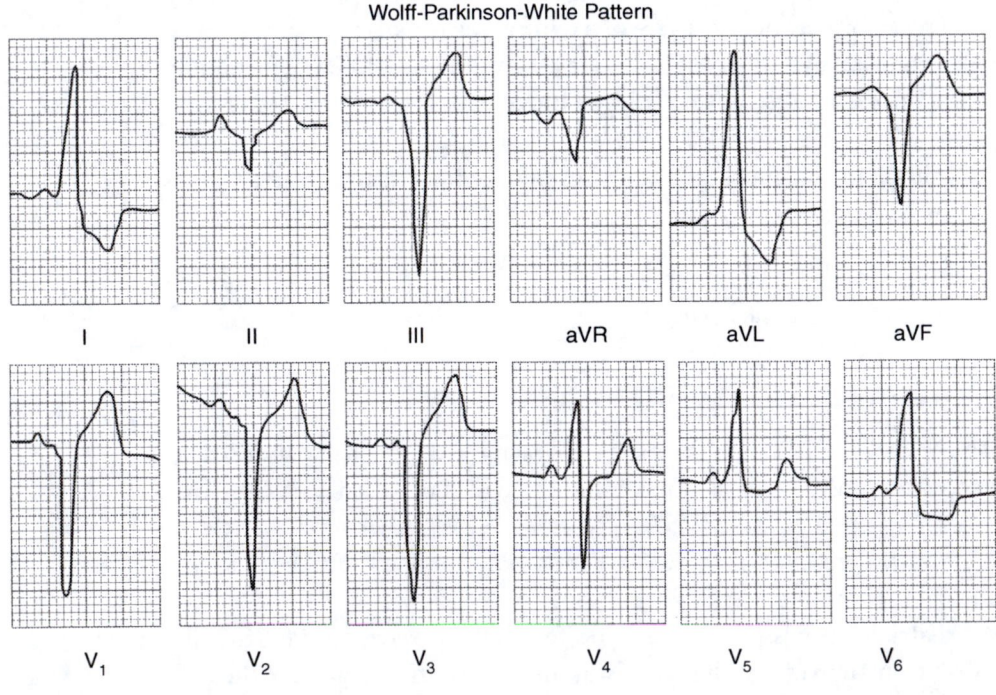

Wolff-Parkinson-White Pattern

Figure 5-58 A 12-lead ECG showing a classic pattern of early activation. Note the short PR interval, and the broad QRS complexes. There are positive delta waves in leads I, aVL, V_4, V_5, and V_6. There are negative delta waves in all the other leads.

Table 5-9 ECG wave forms and characteristics

	Accessory AV Bundle	Intranodal Bypass Tract	Nodofascicular Connection
PR interval	<0.12 second	<0.12 second	normal
QRS duration	>0.10 second	normal*	>0.11 second
Secondary ST-T abnormalities	present	absent	present
Delta waves	present	absent	present
Can mimic myocardial infarction	yes	no*	yes
Can mimic ventricular hypertrophy	yes	no*	yes

*Must rule out prior pathology in the bundle branch system

Patients with persistent complaints of paroxysms of tachycardia should be clinically assessed for active AP. Surgery or transvenous radio frequency or laser ablation may be considered in patients who are becoming intolerant of the arrhythmias or have a predisposition for atrial fibrillation. Table 5-9 summarizes ECG wave forms and characteristics in early excitation using accessory AV bundle, intra-AV nodal bypass tract, and nodofascicular connection.

Summary

This chapter reviews various ECG arrhythmias. Each is explained and, when appropriate, tables are provided to offer a summary of wave forms and their characteristics for each type of arrhythmia. This chapter is not intended to replace ECG rhythm analysis, but rather is a foundation upon which to recognize the salient points necessary for accurate interpretation of the 12-lead ECG.

Self-Assessment Exercises

● ECG Rhythm Identification Practice

For the following rhythms, fill in the blanks and then compare your answers with those found in the back of the book.

Figure 5-59

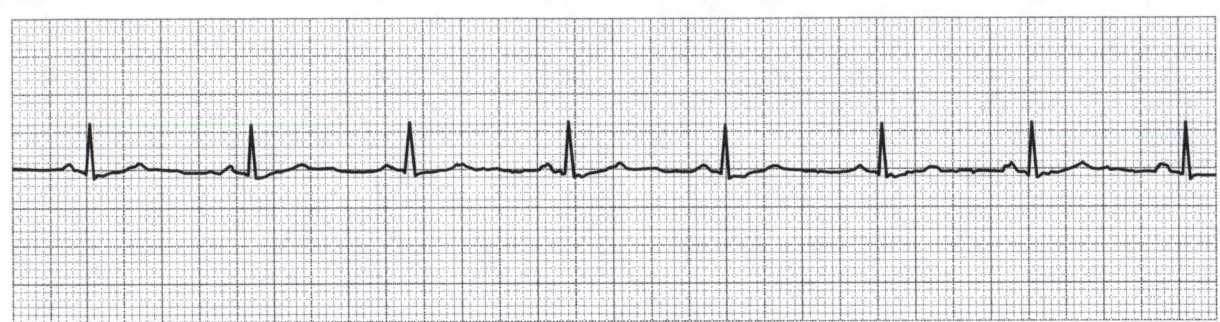

QRS duration _____ QT _____   Identification _____

Ventricular rate/rhythm _____   _____

Atrial rate/rhythm _____   Symptoms _____

PR interval _____   _____

Treatment _____

_____

Figure 5-60

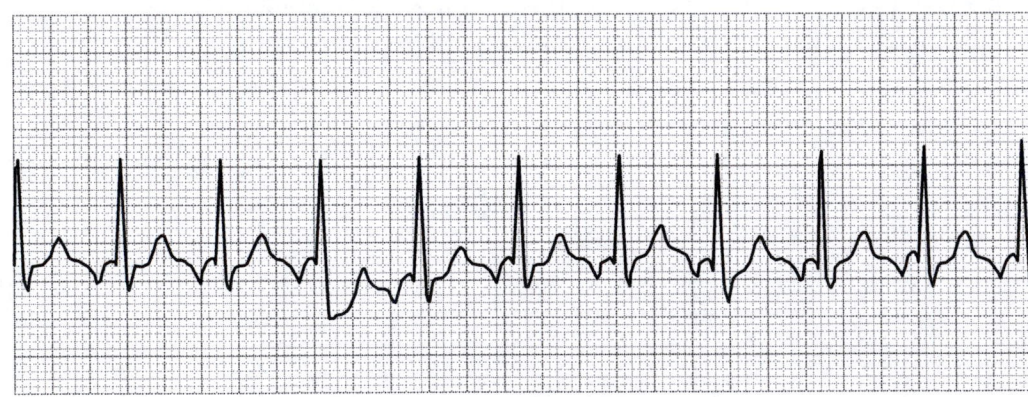

QRS duration _____ QT _____   Identification _____

Ventricular rate/rhythm _____   _____

Atrial rate/rhythm _____   Symptoms _____

PR interval _____   _____

Treatment _____

_____

Figure 5-61

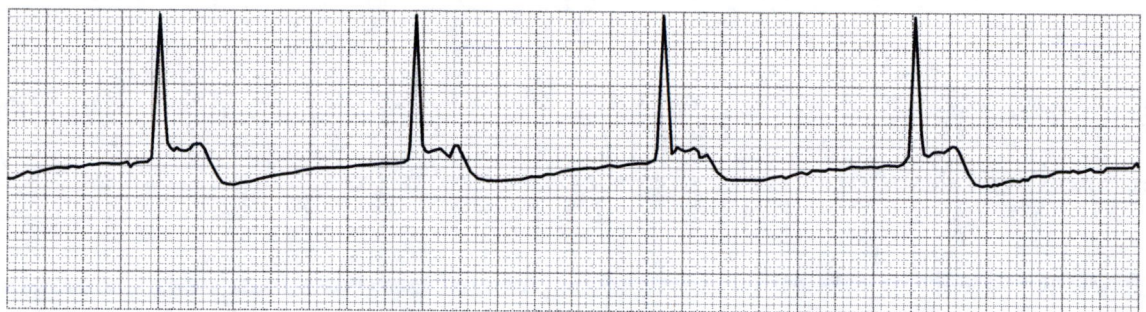

QRS duration _____ QT _____   Identification _____

Ventricular rate/rhythm _____

Atrial rate/rhythm _____   Symptoms _____

PR interval _____   _____

Treatment _____

_____

Figure 5-62

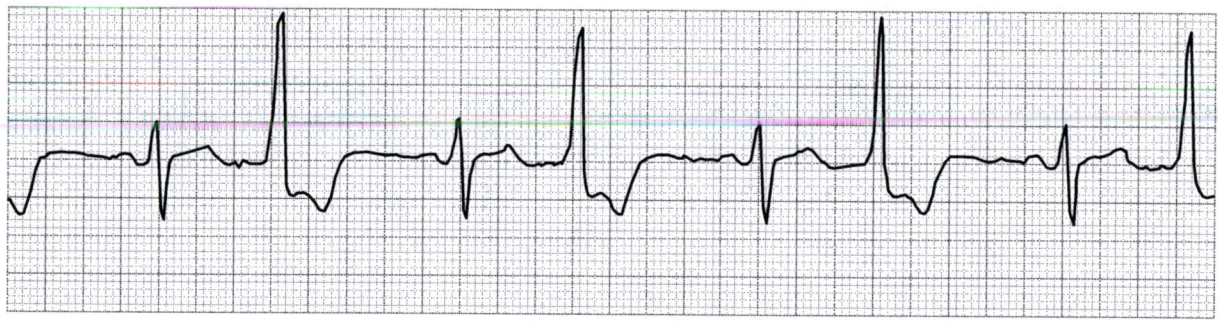

QRS duration _____ QT _____   Identification _____

Ventricular rate/rhythm _____   _____

Atrial rate/rhythm _____   Symptoms _____

PR interval _____

Treatment _____

_____

Figure 5-63

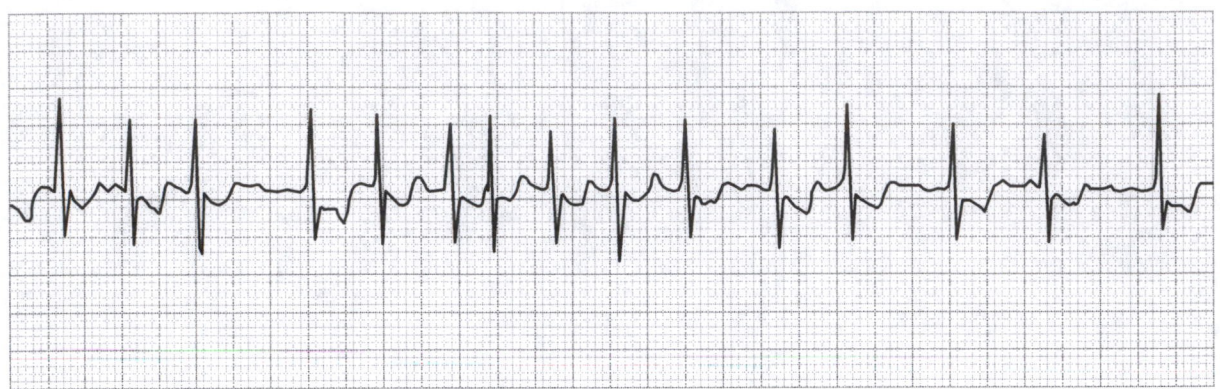

QRS duration _____ QT _____   Identification _____

Ventricular rate/rhythm _____   _____

Atrial rate/rhythm _____   Symptoms _____

PR interval _____   _____

Treatment _____

_____

Figure 5-64

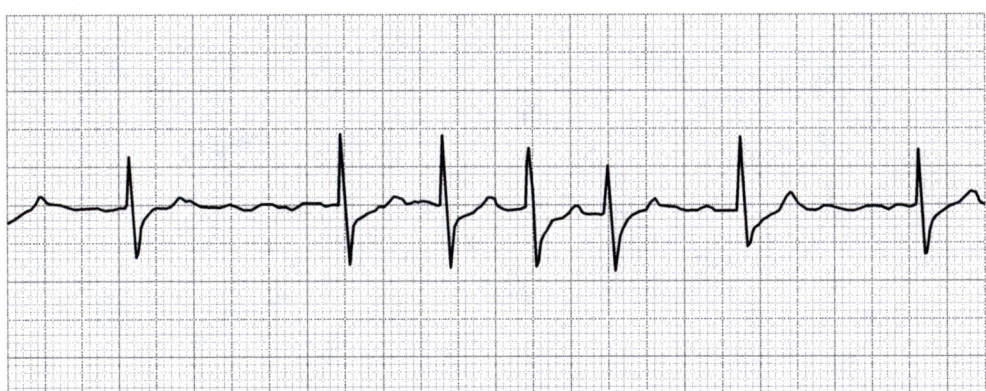

QRS duration _____ QT _____   Identification _____

Ventricular rate/rhythm _____   _____

Atrial rate/rhythm _____   Symptoms _____

PR interval _____   _____

Treatment _____

_____

Figure 5-65

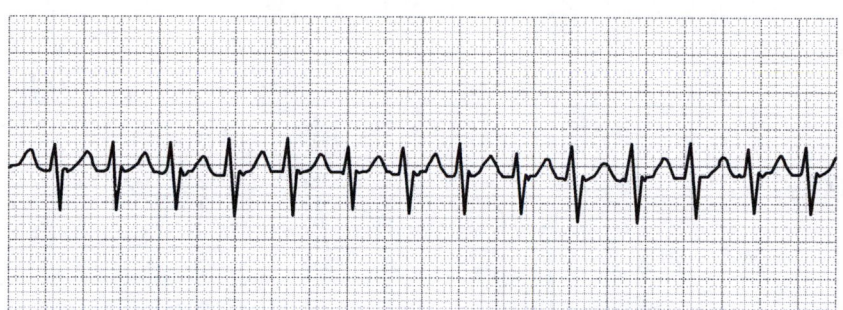

QRS duration _____ QT _____

Ventricular rate/rhythm _____

Atrial rate/rhythm _____

PR interval _____

Identification _____

Symptoms _____

Treatment _____

Figure 5-66

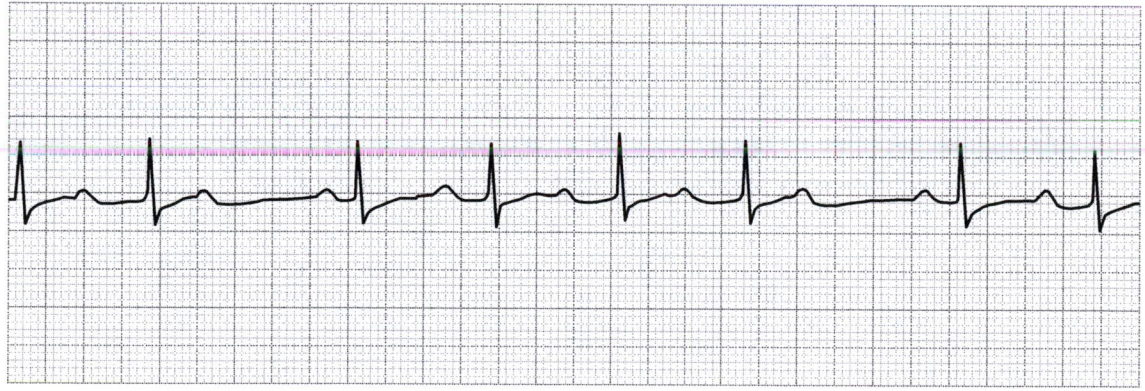

QRS duration _____ QT _____

Ventricular rate/rhythm _____

Atrial rate/rhythm _____

PR interval _____

Identification _____

Symptoms _____

Treatment _____

Figure 5-67

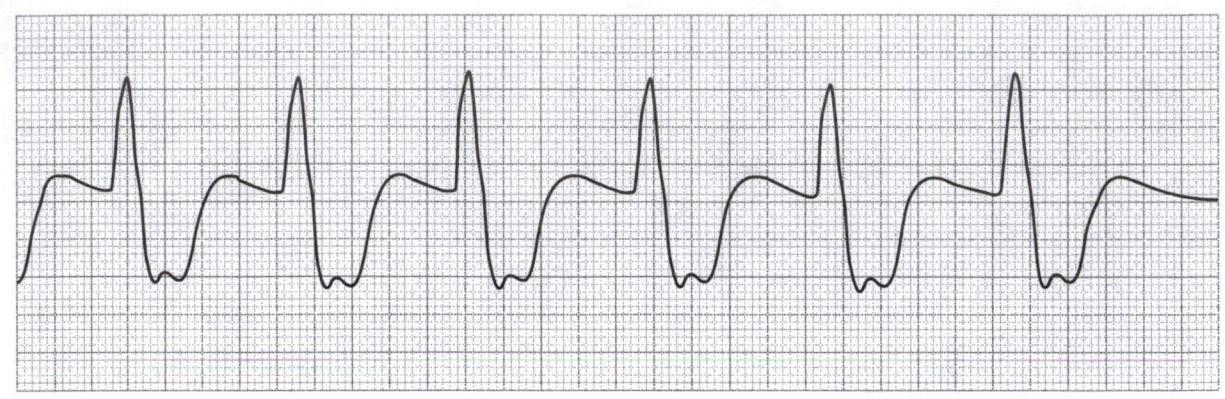

QRS duration _____ QT _____   Identification _____

Ventricular rate/rhythm _____   _____

Atrial rate/rhythm _____   Symptoms _____

PR interval _____   _____

Treatment _____

_____

Figure 5-68

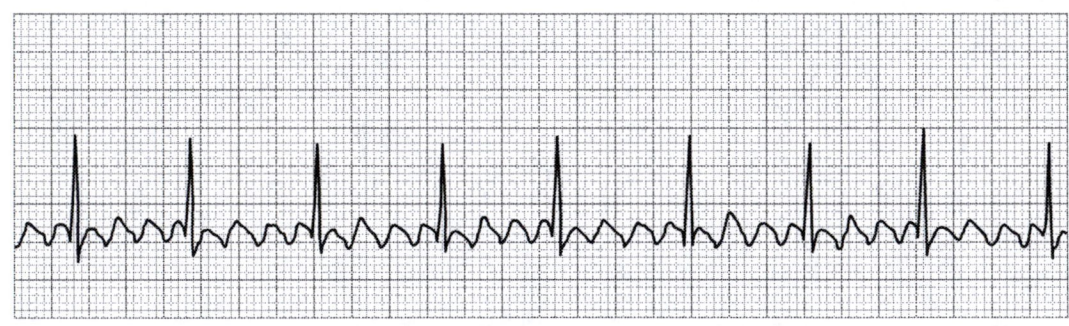

QRS duration _____ QT _____   Identification _____

Ventricular rate/rhythm _____   _____

Atrial rate/rhythm _____   Symptoms _____

PR interval _____   _____

Treatment _____

_____

Figure 5-69

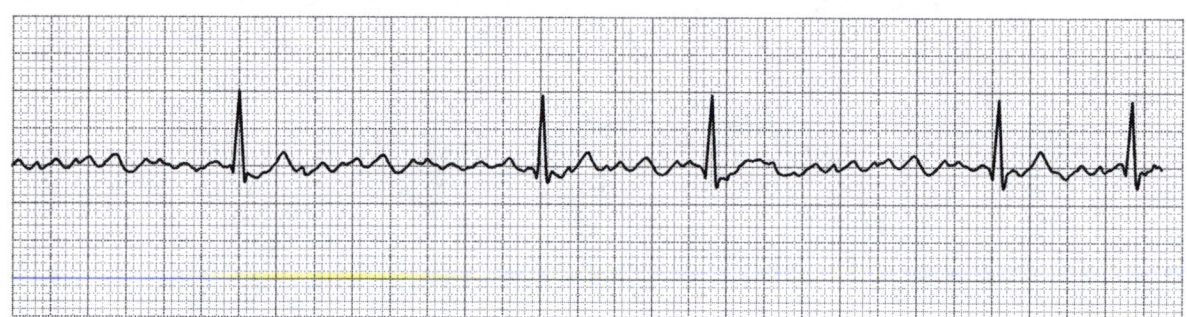

QRS duration _____ QT _____   Identification _____

Ventricular rate/rhythm _____

Atrial rate/rhythm _____   Symptoms _____

PR interval _____   _____

Treatment _____

_____

Figure 5-70

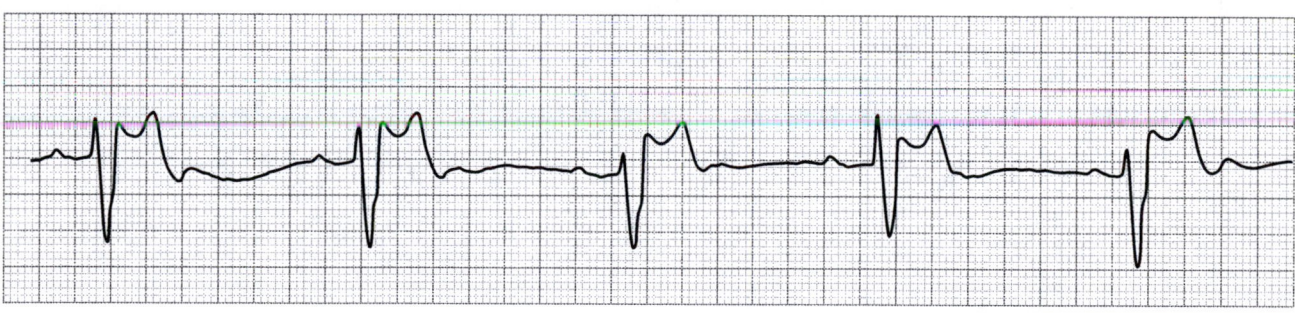

QRS duration _____ QT _____   Identification _____

Ventricular rate/rhythm _____

Atrial rate/rhythm _____   Symptoms _____

PR interval _____

Treatment _____

_____

Figure 5-71

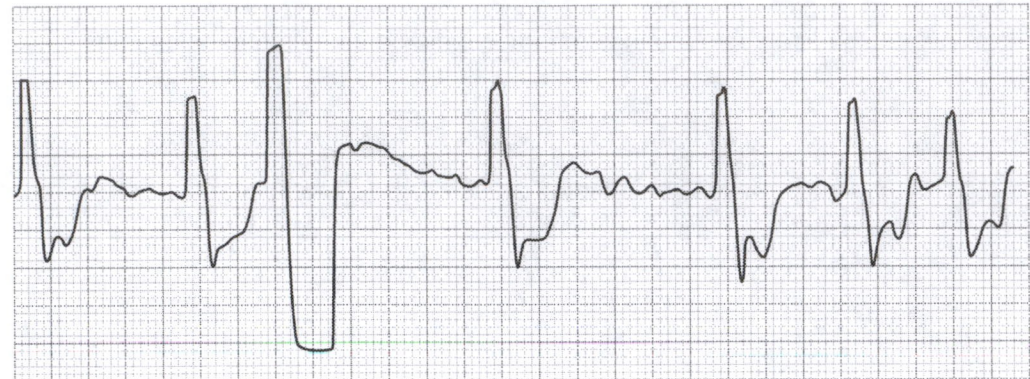

QRS duration _____ QT _____   Identification _____

Ventricular rate/rhythm _____   _____

Atrial rate/rhythm _____   Symptoms _____

PR interval _____   _____

Treatment _____

_____

Figure 5-72

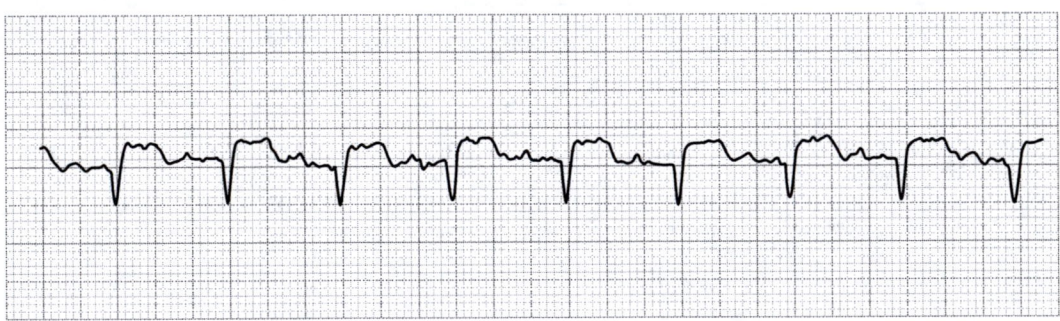

QRS duration _____ QT _____   Identification _____

Ventricular rate/rhythm _____   _____

Atrial rate/rhythm _____   Symptoms _____

PR interval _____   _____

Treatment _____

_____

Figure 5-73

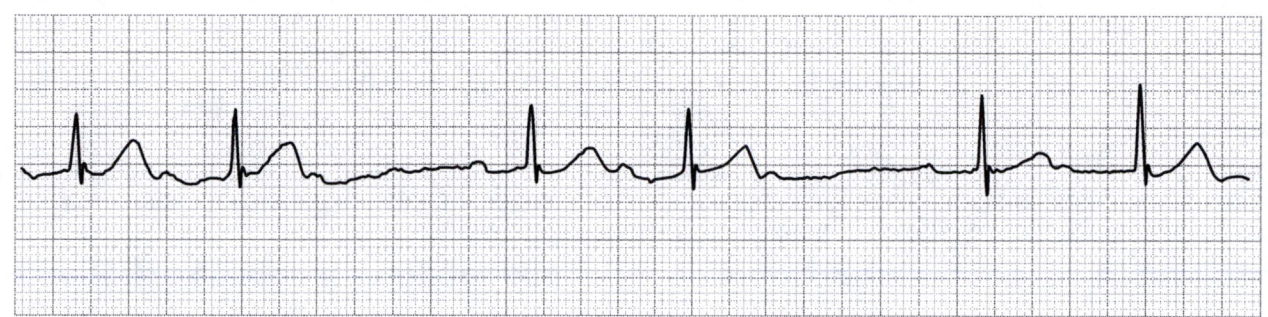

QRS duration _____ QT _____   Identification _____

Ventricular rate/rhythm _____

Atrial rate/rhythm _____   Symptoms _____

PR interval _____

Treatment _____
_____

Figure 5-74

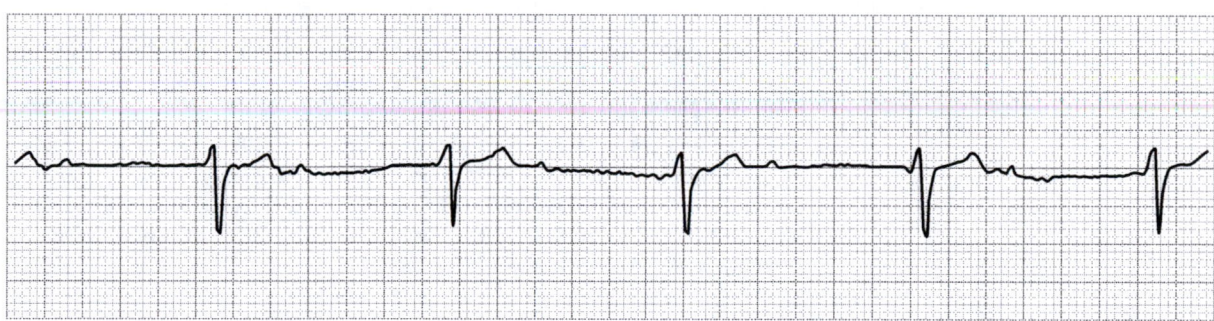

QRS duration _____ QT _____   Identification _____

Ventricular rate/rhythm _____

Atrial rate/rhythm _____   Symptoms _____

PR interval _____

Treatment _____
_____

References

1998 Heart and Stroke Statistical Update. (1998). Dallas, TX: American Heart Association.

Agarwal, J. B., Khaw, K., Aurignac, F., et al. (1999). Importance of posterior chest leads in patients with suspected myocardial infarction; but non-diagnostic, routine 12-lead electrocardiogram. *American Journal of Cardiology*; 1:83(3):323-326.

Barbagelata, A., Califf, R. M., Sgarbossa, E. B., et al. (1997). Thrombolysis and Q-wave versus non-Q wave first myocardial infarction. GUSTO-I substudy. *Journal of the American College of Cardiology*; 15:29:770-777.

Bates, E. R., Clemmensen, P. M., Califf, R. M., et al. (1990). Precordial ST segment depression predicts a worse prognosis in inferior infarction despite reperfusion therapy. *Journal of the American College of Cardiology*; 16:1538.

Boden, W. E., Spodick, D. H. (1989). Diagnostic significance of precordial ST segment depression. *American Journal of Cardiology*; 63:358.

Braat, S. H., Gorgels, A. P. M., Bär, F. W., Wellens, H. J. J. (1988.). Value of the ST-T segment in inferior wall acute myocardial infarction to predict the site of coronary artery occlusion. *American Journal of Cardiology*; 62:140.

Braunwald, E. (1989). Optimizing thrombolytic therapy of acute myocardial infarction. *Circulation*; 82:1510.

Chou, T. C. (1996). Myocardial disease. In *Electrocardiography in clinical practice: Adult and pediatric*. Philadelphia: W. B. Saunders; 257-280.

Cohen, M., Demers, C., Gurfinkel, E. P., et al. (1997). A comparison of low-molecular-weight-heparin with unfractionated heparin for unstable coronary artery disease. *New England Journal of Medicine*; 337(7):447-452.

Conover, M. B. (1996). *Understanding electrocardiography: Arrhythmias and the 12-lead ECG*. (7th ed.). St. Louis: Mosby-Year Book.

Conover, M. B., Wellens, H. J., Hein, J. (1993). *The ECG in emergency decision making*. Philadelphia: W. B. Saunders.

Daviglus, M. L., Liao, Y., Greenland, P., et al. (1999). Association of nonspecific minor ST-T abnormalities with cardiovascular mortality: The Chicago Western Electric Study. *Journal of the American Medical Association*; 281(6):530-536.

Fath-Ordoubadi, F., et al. (1997). Glucose-insulin-potassium therapy for treatment of acute infarction: An overview of randomized placebo-controlled trials. *Circulation*; 96:(8)1152-1156.

Feola, M., Ribichini, F., Gallone, G., et al. (1994). Analysis of right electrocardiographic leads in 195 normal subjects. *Giornal Ital Calriol*; 24: 375-389.

Fesmire, F. M. (1995). ECG diagnosis of acute myocardial infarction in the presence of left bundle branch block in patients undergoing continuous ECG monitoring. *Annual Emergency Medicine*; 26:69-82.

Goodman, S.G., Langer, A., Ross, A. M., Wildermann, N. M., et al. (1998). Non-Q-wave versus Q-wave myocardial infarction after thrombolytic therapy: Angiographic and prognostic insights from the global utilization of streptokinase and tissue plasminogen activator for occluded coronary arteries—I angiographic substudy. GUSTO-I Angiographic Investigators. *Circulation*; 10:97(5):444-450.

GUSTO, ISIS-4 Collaborative Group, (March 18, 1995). *Lancet*; 3, 4, 5, (8951):669.

Kereizker, D. J., et al. (1990). Time delays in the diagnosis and treatment of acute myocardial infarction: A tale of eight cities. Report from the prehospital study group and the Cincinnati Heart Project. *American Heart Journal*; 120:773.

Krucoff, M. W., Green,C. E., Satler, L. F., et al. (1996). Noninvasive detection of coronary artery patency using continuous ST-segment monitoring. *American Journal of Cardiology*; 57:916-921.

Langer, A. et al. (1996). LATE assessment of thrombolytic efficacy (LATE) study: Prognosis in patients with non-Q wave myocardial infarction. (LATE Study Investigators). *Journal of the American College of Cardiology*; 27(6):1327-1332.

Lemery, R., Kleinebenne, A., Nihoyannopoulos, P., et al. (1990). Q waves in hypertrophic cardiomyopathy in relation to the distribution and severity of right and left ventricular hypertrophy. *Journal of the American College of Cardiology*; 16:368-374.

Little, R. C. (1985). *Physiology of the heart and circulation*. (3rd ed.). New York: Year Book Medical.

Mandel, W. J. (1980). *Cardiac arrhythmias: Their mechanism, diagnosis and management.* Philadelphia: Lippincott.

Maeda, S. (1994). Different clinical implications for ST depression and T wave inversion in non-Q wave myocardial infarction. *American Journal of Cardiology*; 24:357-366.

Mehta, M., Jain, A. C., Mehta, A. V. (1999). *Clinical Cardiology*; 22:259-265.

Meier, C., Derby, L., Jick, S., et al. (1999). Antibiotics and risk of subsequent first-time acute myocardial infarction. *Journal of the American Medical Association*; 281:427-531.

Ogawa, H., Hiramori, K., Haze, K., et al. (1985). Classification of non-Q-wave myocardial infarction according to electrocardiographic changes. *Br Heart Journal*; 54:473-478.

Phibbs, B. (1983). "Transmural" versus "subendocardial" myocardial infarction: An electrocardiographic myth. *Journal of the American College of Cardiology*; 1:561-564.

Roth, A., et al (1990). Should thrombolytic therapy be administered in the mobile intensive care unit in patients with evolving myocardial infarction? A pilot study. *Journal of the American College of Cardiology*; 15:932.

Ryan, T. J., Anderson, J. L., Antman, E. M., et al. (1996). ACC/AHA guidelines for the management of patients with acute myocardial infarction: A report of the American College of Cardiology/American Heart Association Task Force on Practice Guidelines. *Journal of the American College of Cardiology*; 28:1328-1428.

The GUSTO Investigators. (1993). An international randomized trial comparing four thrombolytic strategies for acute myocardial infarction. *New England Journal of Medicine*; 329:673.

Weaver, W. D., Cerqueira, M., Hallstrom, A. P., et al. (1993). Prehospital-initiated vs. hospital-initiated thrombolytic therapy: The myocardial infarction triage and intervention trial. *Journal of the American Medical Association*; 270:1211-1216.

Weaver, W. D. et al. (1990). Myocardial infarction triage and intervention project: Phase I patient characteristics and feasibility of prehospital initiation of thrombolytic therapy. *Journal of the American College of Cardiology*; 15:925.

Myocardial Perfusion Deficits and ECG Changes

> *Premise* ⬤ Knowledge of the surfaces of the heart, how they are perfused, and how they are viewed by each of the leads provides the basis of a sensible approach to identifying changes that occur with ischemia, injury, and necrosis, as well as the ability to predict possible outcomes.

Objectives

After reading the chapter and completing the Self-Assessment exercises, the student should be able to:

1. Describe the pathophysiology of acute myocardial infarction
2. Identify the coronary arteries and the structures they perfuse
3. Recognize the ECG changes that occur with ischemia, injury, and necrosis
4. List the complications that can occur with ischemia, injury, and necrosis
5. Identify leads that are reflective and reciprocal of the area involved

Key Terms

acute coronary syndrome (ACS)	infarction	positive ST segment coving
akinesis	injury	reflecting leads
dyskinesia	ischemia	reciprocal leads
fixed atherosclerotic obstruction	necrosis	thrombolysis
	non-transmural (non-Q wave)	trending

Introduction

Myocardial infarction continues to plague society. Nearly 1.1 million people annually experience acute myocardial infarction (AMI), from which about one-third will die. The pathology of AMI is perfusion deficit attributed to occlusion and/or spasm. Initially the patient may experience pain that reflects **ischemia** that will result in a lack of perfusion of oxygenated blood. Prolonged insufficiency of oxygenated blood flow results in **injury**. If the situation persists, **necrosis (infarction)** will occur. For the purpose of this chapter, the term *perfusion deficit* will

⬤ ischemia
Deficiency in perfusion of oxygenated blood

⬤ injury
Damage to tissue; may be reversible

⬤ necrosis
Deadening of tissue as a result of occlusion and lack of oxygenated blood being perfused.

⬤ infarction
Necrosis to heart muscle; usually the result of occlusion of a coronary artery

encompass conditions resulting in AMI due to infection or occlusion because of plaque or clot. The pathology of each will be discussed in turn.

The ECG is the most accessible and widely used diagnostic tool for patients experiencing the signs and symptoms suggestive of acute myocardial ischemia. While the prognostic implications of each of the changes seen on the ECG remain a topic of much investigation, some definitions remain constant.

When acute changes are seen in a monitoring lead in a patient with suggestive signs and symptoms, they are signals with a high index of suspicion that acute changes are taking place. Those changes must be confirmed by multiple-lead ECG analysis and correlated with history, clinical presentation, and lab value analysis.

Signs of ischemia, injury, and necrosis are often not present or recognized initially on the ECG. Trending (repeated ECG recordings with comparison) the patient at specific, frequent intervals, using the 12-lead ECG, lab values, and clinical findings all contribute to early diagnosis and the treatment plan. Trending also monitors the effects of the selected interventions.

● **trending**

Repeated ECG recording with comparison to allow for diagnosis and evaluation of interventions.

Time is a critical factor for successful reperfusion. Therefore, early recognition of the classic signs of ischemia, injury, and necrosis using multiple-lead ECG analysis is vital for successful patient outcomes.

CORONARY ARTERY PERFUSION

Recall that the two primary arteries that supply blood to the myocardium are the left and right coronary arteries. They originate at the sinuses of Valsalva which are located in the aorta just above the cusps of the aortic valve.

As their names imply, the left coronary artery supplies blood to the anterior and left side of the heart while the right coronary artery supplies blood to the right side. The left coronary artery divides almost immediately into two primary branches, the left anterior descending (LAD) and the left circumflex artery. Some hearts have a variant artery with a third branch called the *ramus intermedius* which is located between the LAD and circumflex. The LAD delivers blood to the left ventricular free wall. In addition, several branches of the LAD called *septal perforating arteries* supply the proximal portion of the intraventricular septum and the main trunk of the right bundle branch. The LAD also is responsible for perfusing both major fascicles of the left bundle branch system.

There are arteries and branches of the LAD that furnish blood to the high lateral, lateral, and anterolateral wall of the left ventricle. The left circumflex artery (LCA) supplies blood to the lateral and posterior-lateral walls of the left ventricle. In a left-dominant system, the circumflex winds around the heart and gives rise to the posterior descending artery (PDA). In a right-dominant system, the PDA originates from the dominant right coronary artery and supplies blood to the inferior and posterior walls of the left ventricle.

Recall that the right coronary artery (RCA) supplies blood to the right atrium and the right ventricle. In approximately half of human hearts, a branch of the RCA forms the sinus node artery that supplies the sinus node. In the remaining hearts, the sinus node artery is a branch of the left circumflex. In most hearts (90 percent), the RCA will branch into the AV node artery that supplies the AV node, as the name

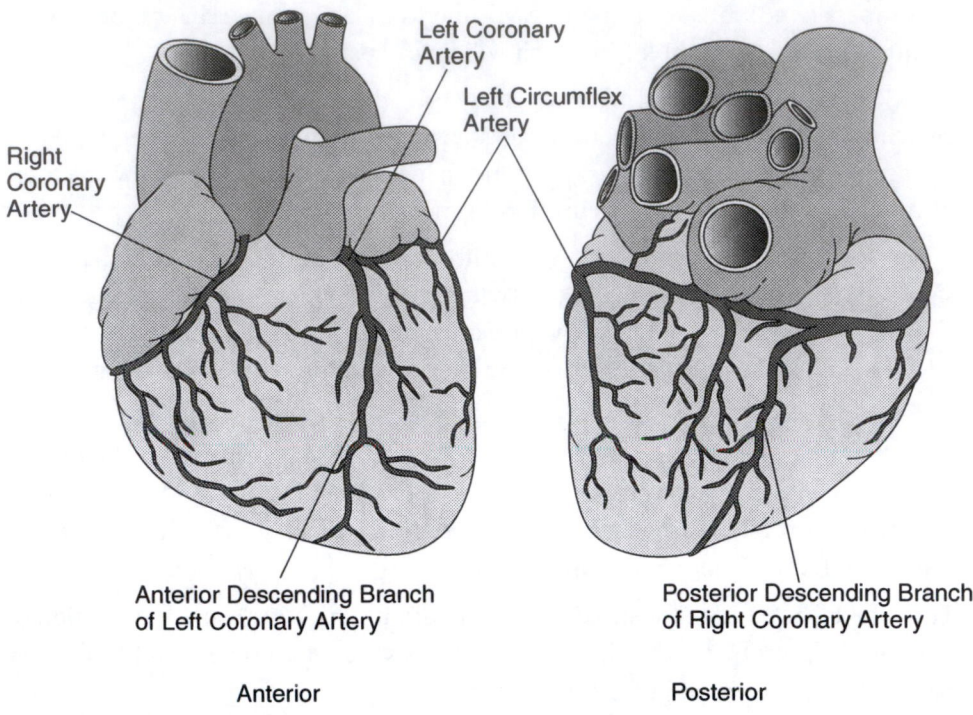

Right Coronary Artery

Left Coronary Artery

Left Circumflex Artery

Anterior Descending Branch of Left Coronary Artery

Posterior Descending Branch of Right Coronary Artery

Anterior

Posterior

Figure 6-1 Coronary artery perfusion (A) anterior view and (B) posterior view.

implies. In the remaining 10 percent, this artery is a branch of the left circumflex. In 90 percent of hearts, the RCA gives rise to the posterior descending artery (right-dominant system). The septal perforating branches of the posterior descending artery profuse the posterior intraventricular septum. Right and left septal perforating arteries often anastomose and provide collateral circulation.

Figure 6-1 is an illustration of the heart's coronary perfusion, anterior, and posterior views.

PATHOPHYSIOLOGY OF
ACUTE MYOCARDIAL INFARCTION

While myocardial infarction is an acute process, it may occur because of a chronic accumulation of atheromatous plaque formation in the coronary arteries. Simply put, the bulging and/or rupture of the plaque may significantly obstruct blood flow. In most cases, without total occlusion, stenosis of a coronary artery can lead to myocardial infarction. The fibrous cap of the atheromatous plaque can fracture or rupture. Subsequently, ulceration of the plaque frequently results in the development of an obstructive thrombus or spasm of the artery. This can cause acute, total occlusion and subsequent myocardial infarction. Thrombus formation resulting from ulceration of the atherosclerotic plaque is stimulated by the exposure of underlying collagen and other thrombogenic substances to blood flow and the subsequent release of thromboplastic elements from the plaque's necrotic core. This exposure is followed by:

- platelet adhesion and aggregation;
- release of thromboplastin which initiates the coagulation cascade;
- formation of platelet plugs; and
- incorporation of fibrins, red blood cells, and plasminogen into the final clot.

DeWood reported the causative role of intracoronary thrombus in acute myocardial infarction. In this study, patients underwent coronary angiography within 24 hours of symptoms to detect the presence or absence of thrombus in the occluded artery. This was felt to be one of the pathophysiological bases for **acute coronary syndrome (ACS)**. In 87 percent of patients who were evaluated within 4 hours after symptom onset, total coronary occlusion was observed. This was confirmed in 88 percent of those patients who subsequently underwent coronary artery bypass surgery.

> **acute coronary syndrome (ACS)**
> A group of signs and symptoms associated with myocardial ischemia and injury in compromised, and hopefully salvageable, tissue

The incidence of observed thromboembolic occlusion decreases with time after onset of symptoms. DeWood first suggested that spontaneous reperfusion may be an important feature in the evolution of myocardial infarction.

Coronary artery spasm can occur in nonoccluded coronary arteries, **fixed atherosclerotic obstruction** (the term that describes a lesion in a vessel with an atheromatous plaque), and the grafts used in coronary bypass surgery. Coronary artery spasm can also result in myocardial infarction due to restriction of blood flow distal to the spasm.

> **fixed atherosclerosis obstruction**
> Localized accumulations of lipid-containing material (atheromas) within or beneath the intimal surfaces of blood vessels

The process of myocardial injury in an acute MI is time-dependent. Necrosis develops over several hours in the presence of coronary occlusion. The evolution of MI follows the "wave front" phenomenon of myocardial ischemia and injury, resulting in necrosis originates in the ischemic subendocardium and progresses outward towards the epicardium to involve an entire area of myocardium perfused by the coronary artery involved. This phenomenon was first described by Reimer and colleagues in 1977.

Initially, the injury is reversible and salvage of myocardial muscle mass is possible if blood flow is restored, but this must occur early. Thromboembolic occlusion is the precipitating cause of most infarctions and with increased duration of the occlusion (necrosis), the area of injury will enlarge and myocardial damage often becomes irreversible. Early recognition and rapid intervention reduces mortality and may improve long-term left ventricular function. The opportunity for reperfusion increases as time-to-treatment decreases. For instance, one intervention, percutaneous transluminal coronary angioplasty (PCTA) may yield the best outcomes when performed within 1 hour after onset of signs and symptoms of the acute event. If there is any delay, **thrombolysis** (use of medication to dissolve components of the occlusion) may be considered.

> **thrombolysis**
> Use of a 'thrombolytic' medication to dissolve components of vascular occlusion.

Current therapy is directed at preventing thrombosis and dissolving the platelet-rich clot with thrombolytics. The PURSUIT trials, that started in 1998 and involved multiple centers, are testing inhibition of platelet factor therapy added to aspirin and heparin therapy for acute coronary syndrome.

Evaluation and research continues to determine the optimal doses of thrombolytic agents. Ultimately, GP IIb/IIIa inhibition (with aspirin and heparin) in combination with other thrombolytic agents may become first-line intervention in all patients, beginning in the prehospital environment. Precise therapies and interventions continue to be the subject of intense clinical research.

Consequences of Coronary Artery Occlusion

Occlusion of the LAD results in anterior wall myocardial infarction. If the occlusion occurs sufficiently high in the vessel at a point where blood flow to the entire bundle branch system is affected, intraventricular conduction disturbances also occur. In addition, loss of a great deal of myocardial wall motion occurs and ventricular failure can ensue. Occlusion of the left circumflex artery will result in lateral wall myocardial infarction. With a left-dominant system, occlusion may result in infero-posterior wall myocardial infarction.

Occlusion of the RCA will result in inferior and/or posterior wall myocardial infarction. Proximal occlusion will result in right ventricular wall myocardial infarction and may affect the electrical conduction system. A major consequence of right ventricular infarction is hemodynamic in nature.

The distinction between myocardial infarction and unstable angina (USA) is at best semantic in most patients. The distinction can rarely be made with confidence early on in presentation. The term *acute coronary syndrome* (ACS) is therefore preferred because it implies a spectrum of disease. The therapy of ACS is divided into patients with persistent ST segment elevation (generally greater than 20 to 30 minutes) and those without ST segment elevation.

In patients with chest pain and ST segment elevation, the possibility of acute evolving MI is very high and they are candidates for thrombolytic-revascularization therapy. If there is no ST segment elevation, patients are unlikely to benefit from thrombolytic therapy, with few exceptions. In fact, outcomes may be worse. Patients without ST segment elevation in leads I and aVL generally get the same initial therapy whether they are ultimately diagnosed with MI or unstable angina.

For the purposes of this book, *chest pain* describes a wide range of subjective terms that patients may use. These include but are not limited to: abdominal or stomach discomfort, aching, belly pain, burning, difficulty getting one's breath, fullness, grasping pain, hard to breathe, heaviness, pain, point tenderness over an area of the chest or epigastrium, pressure, shoulder aches, tightness and tingling or pain in the arm or jaw.

The initial ECG in 25 percent of patients who subsequently have the diagnosis of acute MI have nondiagnostic changes. Classically, these nonspecific ST-T changes are scattered among various leads but do not show a pattern that can readily be equated with a specific focus.

Through alterations in wave forms, the ECG allows for visualization of the myocardial disease continuum. Impaired blood flow through coronary arteries results in varying degrees of myocardial damage, depending on the duration and extent of flow reduction. Acute interruption of blood supply to the myocardium is followed by depletion of the myocardial metabolic reserve, when the process of necrosis or infarction begins. This process is seen in the leads that explore the damaged area.

In transmural cardiac injury the duration of ECG manifestations vary. Those observed during coronary angioplasty or in patients with coronary spasm may change or disappear rapidly when the coronary occlusion is removed. Transmural injury secondary to coronary thrombosis resolves gradually following spontaneous or therapeutic restoration of flow. It is critical for rapid restoration of perfusion to salvage myocardium and minimize irreversible injury.

Reflecting and Reciprocal Leads

ECG signs of ischemia, injury and necrosis are best seen in the leads facing the affected surface of the heart. These leads are called the **reflecting leads**. **Reciprocal leads** are those that are in the same plane but the event is a reflection, or mirror image. Events that reflect the inferior surface are leads II, III, and aVF and the reciprocal leads are I and aVL. Similarly, leads I, aVL and V_6 reflect the lateral surface, and leads II, III, and aVF are the reciprocal leads.

> ⦿ **reflecting leads**
> Leads that are facing the affected surface of the heart
>
> ⦿ **reciprocal leads**
> Leads that are in the same plane but show a reflection or mirror image

The standard 12-lead ECG is limited in that it neither monitors the true posterior surface nor provides much information about the right ventricle. It is clinically necessary to do additional leads on the right side of the heart, because inferior wall myocardial infarction may be complicated by extension to the right ventricle or to the posterior wall.

Lead V_{4R} is very informative. ST elevation in V_{4R} is 90 percent predictive of right ventricular wall myocardial infarction. This lead will also help the clinician to identify:

1. The site of coronary occlusion

    - ST elevation and positive T waves indicate proximal occlusion of the RCA

    - Normal ST segments and positive T waves may indicate distal RCA occlusion

    - Normal ST segment and negative T waves implicate the occlusion of the circumflex artery

2. Patients at risk for AV conduction defects

3. Patients who would benefit most by aggressive reperfusion techniques

In a normal heart, V_{4R} through V_{6R} resemble the ECG complexes seen in lead V_1, but are lower in amplitude. The posterior leads resemble V_6, but are also of lower amplitude. Remember, posterior infarction accompanies inferior wall myocardial infarction in perhaps 30 percent of the patients. Right ventricular involvement may occur in as many as one-third of inferior wall myocardial infarction.

Finally, while the posterior surface is reflected by leads V_7 and V_8, the reciprocal leads are V_1 through V_4. Table 6-1 is a summary of the reflecting leads. Figure 6-2 provides illustrations of the surfaces of the heart as seen by the reflecting and reciprocal leads.

MONITORING MYOCARDIAL ISCHEMIA, INJURY, AND NECROSIS ON THE ECG

The phrase *time is muscle* seems trite and overused, but the concept of time is crucial. When blood flow is compromised, the affected area of the heart is unable to conduct electrical impulses normally and contractility is impaired. The characteristic changes on the ECG will represent the degree of functional insult in the lead system facing that insult. Direct patient assessment will provide insight into deficits in cardiac output.

Table 6-1 The surface of the heart as seen by the reflecting ECG leads.

Surface of the Heart	Reflecting Leads
Anterior	V_3 and V_4
Anterolateral	I, aVL; V_3–V_6
Anteroseptal	V_1–V_4
High lateral	I and aVL, V_5 and V_6
Inferior (and distal posterior wall)	II, III, and aVF
Posterior	V_1–V_4 (R waves and marked ST) segment depression; V_7, V_8, V_9
Right ventricular	V_4R, II, III, and aVF

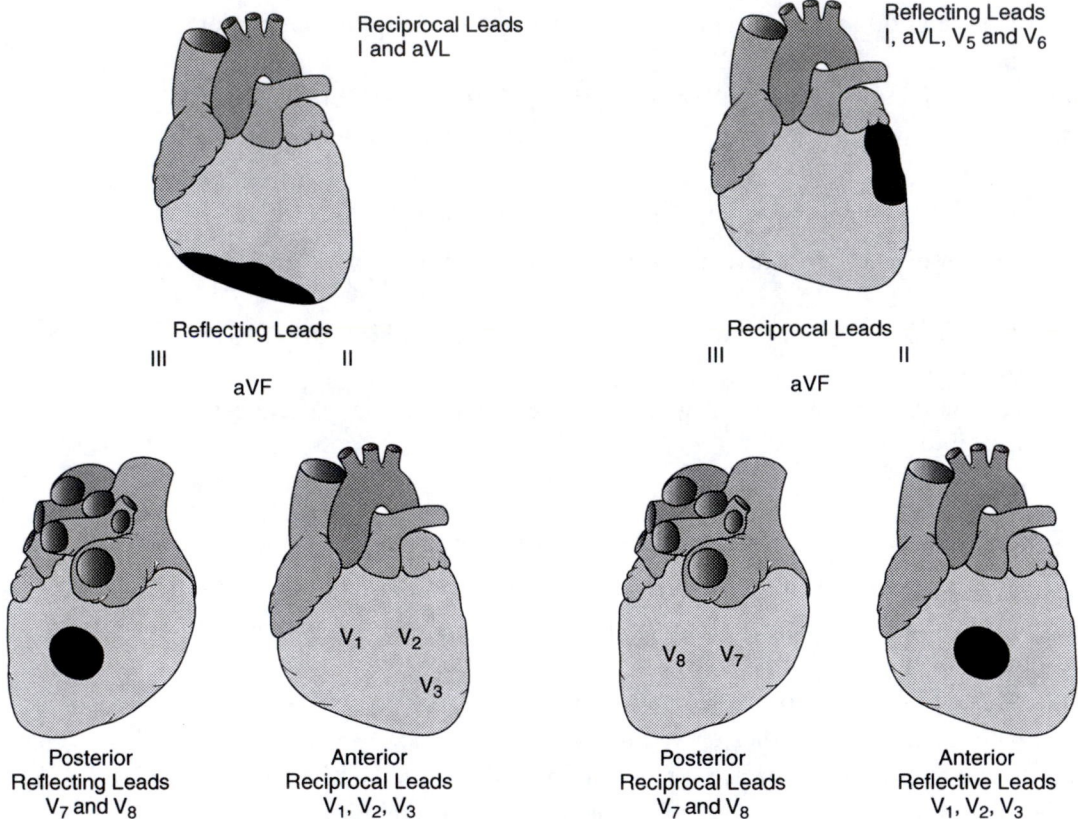

Figure 6-2 Reflecting and reciprocal leads highlighting the area of the heart the lead sees: (A) inferior surface reflecting leads II, III, and aVF and the reciprocal leads I and aVL; (B) high lateral surface reflecting leads I, aVL, V_5, and V_6 and the reciprocal leads II, III, and aVF (C) posterior reflecting leads, V_7, V_8, and V_9 and the reciprocal leads V_1, V_2, and V_3; and (D) anterior reflecting leads V_1, V_2, and V_3 and the reciprocal leads V_7 and V_8.

In ischemia the ECG changes include T wave inversion and ST segment depression in the lead facing or reflecting the ischemic tissue. With injury the ECG changes include ST segment elevation in the lead reflecting the injured muscle. In necrosis the significant ECG change is the development of Q waves greater than 0.04 second in the lead reflecting the necrotic tissue.

Changes in Wave Forms

The process of ischemia, injury, and infarction is represented by ST segment elevation, T wave inversion, or the presence of Q waves in the leads facing the surface of the heart that is affected.

ST Segment Depression. ST segment depression may be nonspecific, as well as an important index of myocardial ischemia. ST segment depression may indicate subendocardial (non-Q wave) infarction or may be present as a reciprocal change in leads opposite the area of acute injury. ST segment depression can be seen during anginal attacks or during a positive stress test. Identical ST segment alteration in the lateral as well as inferior leads can be produced by the effects of antiarrhythmic medications, such as digitalis and quinidine.

Other conditions such as hypothermia and electrolyte imbalances, principally hyperkalemia or hypokalemia, affect wave forms and segments. (See Chapter 3 for more details.) Left ventricular hypertrophy is seen on the lateral leads of the 12-lead ECG as ST segment depression. Such changes over the right precordial leads are slightly more reliable for specific pathologic conditions, present with right ventricular hypertrophy and infarction of the true posterior wall.

ST segment abnormalities may also be a normal variant in up to 20 percent of otherwise healthy females.

ST Segment Elevation. ST segment elevation (J point elevation) is also a normal variant, but new ST segment elevation in a lead facing a surface of the heart greater than 1 mm is an acute sign. ST segment elevation is also known as the *current of injury pattern.* Again, ST segment elevation greater than 1 mm in the limb leads and greater than 2 mm in the precordial leads indicates an evolving AMI till proven otherwise. ST segment elevation is usually evident soon after transmural injury is recognized so that steps in reperfusion can be implemented as quickly as possible.

The ST segment elevation associated with infarction usually encompasses the T wave in its contour. This is to be contrasted with other minor causes for alterations in ST segment contour. One such change, called *early repolarization,* is a normal variant to the ST segment often seen in about 1 to 2 percent of younger, male patients. Elevated, concave ST segments are commonly located in the precordial leads. Figure 6-3 is a representation of the injured myocardium and the accompanying ECG changes in the lead reflecting the injury.

Recall that myocardial ischemia may be indicated by ST depression in a reciprocal lead. It is critical to assess clinical presentation and the ECG is one of the valuable tools in making the diagnosis of ischemia, injury, and infarction. The clinician must be vigilant and maintain a high index of suspicion for any patient who presents with chest pain of any description. Figure 6-4A is a generic illustration of nonspecific ST-T changes and a 12-lead ECG with nonspecific ST-T changes. Later, it was confirmed to be an early manifestation of an infarction. The patient reportedly described a "feeling of agita low in the belly." This is further evidence that ECG confirmation of an MI requires 12-lead ECG analysis and trending the patient from baseline. ECG analysis at the time of chest pain is critical.

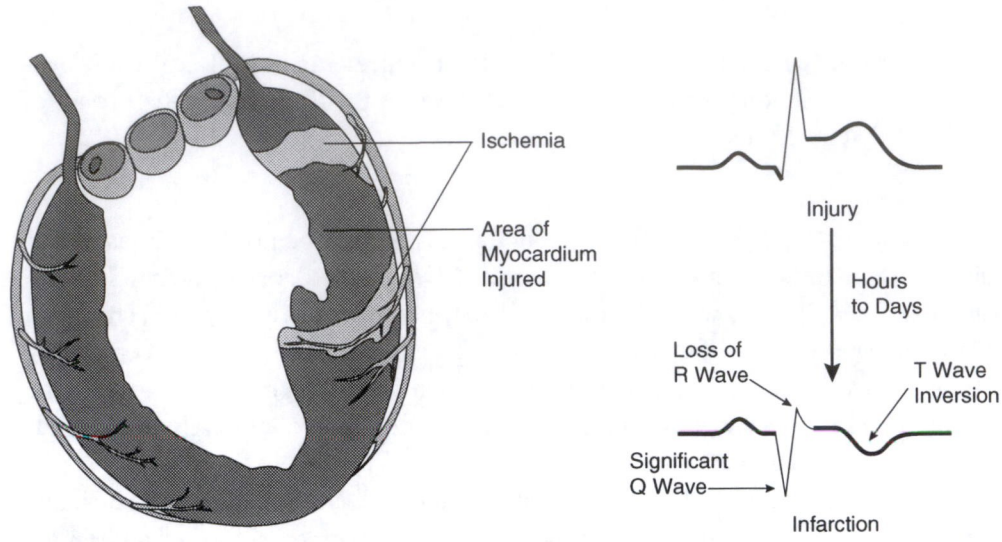

Figure 6-3 The injured myocardium and the accompanying acute changes: the Q wave and ST-T changes initially and after time has passed.

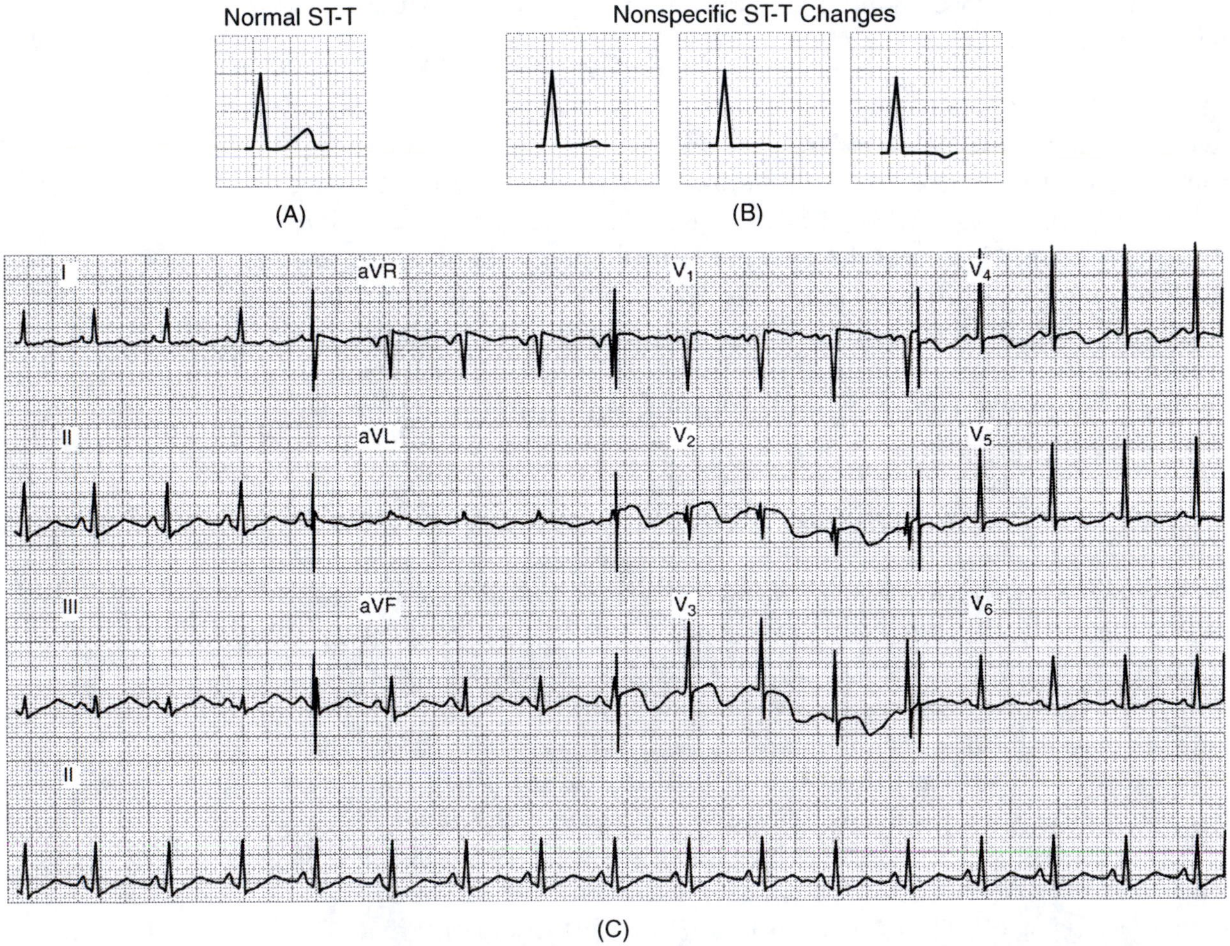

Normal ST-T

Nonspecific ST-T Changes

(A)

(B)

(C)

Figure 6-4 (A) is an illustration of normal and (B) nonspecific ST-T. (C) is a 12-lead ECG showing nonspecific ST-T changes on a 12-lead tracing that was later confirmed as an early manifestation of MI. The patient reportedly described a "feeling of agida low in the belly."

Figure 6-5 is an ECG tracing from a patient who presented with substernal chest pain radiating to the left arm, shortness-of-breath, pallor, and diaphoresis. Changes in ST segments occurred from time of the initial encounter to 14 minutes after oxygen therapy and nitroglycerin.

ST segment elevations related to myocardial injury usually appear convex or curved. Sometimes this is referred to as a **positive ST segment coving**. Following acute infarction, or when resolution of ischemia has taken place, the ST segment usually returns toward baseline; this usually occurs in the first 72 to 96 hours after damage.

To summarize, one of the following criteria is necessary to make the diagnosis of **transmural injury**:

- Elevation of the origin of the ST segment at 0.04 second past the J point and of greater than or equal to 1 mm in two or more limb leads or precordial leads V_4 to V_6, or greater than or equal to 2 mm in two or more precordial leads V_1 to V_3.

- Depression of the origin of the ST segment at the J point of greater than or equal to 1 mm in two or more leads V_1 to V_3, with ST segment elevation greater than 1 mm in two or more leads V_7 to V_9.

positive ST segment coving

ST segment elevations that are convex or curved in appearance as a result of myocardial injury

13:11:42

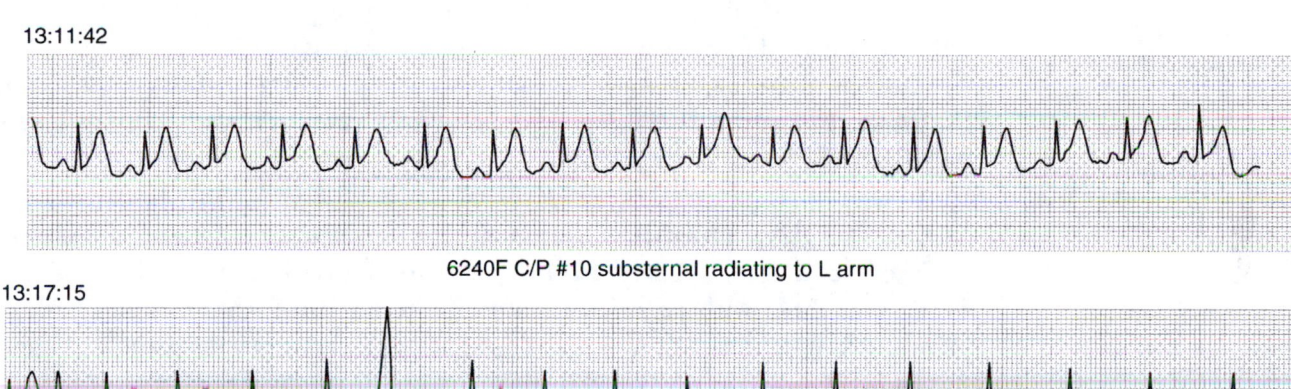

6240F C/P #10 substernal radiating to L arm

13:17:15

13:23:04

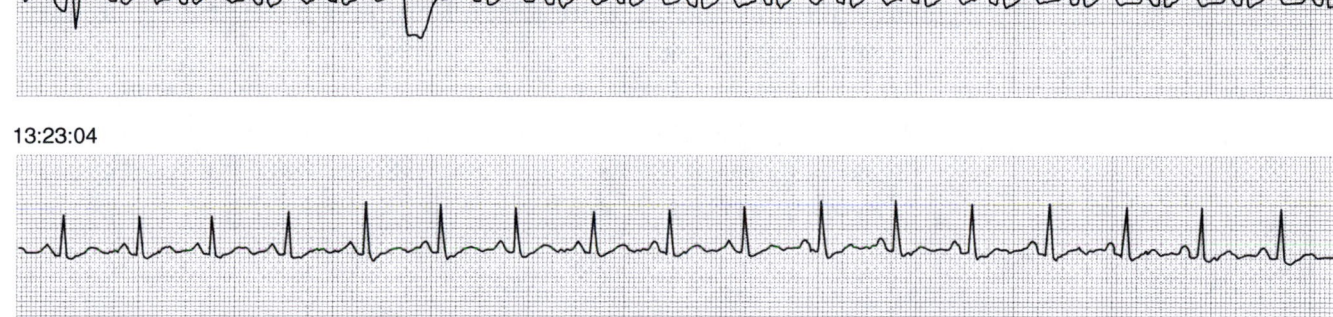

$\overline{p}$ O_2 + nitro x 1

Figure 6-5 Prehospital ECG tracings from a patient who presented with substernal chest pain reported as 10 (on a scale of 1-10, 10 being the worst), radiating to the left arm, shortness-of-breath, pallor, and diaphoresis. In the first tracing (13:11:42), the ECG shows sinus at 100 beats per minute with 2 mm ST segment elevation. At 13:17:15, ST segment is at baseline and the rate is 93 beats per minute; pain was reported as a 7. At 13:23:04, ST segment shows 1 mm depression. The patient reported relief from pain (a 3), color improved, respiratory effort was unimpaired. The patient was later successfully reperfused.

Other cardiac conditions that cause ST segment elevation include:

- Pericarditis: ST elevation is marked by a flat or concave ST segment and usually accompanied by T wave elevation and depressed PR segments. (See Chapter 3.)

- Ventricular Aneurysm: ST segment elevation that does not return to baseline over time.

Ventricular aneurysm is a condition where a portion of infarcted myocardial tissue does not contract nor expand normally. During ventricular systole, that portion of the myocardium bulges outward instead of contracting. This major wall motion disorder is usually seen on the ECG as the persistent ST segment elevation that continues well after the infarction, lasting for months or even years. However, it should be noted that wall motion disorders can be present without ECG changes. Left ventricular aneurysm following extensive infarction may show persistent ST segment inversion over the damaged muscle. This ST segment elevation may be present for years and may be confused with acute necrosis or may mask future ischemic episodes.

Akinesis describes the lack of motion, and **dyskinesia** the paradoxical bulging during ventricular systole. Patients with suspected wall motion disorders are chronically fatigued due to the low cardiac output.

ST elevation associated with ventricular aneurysm also exhibits an upward convex form that is usually seen with accompanying deep Q waves. Clinical presentation and matching of ECG changes over time is necessary. Remember that ECG signs which support a diagnosis of acute myocardial infarction are ST elevation in the presence of reciprocal ST depression and/or Q waves in leads opposite the suspected surface.

Minor ST-T Abnormalities. Daviglus, Liao, Greenland, completed a long-term study of trending the 12-lead ECG of men without overt cardiac disease. They found that those with persistent nonspecific minor ST-T abnormalities had an increased long-term risk of mortality due to MI, coronary heart disease (CHD), and cardiovascular disease (CVD). This study underscores the potential value of including nonspecific ECG findings, especially ST-T abnormalities, in the overall assessment of cardiovascular risk.

Criteria for minor ST-segment depression are either of the following:

- No ST-J depression as much as 0.5 mm. ST segment downward sloping and segment or T-wave nadir at least 0.5 mm below P-R baseline, in any leads I, II, aVL, or V_2 to V_6;

  OR

- ST-J depression of 1 mm or greater and ST segment upward sloping or U-shaped, in any of leads I, II, aVL, or V_1 to V_6.

T Wave Changes. The T wave contour is susceptible to many extracardiac factors. T wave inversion or flattening is nonspecific for ischemic heart disease, but the presence of deep, symmetric T wave inversion is somewhat more suggestive of the diagnosis of ischemia. T wave contour is not only affected by many pathologic car-

● **akinesis**

Lack of motion in the muscle wall of the heart

● **dyskinesia**

The paradoxical bulging of the heart wall during ventricular systole

diac conditions but may also be altered by exercise, hyperventilation, food ingestion, smoking, or significant electrolyte disturbance.

The normal amplitude for T wave excursion has never been firmly established. In precordial T waves that are greater than 10 mm in deflection, however, hyperkalemia should be highly suspected. They may also be seen in the right precordial leads in patients with left ventricular hypertrophy. It is because of these considerations that ST segments and T waves should only be interpreted after the QRS has been carefully analyzed.

Symmetrical T wave inversion in a lead that normally has an upright T wave is an acute sign and may be clinically associated with ischemia. T wave inversion that is symmetrical and greater than 5 mm in depth is called *nadir T waves*. Figure 6-6 is a graphic illustration of the nadir T waves and an ECG tracing showing both ST segment elevation and nadir T waves.

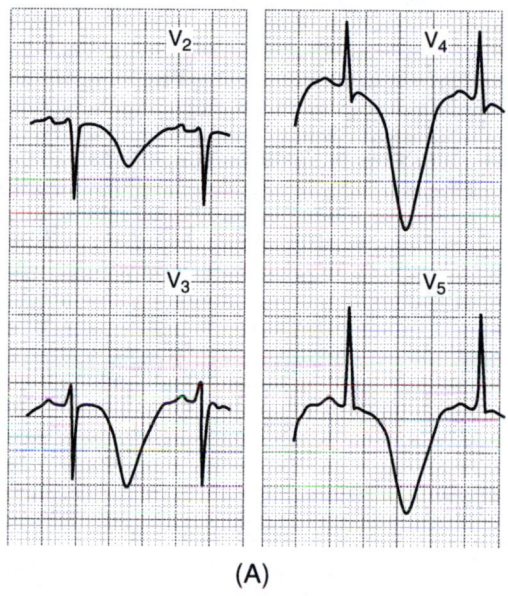

(A)

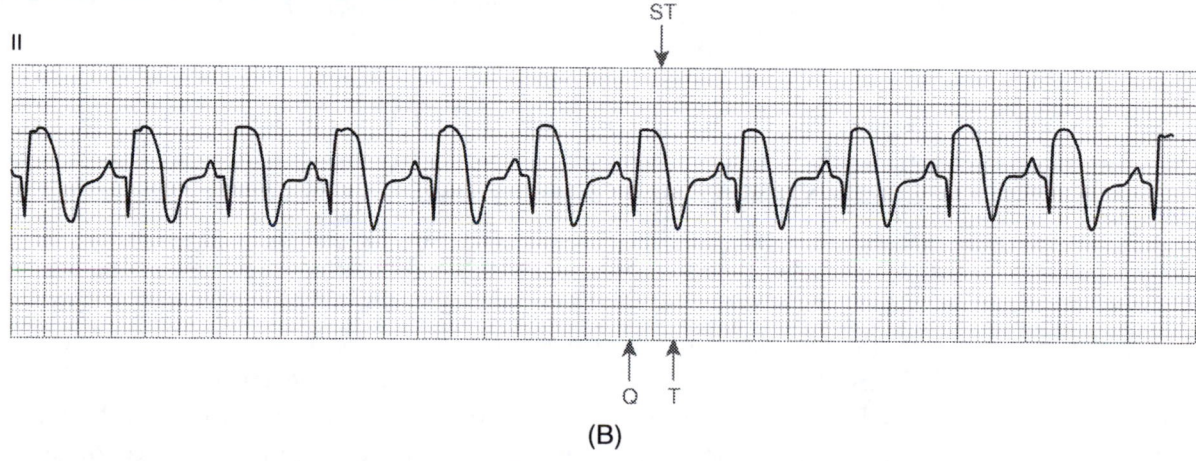

(B)

Figure 6-6 View A is an illustration of T wave inversion and nadir T waves. View B is an ECG tracing of sinus at 100 beats per minute with acute changes reflecting inferior myocardial infarction: Q waves 5 mm, 6 mm ST segment elevation, and nadir T waves.

Because T wave inversion may be due to other causes, it is vital that the clinician compare clinical history and patient presentation to the changes as they are noted. Cardiac causes of T wave inversion include:

- bundle branch block;
- ventricular hypertrophy; and
- pericarditis.

Noncardiac causes of T wave inversion include:

- electrolyte disorders;
- shock;
- positional changes such as posturing with dyspnea, or the patient is seated in the upright rather than supine position; and
- central nervous system disorders such as subarachnoid hemorrhage and stroke.

Minor T Wave Abnormalities. Minor T wave abnormalities may be associated with occult cardiac events. They may accompany other minor wave form abnormalities such as changes in ST segments. Accepted criteria for minor T wave abnormality are either of the following:

- T-wave amplitude zero (flat), negative, or diphasic (negative-positive type only) with less than 1 mm negative phase in leads I, II, V_3 to V_6, or in lead aVL when R wave amplitude is 5.0 mm or greater; or
- T-wave amplitude positive and T- to R-wave amplitude ratio of less than 1:20 in any leads I, II, aVL, or V_3 to V_6 when R-wave amplitude in the corresponding leads was 10 mm or greater.

Abnormal U Waves. An abnormal U wave is a frequent mark of ischemic heart disease. It is most often recorded in lead I, II, and precordial leads V_5 and V_6. A negative U wave is seen in from 10 to 60 percent of patients with anterior myocardial infarction, and in up to 30 percent of patients with inferior myocardial infarction. Appearance of a negative U wave may precede other ECG changes of infarction by up to several hours.

Q Waves. Q waves are absent in most leads in the normal ECG. A word of caution, however; there are small Q waves commonly present in leads I, aVL, aVF, V_5 and V_6; Significant, pathologic Q waves are wide, greater than 0.04 second in duration and at least one-quarter of the amplitude of the entire QRS.

In AMI the foremost change of the QRS complex is the development of a Q wave. The new Q waves will be seen in those leads that explore the particular area of infarction. Necrotic tissue has no polarity; thus with acute myocardial necrosis, the forces of depolarization are no longer generated in the damaged areas. The remaining forces of ventricular depolarization are accentuated, displacing the mean QRS vector in each lead system away from the zone of necrosis. The forces of depolarization will be seen moving away, and a Q wave or negative deflection will be recorded. The lead system closest to the infarcted tissue will record the most significant Q waves. At the same time, the reciprocal leads will show initial positive deflection.

While the necrotic area is no longer capable of depolarization, contraction or repolarization, it is still surrounded by an area of ischemic myocardium, incompletely depolarized with each ventricular activation.

Figure 6-7 illustrates the flow of current as it is affected by necrosis.

In the patient who presents with chest pain, a detailed clinical history including history of present illness, past medical conditions, and a family history of risk factors and accurate reporting of the ECG to include ST-T and QRS configuration are necessary. Prompt application of the 12-lead ECG on any patient with chest pain is necessary to ensure that transmission of data, accurate reporting, and diagnosis are available for rapid intervention.

Transmural infarctions (full thickness infarction) produce Q waves. While the presence of Q waves is the hallmark of infarction, there is no way to determine whether Q waves represent an evolving event, a recent event, or are a historical sign of old infarction. Thus, a detailed clinical history and accurate reporting of the QRS configuration are critical. A request for previous ECGs for comparison is always advisable.

Q waves will persist over time. While they occasionally decrease in size, rarely do they resolve completely. Other conditions can produce pathologic Q waves, including ventricular hypertrophy, diffuse myocardial disease, and the fascicular blocks.

Absence of Q waves does not rule out myocardial infarction. Myocardial infarction that does not involve all 3 layers of the heart is called **nontransmural** and often Q waves are not present in the leads reflecting the infarction (see Non-Q wave Myocardial Infarction on page 148).

● **nontransmural**

Myocardial infarction that does not involve all 3 layers of the heart

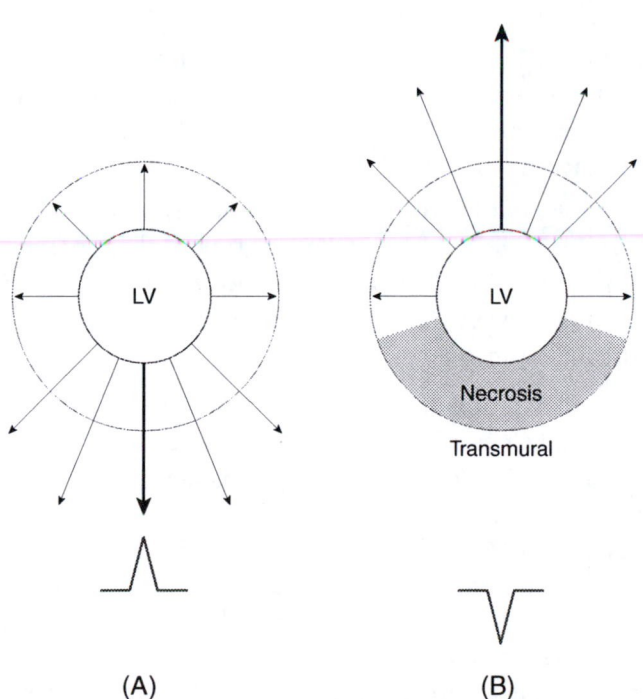

(A) (B)

Figure 6-7 Illustrations showing (A) the flow of current towards the reflecting lead and the resulting positive deflection; and (B) transmural necrosis and the deflection away from the necrotic area and the subsequent negative deflection.

ECG Indicators of Perfusion Deficits

ST segment elevation and Q waves are reliable indicators of the anatomic location of injury and infarction in the heart. The depth of ST depression and the number of leads demonstrating ST segment depression and/or T wave inversion reflects the amount of heart muscle that is ischemic. Q waves are the hallmark of infarction; however, Q waves may not appear on the ECG until late in the course of infarction indicating necrosis has occurred. Early in the course of myocardial infarction, the most prominent ECG finding is ST segment elevation in the lead reflecting the injured tissue. A confirming feature is ST depression (reciprocal changes) in the lead opposite the injury. Presence or absence of reciprocal changes helps to differentiate between conditions with diverse etiologies for chest pain such as pericarditis, ischemia, aneurysm, and gastrointestinal problems. ST segment elevation, with reciprocal changes, indicates the myocardium is in immediate danger. Without intervention, necrosis, that is, irreversible loss of functioning muscle, will occur. Therefore, when evaluating a suspected MI patient, the clinician must observe for ST segment elevation in all leads to establish the correct diagnosis.

INFERIOR WALL (DIAPHRAGMATIC) MYOCARDIAL INFARCTION

Inferior wall myocardial infarction (IWMI) usually results from occlusion of the RCA. In the acute phase ST segment elevation and/or Q waves is seen in leads II, III, and aVF. There is reciprocal ST segment depression in leads I and aVL, and the lateral precordial leads V_5 and V_6. With further evolution, the ST depression resolves, the T wave is less inverted, but the Q waves persist. Eventually, the T waves return to normal, and the fibrotic scar on the inferior wall is represented by Q waves. There are two aspects of inferior wall myocardial infarction that deserve emphasis at this point:

1. With Q waves in leads II, III, and aVF, the mean axis of depolarization may be shifted to the left, more negative than −30 degrees. In the setting of inferior wall infarction with leftward shift of axis, left anterior hemiblock cannot be diagnosed (Chapter 7).

2. A Q wave in standard lead III may be entirely normal and thus must always be interpreted in light of electrocardiographic changes seen in standard leads II and aVF. The Q wave in these two leads must be 0.04 second in duration, and 25 percent of the amplitude of the R wave to be considered diagnostic for myocardial damage.

Figure 6-8 is an illustration of the surface of the heart affected by inferior wall MI. The accompanying ECG patterns reflect the Q waves and ST segment elevation in limb leads II, III, and aVF. Note the reciprocal changes in lead I.

Approximately half of all inferior myocardial infarctions may lose criteria for significant Q waves in about 6 months following necrosis. Therefore, small Q waves in the inferior leads that do not fulfill criteria for significant Q waves must still be interpreted with caution and should alert the observer that an acute inferior myocardial infarction pattern might once have been present.

Occlusion of a dominant circumflex artery can cause inferior wall myocardial infarction. In this case, ST segment elevation is present in one or more of the lateral leads aVL, V_5, and V_6. Also, conduction defects secondary to inferior wall myocardial infarction are transient and include first-degree AV block and Type I second-degree AV block.

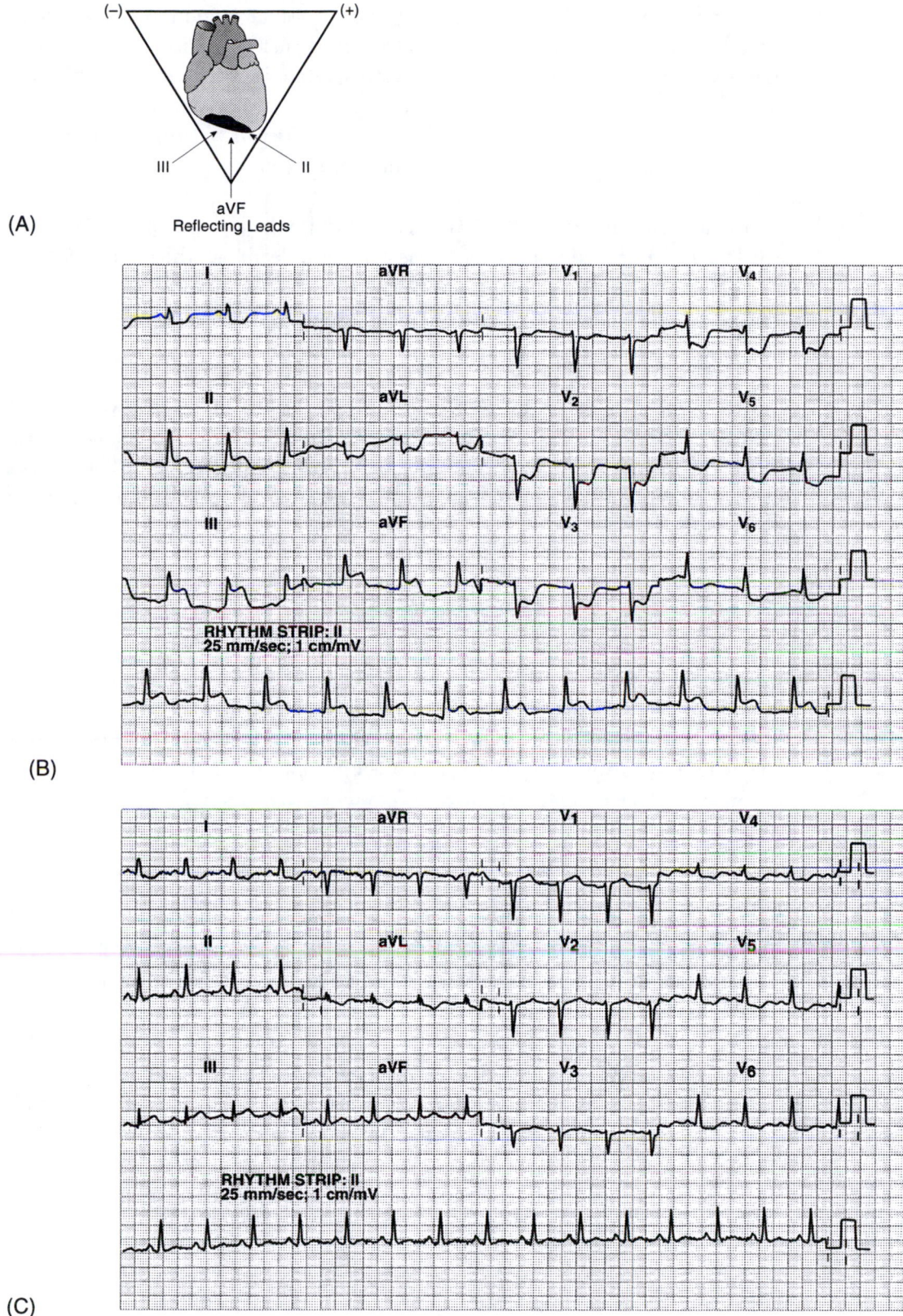

Figure 6-8 (A) is an illustration of the leads that face the inferior surface of the heart. (B) is a 12-lead ECG showing the changes in the injury pattern in the limb leads. Note the changes in leads II, III, and AVF that include ST segment elevation. (C) is the 12-lead ECG on the same patient, after reperfusion. Note in this case the return of the ST segment to baseline 6 minutes after treatment.

Although inferior infarction typically involves a small amount of left ventricular myocardium, these infarctions should be taken just as seriously in terms of diagnosis and treatment. Inferior wall myocardial infarctions may extend to the posterior left ventricular wall particularly in a right-dominant coronary artery system. Right ventricular involvement occurs in one-third of inferior wall myocardial infarctions. Unfortunately right ventricular wall myocardial infarction is recognized infrequently.

All abnormal inferior wall ECG tracings require the analysis of the right precordial leads. Of critical importance is the analysis of lead V_{4R} which identifies:

- the affected coronary artery;
- presence of right ventricular wall infarction; and
- presence of AV nodal conduction defect.

ECG changes are specific for the level of vascular occlusion. ST segment elevation in the inferior leads only occurs when proximal right coronary disease exists. Elevated T waves in the inferior leads are seen in distal right coronary disease. Inverted T waves appear in inferior leads with distal left circumflex disease. Table 6-2 summarizes the characteristics of IWMI.

Clinical Implications of Inferior Wall Myocardial Infarction

Once IWMI has been confirmed, the clinician must be vigilant for changes in sinus rate and AV conduction defects. Parasympathetic activity is common with IWMI and bradycardia. Further potential complications are hypotension and hypoperfusion. In addition, leads V_2, V_3, and V_4 should be monitored for anterior involvement and reciprocal changes reflecting extension to the posterior surface.

ANTERIOR WALL MYOCARDIAL INFARCTION

A QS or QR complex in leads V_1 to V_4 is diagnostic of an acute anterior wall myocardial infarction. A decrease in the R wave height (excursion) over the anterior precordial leads is also consistent with acute anterior necrosis. Reversed R wave progression, the R wave diminishing from V_1 to V_4, is often overlooked as a criterion for anterior wall damage. In addition, absent or poor R wave progression over the anterior precordial leads may be seen in left ventricular hypertrophy or right ventricular hypertrophy (see Chapter 8). It is important to remember that T wave inversion

Table 6-2 Summary of the ECG characteristic found in inferior wall MI

ECG Changes	Early	Late
ST segment	up in II, III, aVF down in I and aVL	
T wave	↓ can be an initial change	deep, inverted II, III, aVF
Q wave		II, III, aVF

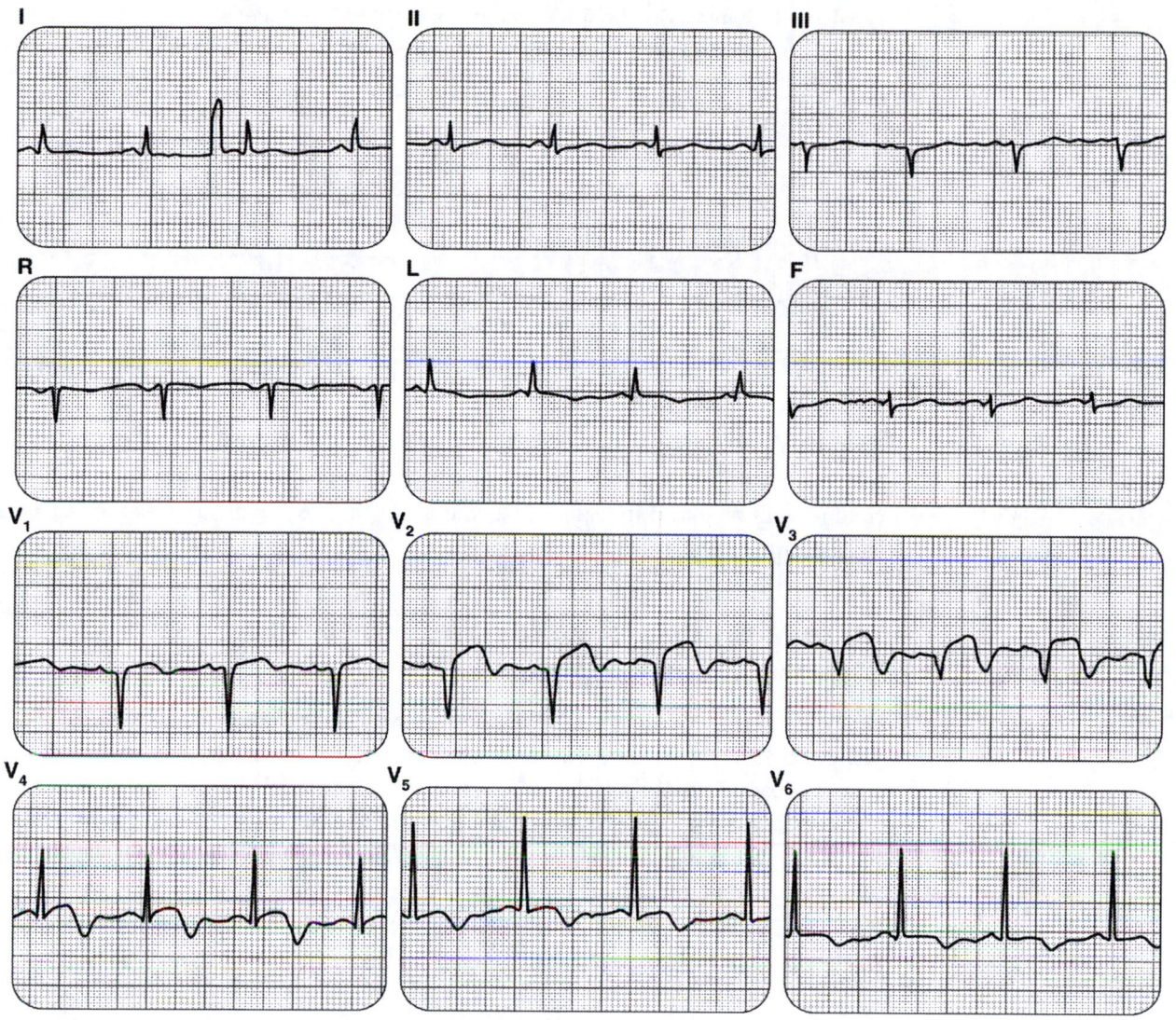

Figure 6-9   The 12-lead evidence of anterior myocardial infarction. There are no significant changes in lead II, however, the 12-lead ECG demonstrates acute changes: Q waves, ST elevation, and inverted T waves in the precordial leads V_2 and V_3. V_4 and V_5 show ST elevation and inverted T waves, and . V_6 shows horizontal ST segments with inverted T waves. Interpretation: sinus rhythm at 78 beats per minute with acute signs supporting the anteroseptal wall myocardial infarction and anterolateral ischemia.

over the anterior precordial leads may be a normal variant, most often seen in younger females under 30 years of age.

In acute non-Q wave anterior wall myocardial infarction, there is ST segment depression with T wave inversion in leads I, aVL, and V_6 but no significant alteration of the QRS configuration. These changes slowly return to baseline as acute necrosis resolves. Figure 6-9 is a 12-lead ECG of anterior wall myocardial infarction.

In summary, the magnitude of anteroseptal or anterior myocardial infarction may be judged by the extent of the precordial leads involved. Sequential ECGs should be carefully scrutinized for evidence of an altered and unstable conduction system.

Acute obstruction of the LAD will result in anterior wall myocardial infarction (AWMI). ST segment elevation and/or Q waves in one or more leads from V_1

Table 6-3 Summary of the ECG characteristic found in anterior wall MI

ECG Changes	Early (Ischemia)	Late (Necrosis)
ST segment	up in I, aVL, V_5–V_6	
	little or no change in II	
T wave		Inverted I, aVL, V_1–V_6
Q wave		+I, aVL, V_5–V_6
QS complex		V_5-V_6
R wave	poor R wave progression	

through V_4 are are significant signs of an anterior wall myocardial infarction. There may be small Q waves in V_5 and V_6 that were there normally; however, reciprocal changes will be found in leads II, III, and aVF. Table 6-3 summarizes the characteristics of anterior wall MI.

Clinical Implications for Anterior Wall Myocardial Infarction

Because anterior infarctions frequently involve a large area of myocardium, cardiogenic shock is very common in the acute phase of this infarction area. Some patients may have sympathetic hyperactivity resulting in sinus tachycardia and hypertension.

Once AWMI has been diagnosed, the clinician must also be vigilant for changes in AV conduction defects such as Type II second-degree AV block or complete AV block. Signs of left anterior fascicular block may be visible in leads II, III, and aVF. In addition leads V_5 and V_6 should be carefully monitored for signs of extension to the left lateral wall.

ANTEROSEPTAL MYOCARDIAL INFARCTION

Anteroseptal myocardial infarction is sometimes called *midanterior* myocardial infarction. Specific ECG changes are ST elevation, circumscribed to aVL and V_2, with ST segment depression in leads III, aVF, and V_4. Figure 6-10 is a 12-lead ECG with evidence of anteroseptal myocardial infarction.

ANTEROLATERAL MYOCARDIAL INFARCTION

There may be instances when there is ECG evidence of acute necrosis in leads I and aVL, but absent in V_5 or V_6. This represents an infarction on the high lateral wall of the left ventricle (high lateral infarction) not seen in conventional leads V_5 and V_6, for the explore ventricular tissue in a horizontal plane below the damaged area. In such instances, all precordial leads should be moved up one intercostal space (high lateral leads). This simple manipulation may unmask acute infarction changes in V_5 and V_6 that would otherwise be missed. These criteria are important because small, insignificant Q waves may be generated in the normal lateral precordial leads, representing septal depolarization in a left-to-right direction. Significant Q waves in

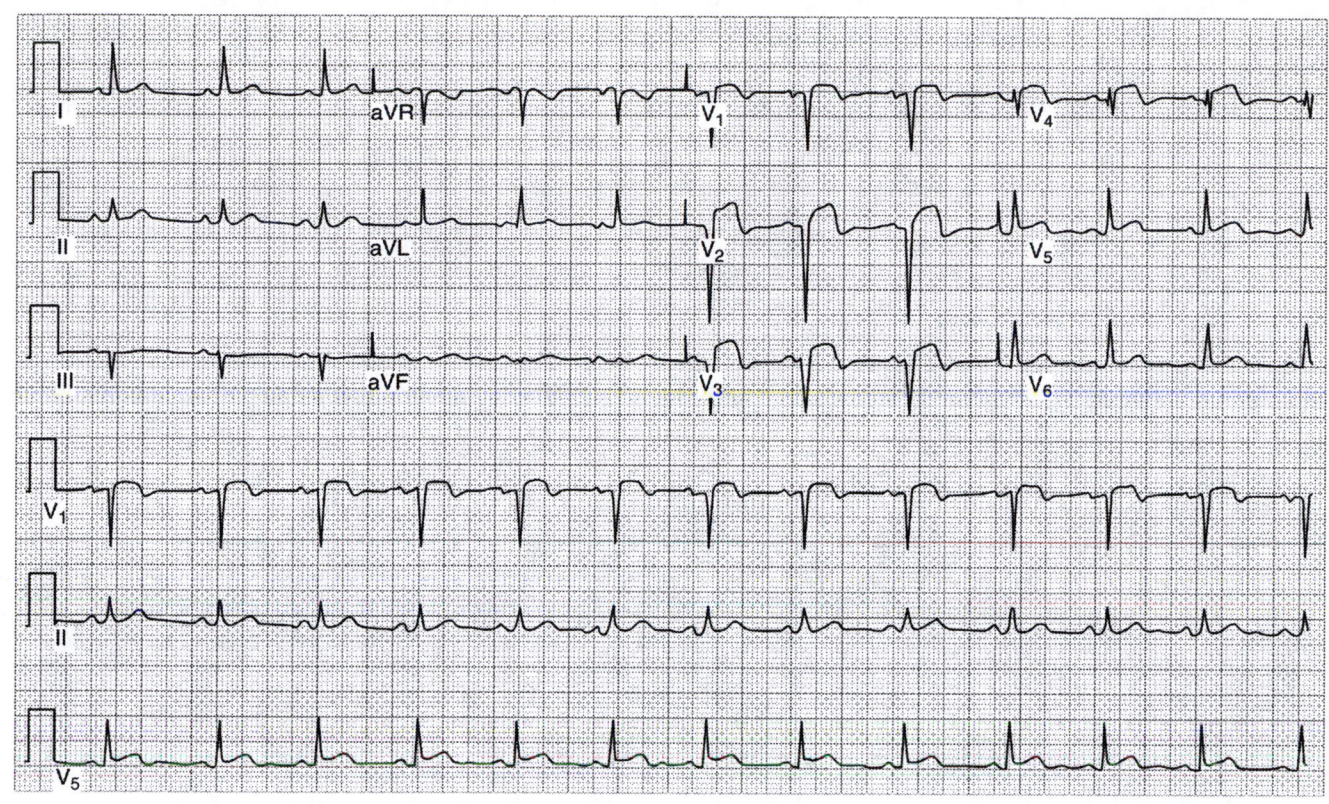

Figure 6-10 A 12-lead ECG with evidence of anteroseptal myocardial infarction. The QRS in lead V_1 is essentially negative; deep Q waves in V_1, V_2, and V_3 with ST segment elevation from V_1 to V_5. Interpretation: sinus at 75 beats per minute with acute signs supporting the anteroseptal wall myocardial infarction and anterolateral ischemia.

the lateral precordial leads V_2 to V_5 are at least 25 percent of the total amplitude of the QRS complex.

Figure 6-11 is an illustration of the surface of the heart affected by anterolateral wall MI. The accompanying ECG patterns reflect the Q waves, ST segment elevation in precordial leads V_5 and V_6.

Clinical Implications of Anterolateral Wall Myocardial Infarction

Patients may be more prone to ventricular ectopics and arrhythmias. In addition, limb leads should be observed for fascicular block.

LATERAL WALL MYOCARDIAL INFARCTION

Lateral wall myocardial infarction most often results from occlusion of the circumflex artery. ST segment elevation and Q waves are seen in leads I, aVL, V_5, and V_6. A drop in QRS amplitude in these leads may indicate lateral wall myocardial infarction. Reciprocal ST segment depression may be seen in V_1. Lateral wall myocardial infarction usually results from extensions of anterior or inferior wall myocardial infarction. Conduction defects are rare. Figure 6-12 is an illustration of lateral wall myocardial infarction and the resulting ECG changes. Table 6-4 summarizes the characteristics of lateral wall myocardial infarction.

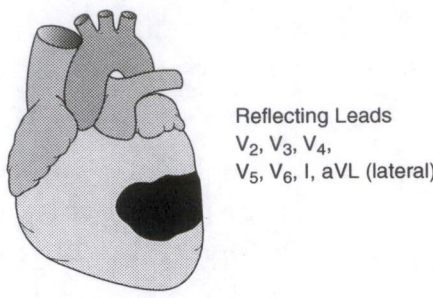

Reflecting Leads
V₂, V₃, V₄,
V₅, V₆, I, aVL (lateral)

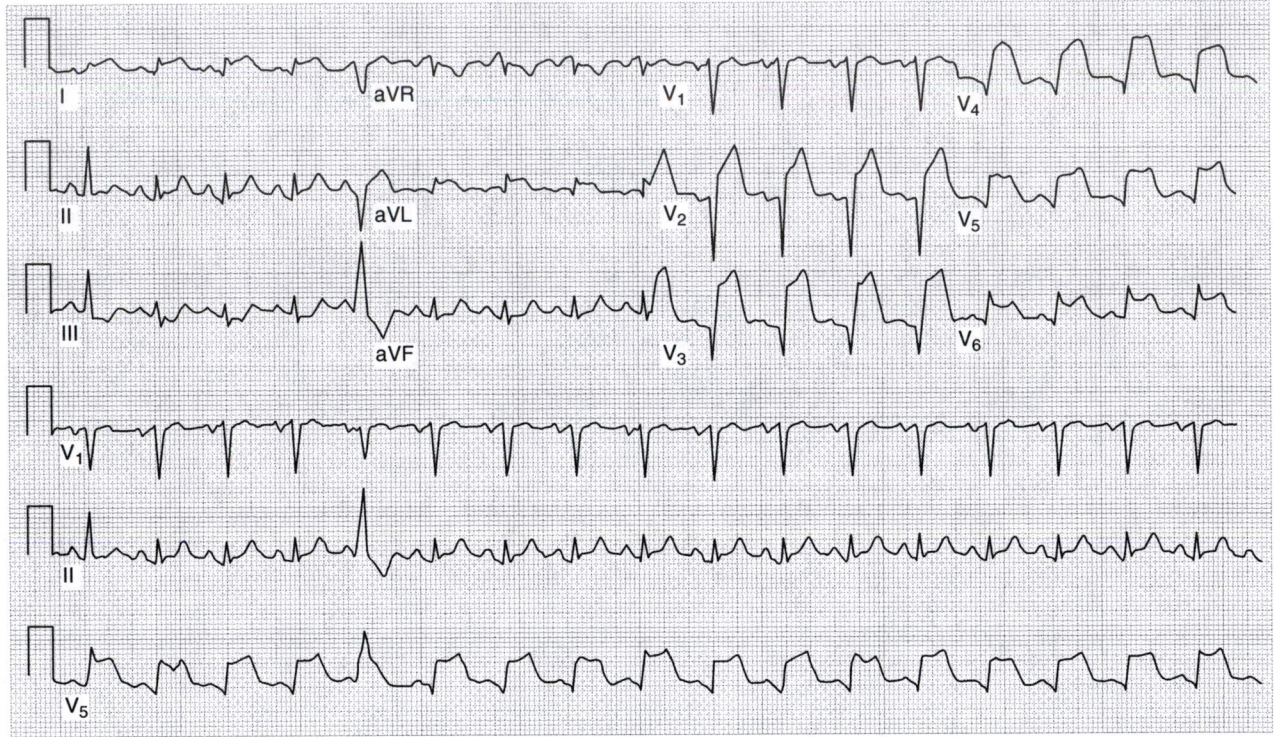

Figure 6-11 View A is an illustration of the surface of the heart affected by anterolateral wall MI. View B is the 12-lead ECG showing sinus at 100 beats per minute with 2 mm ST segment elevation is I and aVL, with reciprocal ST depression in III and perhaps aVF. There are Q waves in V_2-V_6. There is progressive ST elevation in V_2-V_4; 5 mm ST elevation in V_5 and 4 mm ST elevation in V_6. Interpretation: sinus at 100 beats per minute with acute signs supporting the anterolateral infarction.

Clinical Implications of Lateral Wall Myocardial Infarction

Once lateral wall myocardial infarction has been diagnosed, the clinician should be vigilant for changes that indicate cardiogenic shock or congestive heart failure.

POSTERIOR WALL MYOCARDIAL INFARCTION

Posterior wall myocardial infarctions are caused by occlusion of the dominant RCA or the circumflex artery. As explained earlier, posterior wall myocardial infarctions are particularly common in conjunction with inferior wall myocardial infarction.

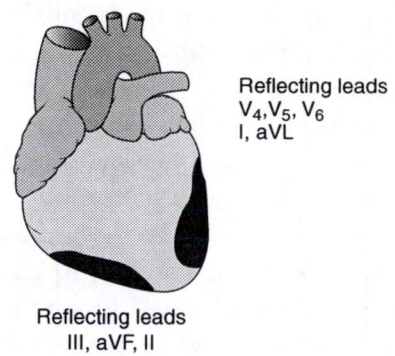

Reflecting leads
V₄,V₅, V₆
I, aVL

Reflecting leads
III, aVF, II

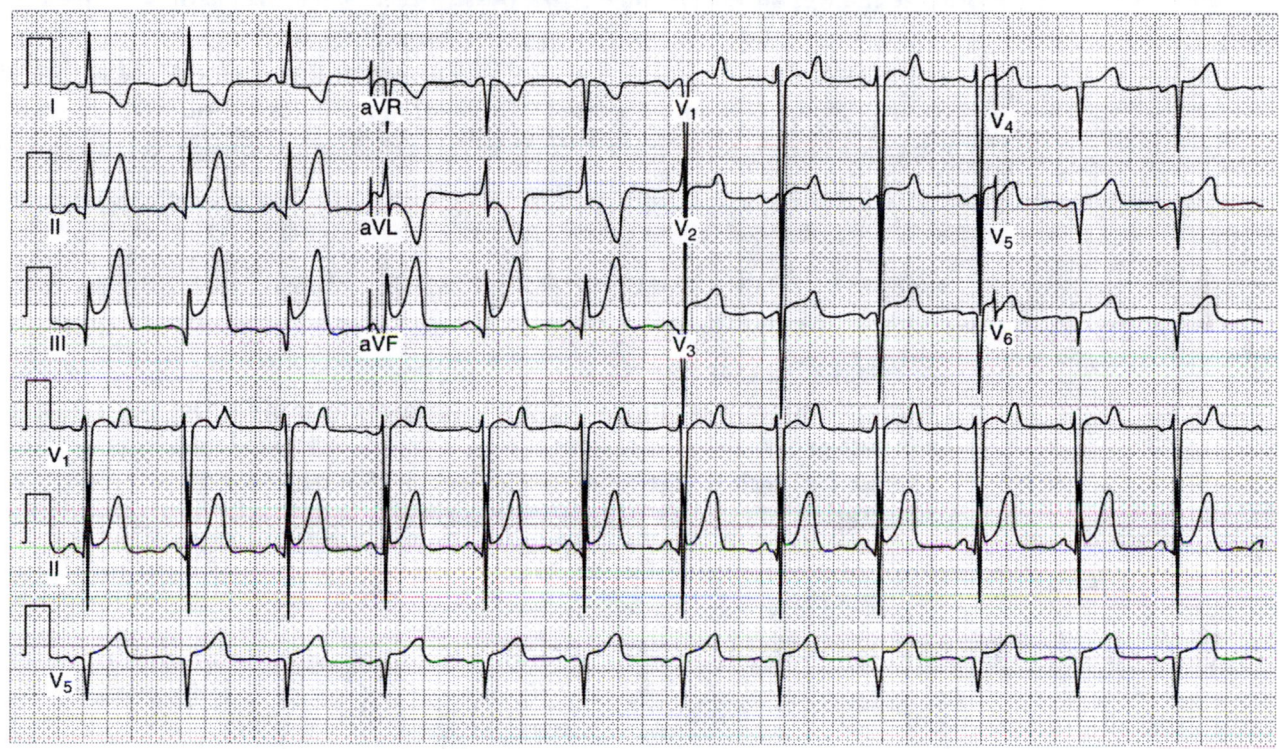

Figure 6-12 View A is an illustration of lateral wall MI, and in this patient inferior wall MI. Sinus rhythm at 76 beats per minute with Q waves and ST elevation in V_4-V_6, significant for lateral wall MI. There are Q waves, ST elevation in the inferior leads II, III, and aVF, indicating inferior MI. Interpretation: sinus rhythm at 76 beats with acute signs supporting the lateral and inferior wall myocardial infarction.

Table 6-4 Summary of the ECG changes for lateral wall MI

ECG Changes	Early (Ischemia)	Late (Necrosis)
ST segment	up in I, aVL	
	up in , V_5 and V_6	
T wave	down in I, aVL, V_5	
Q wave		I, aVL, V_5–V_6
QS complex		I, aVL, V_5–V_6

Characteristic ECG changes are tall R waves and ST segment depression in leads V_1 or V_2, with R wave height greater than S wave depth in lead V_1. In posterior myocardial infarction there are tall R waves in leads V_1 and V_2.

While there is ST segment depression in leads V_1 and V_2, a true posterior lead will display ST elevation. These are considered reciprocal changes because the lead directly reflecting the posterior wall is not commonly monitored.

The posterior ventricular leads, V_7-V_9, are true views of the posterior surface and should be recorded in clinically suspect patients without 12-lead ECG changes. However, since criteria for reperfusion therapy require ST segment elevation in two contiguous leads, the value of a posterior ECG can be significant. If acute changes are documented in the posterior leads, there is justification for reperfusion intervention. Be aware that positioning the patient for these leads may be uncomfortable, and resulting artifact and patient movement may complicate the tracing. Figure 6-13 contains two ECGs illustrating inferoposterior wall myocardial infarction and the resulting ECG changes. Table 6-5 summarizes ECG changes associated with posterior wall myocardial infarction.

Clinical Implications for Posterior Wall Myocardial Infarction

Because the RCA supplies the sinus and AV nodes in most hearts, posterior infarctions are frequently identified with AV conduction disturbances and changes in sinus rate and rhythm. Also, since a posterior wall myocardial infarction may result in papillary muscle dysfunction, the clinician must observe for signs and symptoms of cardiogenic shock, heart failure, and signs of AV conduction defects.

RIGHT VENTRICULAR MYOCARDIAL INFARCTION

Right ventricular myocardial infarction (RVI) is caused by proximal occlusion of the right coronary artery. Although a true right ventricular wall myocardial infarction can occur independently, it is more commonly associated with inferior wall myocardial infarction because the right ventricle is not well represented on a standard ECG. It is critical to perform and interpret right side precordial leads in all suspected inferior wall myocardial infarctions. In a right ventricular wall myocardial infarction ST

Table 6-5 Summary of ECG changes with posterior wall MI

ECG Changes	Early (Ischemia)	Late (Necrosis)
R wave		tall in V_1 and V_2
		R>S in V_1
ST segment	depressed in V_1 and V_2	
T wave	up in V_1 and V_2	
Q wave		V_7 and V_8
QS complex		V_7 and V_8

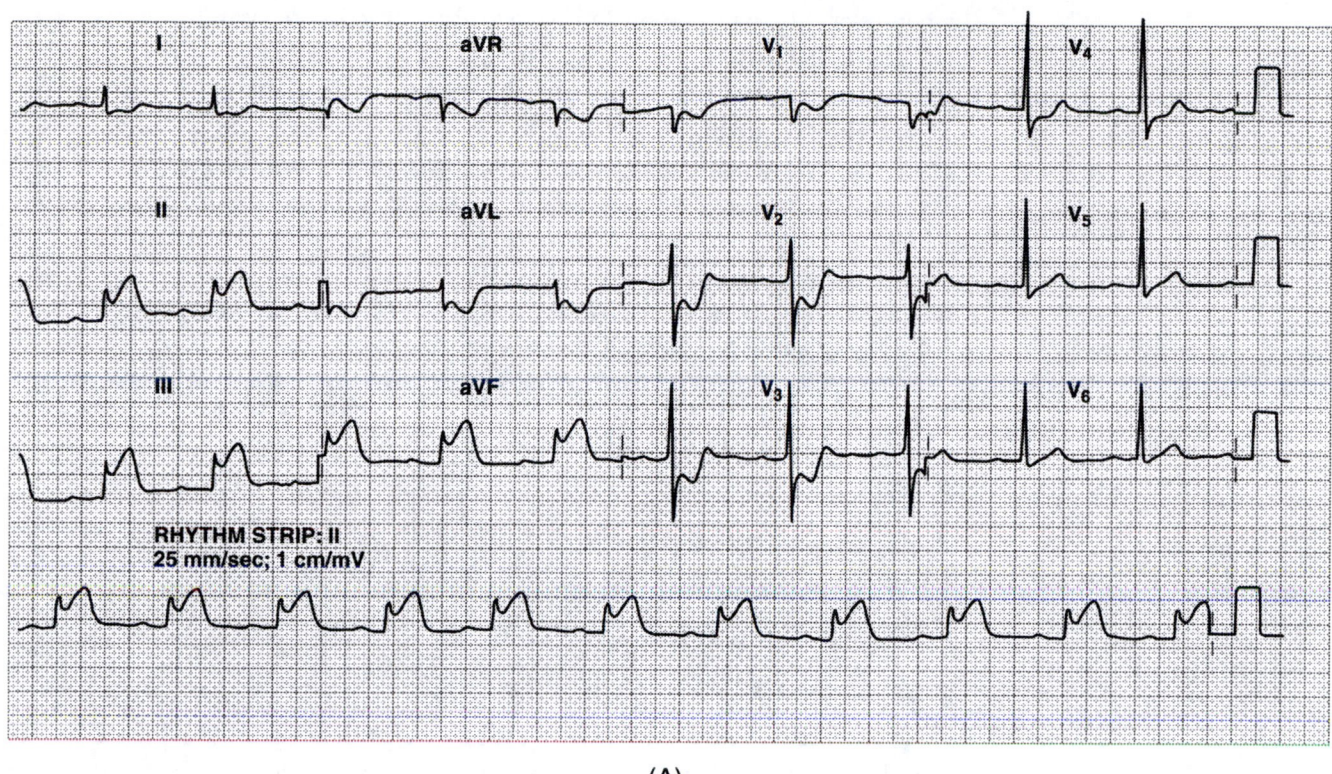

(A)

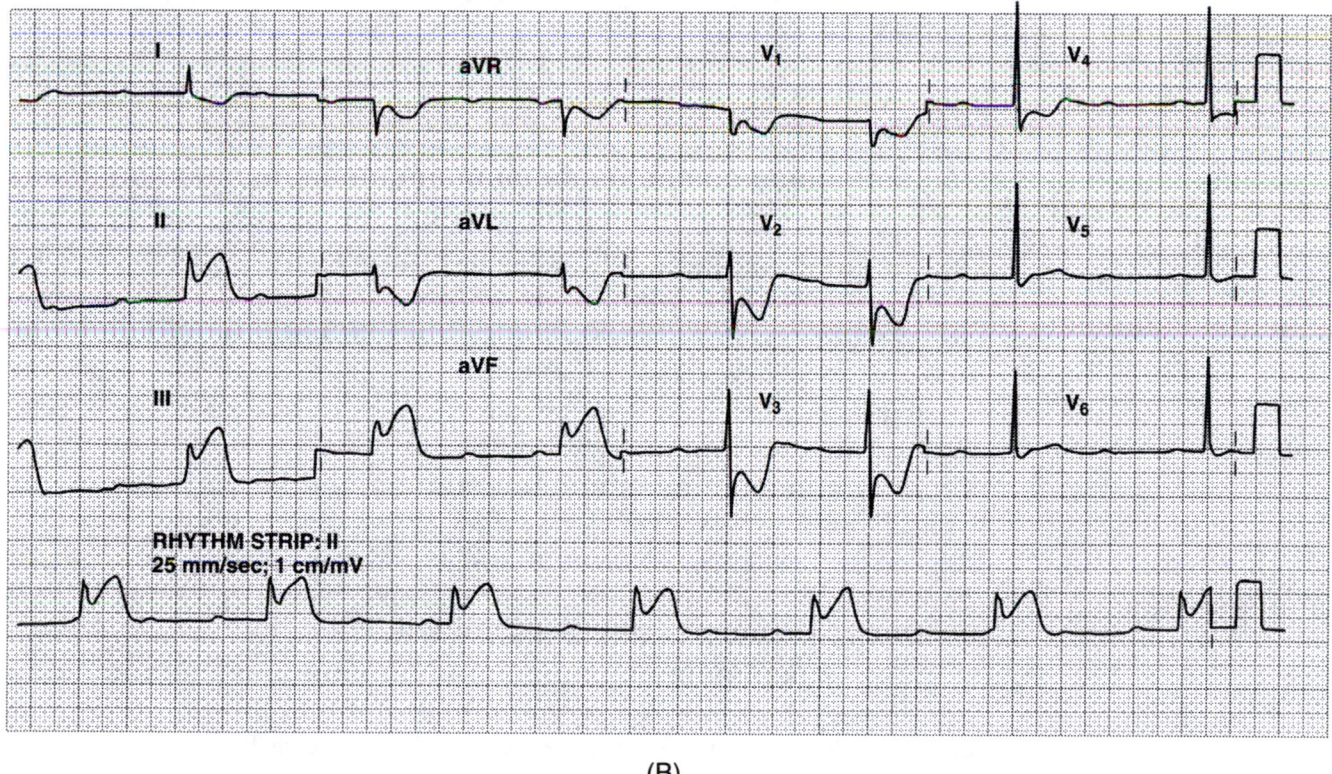

(B)

Figure 6-13 Two 12-lead ECGs from a patient with acute inferior-posterior MI. Note the acute changes in the limb leads II, III, and AVF (inferior). Note the R waves, ST depression in V_2 and V_3, the reciprocal of the posterior surface. Interpretation: sinus rhythm at 67 beats per minute with first-degree AV block (50 beats per minute (B) with acute signs supporting inferior-posterior myocardial infarction) complete AV block.

segment elevation will present in right-sided chest leads. A useful ECG indicating right ventricular involvement shows 1 mm or greater ST elevation in lead V_{4R} which is the mirror image of lead V_4 but it is obtained from the right chest.

A right-side set of precordial leads (the mirror image of the left-side leads) is very useful in diagnosing inferior wall myocardial infarctions because right ventricular infarction may be life-threatening and is treated differently from the more common left ventricular wall MI.

Clinical Implications of Right Ventricular Wall Myocardial Infarction

Complications of right ventricular MI include hypotension, decreased cardiac output, and cardiogenic shock. Signs and symptoms of right ventricular MI include:

- hypotension;
- jugular venous neck distension;
- ventricular gallop: S_3;
- summation gallop: $S_3 + S_4$; and
- diminished urine output.

It is critical to note that these signs may be present without evidence of pulmonary congestion. Figure 6-14 is an illustration of a right ventricular wall MI from right coronary artery disease. Table 6-6 summarizes the characteristics found in right ventricular wall myocardial infarction.

NON-Q WAVE MYOCARDIAL INFARCTION

Absence of Q waves does not rule out myocardial infarction. Subendocardial infarction may occur without Q waves on the ECG. The designation of nontransmural is made when all three layers of the myocardium are not involved; this is also called non-Q wave myocardial infarction. Non-Q wave infarctions clinically are smaller than Q wave infarctions as measured by cardiac serum enzyme markers (CPK criteria). They may be associated with a higher frequency of postinfarction angina and recurrent ischemic events. (At this printing, the literature makes conflicting distinctions in this regard.)

Angiographies of patients often show a recanalized vessel. Subendocardial injury causes ST-T wave changes. Specifically ST segment depression drags down the T wave or the T wave becomes inverted as a result of delayed repolarization in the ischemic myocardium. In some cases only small Q waves (less than 5 mm in depth) or diminished R wave amplitude (less than 10 mm) may appear.

The characteristic changes seen in non-Q wave myocardial infarction involve repolarization abnormalities. Patients may present with ST segment elevation, depression, or both, with isolated T wave inversion. No early ECG changes can predict the evolution of a non-Q wave MI.

In non-Q wave MI, the location of the ST segment depression is not always an accurate indicator of the specific site of the ischemia. Recall that ST segment depression seen in 1 lead can reflect the mirror-image (reciprocal) sign of ischemia occurring elsewhere in the heart.

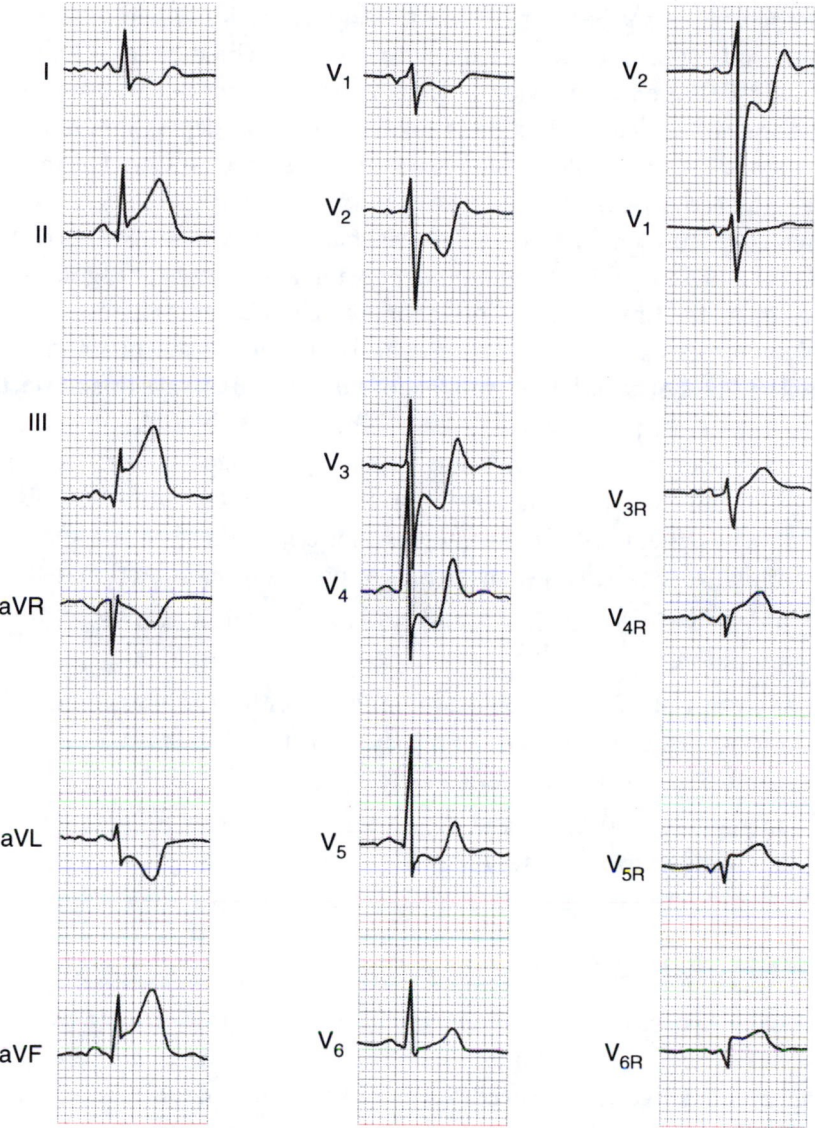

Figure 6-14 Acute infero-posterior wall myocardial infarction and right ventricular infarction. Note the elevated ST segment in lead V_{3R} indicating an occlusion in the proximal right coronary artery and right ventricular involvement. (From Wellens, H.J.J. and Conover, M.B. *The ECG in Emergency Decision Making*, W.B. Saunders Company, 1992.)

Table 6-6 Summary of ECG characteristics of right ventricular wall MI

ECG Changes	Early (Ischemia)	Late (Necrosis)
R waves		
ST segment	up in V_1–V_4 up in II, III, aVF	
T wave		
Q wave		V_1–V_{4R}
QS complex		V_1–V_{4R}

In approximately 9 percent of non-Q wave infarctions there is transmural injury to the inferoposterior wall of the left ventricle. These patients will present with isolated ST segment depression in leads V_1 to V_4. A representative ECG finding of anterior non-Q wave infarction is a downsloping ST depression, not the typical horizontal ST segment depression seen with posterior myocardial infarction. There is also an accompanying T wave inversion.

Patients who present with only T wave changes have a lower mortality rate than those who present with ST segment depression and T wave changes.

To estimate the timing of the infarction, the clinician must assess all changes and trending at specific intervals. The prognosis of non-Q wave infarction among patients with thrombolysis is better than that of a diagnosed Q wave infarction, therefore a high index of suspicion should prevail. There should be close observation for ST segment elevation or depression, T wave inversion, changes in heart rate, rhythm, QRS duration, and changes in the PR interval. ECG changes must be weighed in conjunction with patient history, clinical presentation, and cardiac enzyme analysis.

To summarize, ECG changes suspicious of non-Q wave infarction include:

1. Inferior wall; leads II, III, and aVF; symmetrical convex ST segment depression.

2. Anterior wall; V_1 to V_4; ST elevation in V_1 with ST depression in V_2 to V_4 without associated posterior wall MI. Inverted or diphasic T waves with a terminal inverted segment in V_2 and V_3.

3. Lateral wall; I, aVL, V_5, and V_6; symmetrical convex ST segment depression; inverted or diphasic T waves.

PSEUDO-INFARCTION PATTERNS

Left ventricular hypertrophy generates poor R wave progression over the anterior precordial leads, suggesting an anterior wall myocardial infarction. Such poor R wave progression is due to enhanced forces of ventricular depolarization over the lateral wall of the left ventricle. This pseudo-infarction pattern is of particular importance in a patient with aortic valve disease, whose initial clinical presentation may include significant anginal pain.

Pulmonary embolus, emphysema, and chronic obstructive pulmonary disease with right ventricular hypertrophy may also present with poor precordial R wave progression. In this instance, the right axis deviation, if present, may be adequate to differentiate anterior wall myocardial infarction from right ventricular hypertrophy.

Pneumothorax is another common etiology of a pseudo-infarction pattern on ECG. Because of displacement of the heart and mediastinum, the QRS voltage is reduced and the QRS axis significantly shifted, generating what is interpreted as pathologic appearing Q waves.

As noted earlier, hyperkalemia classically causes peaked T waves, which may incorporate some ST segment elevation. This is easily confused with the acute current of myocardial injury.

Wolff-Parkinson-White (WPW) preexcitation syndrome can cause what may appear to be pathologic Q waves in both the inferior and anterior leads due to initial aberrant forces of depolarization through the accessory bypass tract. In patients with WPW, conduction down the accessory tract often creates a delta wave on many of the ECG leads. This makes further conclusions regarding the QRS morphology as it relates to infarction difficult and at times impossible.

Patients with hypertrophic cardiomyopathy (HCM) often have significant Q waves on their ECG. Rather than infarction, these Q waves represent hypertrophied asymmetric ventricular muscle with distortion of the normal patterns of depolarization. Always suspect a pseudo-infarction pattern when the clinical setting and laboratory data do not correlate with electrocardiographic suggestion of infarction.

There may also be dramatic alterations to the T waves and ST segments with sudden increases in intracranial pressure. In these patients, changes do not reflect a primary myocardial problem, but rather changes in repolarization due to enhanced sympathetic nervous system activity. (See Chapter 2.)

Early Repolarization

Early repolarization with ST segment elevation in the anterior leads can be a normal variant. More pronounced in some, a 1 to 2 mm ST segment elevation can lead to the erroneous diagnosis of either pericarditis or acute myocardial necrosis. In instances of early repolarization, there is usually a notch at the end of the R wave with an upward concavity to the ST segment. In addition, the T wave morphology remains distinct and separated from the ST segment.

NONCLASSIC ECG PRESENTATION OF ACUTE MYOCARDIAL INFARCTION

In the elderly suffering an acute myocardial infarction, the classic ECG changes of ST elevation and reciprocal depression may not be evident early on. New onset atrial fibrillation, with or without chest pain, may herald the infarction. If there is any suspicion following the acute rhythm disturbance, classic changes such as ST elevation on 12-lead ECG and associated elevated enzyme studies confirm the diagnosis.

ECG complications such as left bundle branch block may mask the ability of the 12-lead ECG to confirm a myocardial infarction. In left bundle branch block the initial forces of left-to-right septal activation are no longer intact. So, when anterior wall myocardial infarction occurs the resulting Q wave and ST elevation are not visible in the precordial leads. The left current of flow overshadows the Q waves seen with inferior and anterior wall myocardial infarction. Correlation among clinical presentation and present and previous 12-lead tracings is vital in making this diagnosis.

CONTINUOUS ST SEGMENT MONITORING

As stated previously, there are limitations to the absolute diagnostic value of the standard 12-lead ECG in initially confirming an acute or recent infarction. In fact, the initial ECG that is diagnostic of acute injury is seen only in approximately a quarter of the patients who have a final diagnosis of an acute MI. Trending or taking subsequent ECGs can assist in establishing the diagnosis of MI, but valuable time may be lost in the process because serial ECGs are frequently not performed for several hours unless the patient's condition changes. Occasionally, ST segment changes go undetected until late in the course of infarction after the opportunity for optimal treatment and reperfusion has passed. Continuous ST segment monitoring is thus an important tool for detecting early signs of injury and infarction. Continuous ST segment monitoring can be done noninvasively to detect reperfusion in patients who receive thrombolytic therapy.

Continuous ECG monitoring using a single-lead system should never be used to confirm or rule out infarction. Trending the patient using 12-lead ECG is valuable to confirming other ECG changes suggestive of acute MI, such as loss of R wave progression and the presence of T wave inversion. Some facilities employ a computerized 12-lead ECG that is updated every 20 seconds. The ECGs are simultaneously analyzed and compared with previous readings. If 4 sequential tracings meet a predetermined threshold criteria an alarm will sound alerting the clinician to new changes. Changes in the 12-lead may indicate a cardiac event in advance of patient complaint. In lieu of such a system, it may be advisable to perform 12-lead ECG every 30 minutes and whenever the patient has:

- recurrent pain;
- signs and symptoms of heart failure; or
- any new ectopy.

Figure 6-15 is a quick reference to the surfaces of the heart as seen in the leads reflecting those surfaces. Table 6-7 outlines the most effective lead systems for observation and anticipated complications.

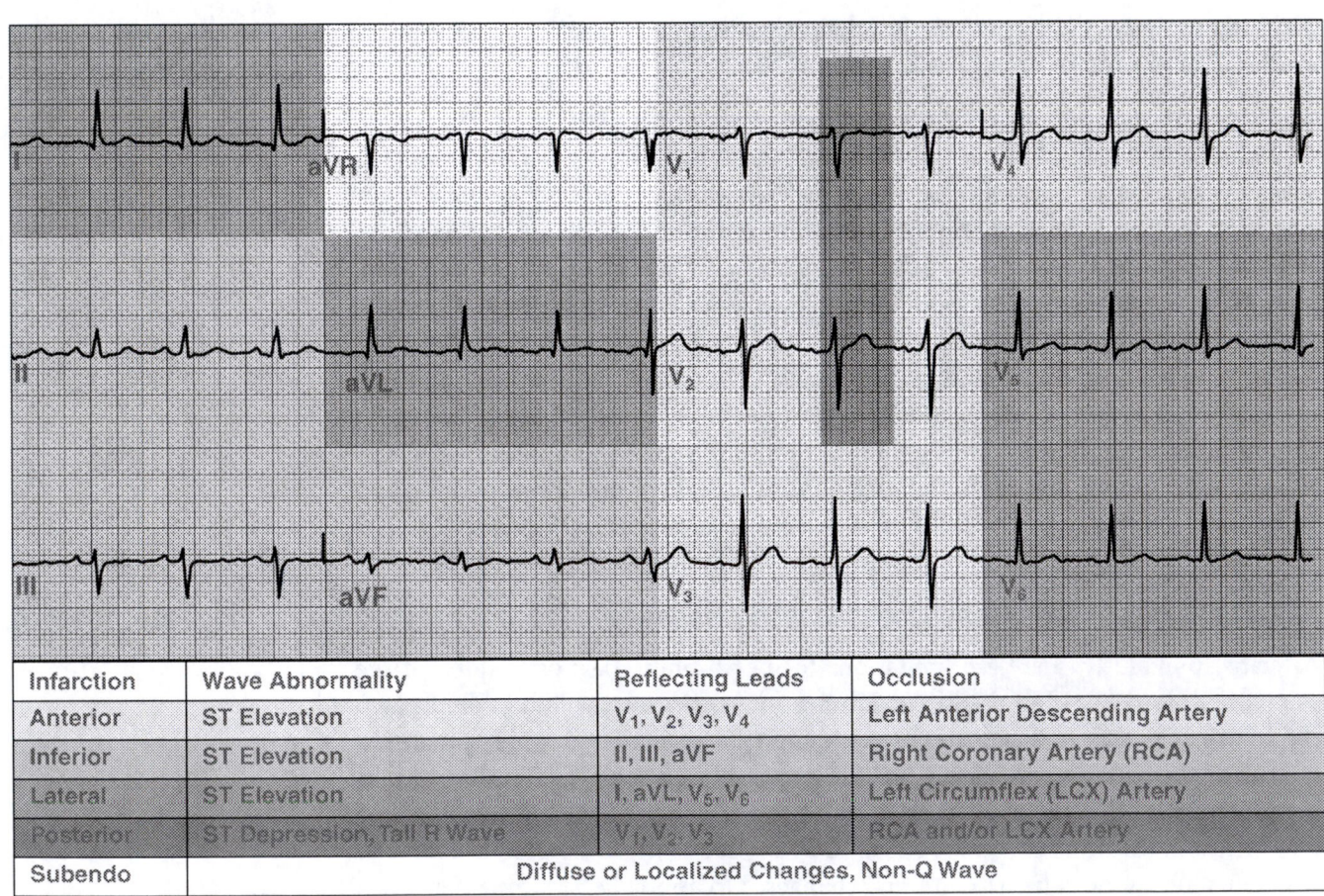

Infarction	Wave Abnormality	Reflecting Leads	Occlusion
Anterior	ST Elevation	V_1, V_2, V_3, V_4	Left Anterior Descending Artery
Inferior	ST Elevation	II, III, aVF	Right Coronary Artery (RCA)
Lateral	ST Elevation	I, aVL, V_5, V_6	Left Circumflex (LCX) Artery
Posterior	ST Depression, Tall R Wave	V_1, V_2, V_3	RCA and/or LCX Artery
Subendo	Diffuse or Localized Changes, Non-Q Wave		

Figure 6-15 A quick reference to the surfaces of the heart as seen on the ECG, including ECG wave form abnormalities common to coronary artery occlusion.

Table 6-7 The relationship of coronary artery perfusion to the sites of myocardial infarction and the most effective lead systems for observation.

Coronary Artery	Primary Area of Distribution	Site of Infarction and Lead System Visualization	Anticipated Complications
Right	1. 55% of the SA node 2. 90% of the AV node 3. Penetrating portion of the bundle of His 4. Right atrium and ventricle 5. Left inferior surface 6. Posterior IV septum 7. Left inferior-posterior fascicle	Inferior wall infarction Leads II, III, aVF	1. Sinus bradycardia, blocks, and arrest 2. AV junctional rhythm 3. First-degree AV block 4. Second-degree AV block, Type I, Wenckebach 5. Complete AV block 6. Papillary dysfunction
Left Anterior Descending	1. Left anterior wall 2. Anterior two-thirds of the IV septum 3. Bundle of His 4. Right bundle branch 5. Left anterior-superior fascicle	Left anterior infarction Precordial leads to demonstrate the MI V_1 for RBBB Limb leads to observe for conduction defects	1. Bundle branch blocks 2. Type II AV block 3. Complete AV block 4. Septal defect
Left Circumflex	1. 45% of the SA node 2. 10% of the AV node 3. Left inferior surface 4. Left lateral wall 5. Left infero-posterior fascicle	Left lateral wall infarction Leads I, aVL, and V_6	1. As in inferior wall MI 2. Rupture of the left ventricular free wall 3. Ventricular aneurysm 4. Papillary dysfunction

Source: Little, R. C. (1985). *Physiology of the Heart and Circulation* (3rd ed.) New York: Year Book Medical;
Mandel, W. J. (1980). *Cardiac arrhythmias: Their mechanisms, diagnosis and management.* Philadelphia: Lippincott.

Summary

By current estimates, approximately 1.1 million people in the United States have a new or recurrent acute myocardial infarction each year; one-third of which prove fatal. Among patients with nonfatal myocardial infarction, many experience debilitating loss of cardiac muscle because of delay in recognition, diagnosis, and successful reperfusion.

Despite two decades of pharmacologic and percutaneous reperfusion, supported by advances in resuscitation technology, the principal cause of myocardial infarction morbidity and mortality is still delay from onset of signs and symptoms to recognition and treatment.

Enhancement of prehospital recognition and 12-lead transmission is becoming the standard, with the goal being to recognize and intervene in a timely fashion to prevent cardiac death. Braunwald suggests that paramedics and nurses, as well as physicians, be educated in the recognition of candidates for thrombolytic therapy. The concept has been supported since 1990. An algorithm has been developed supporting the use of thrombolytic agents by paramedics in the field and under the direction of a hospital-based physician. There are other studies that support that premise.

The 12-lead ECG is a valuable tool in the hands of an educated and discriminating medical professional. As with any other diagnostic tool, the 12-lead ECG is a beneficial adjunct to thorough history taking, physical examination, and monitoring clinical course. The clinician must always treat the patient, not only the ECG.

Self-Assessment Exercises

● Matching

Match the term in the left column with the definition in the right column and compare your answers with those in the back of the book.

Term	Definition
_____ 1. Anterior wall MI	A. ST elevation 3 to 4 weeks post-MI
_____ 2. Current of injury	B. ST elevation
_____ 3. Inferior wall MI	C. Q wave, ST elevation II, III, and aVF
_____ 4. Transmural MI	D. Q wave, ST elevation V_3, V_4, V_5, V_6
_____ 5. Ventricular aneurysm	E. Q, ST elevation, hyperacute T wave

● ECG Rhythm Identification Practice

Identify the ECG criterion listed below each 12-lead ECG, and then compare your answers with those in the back of the book.

Figure 6-16

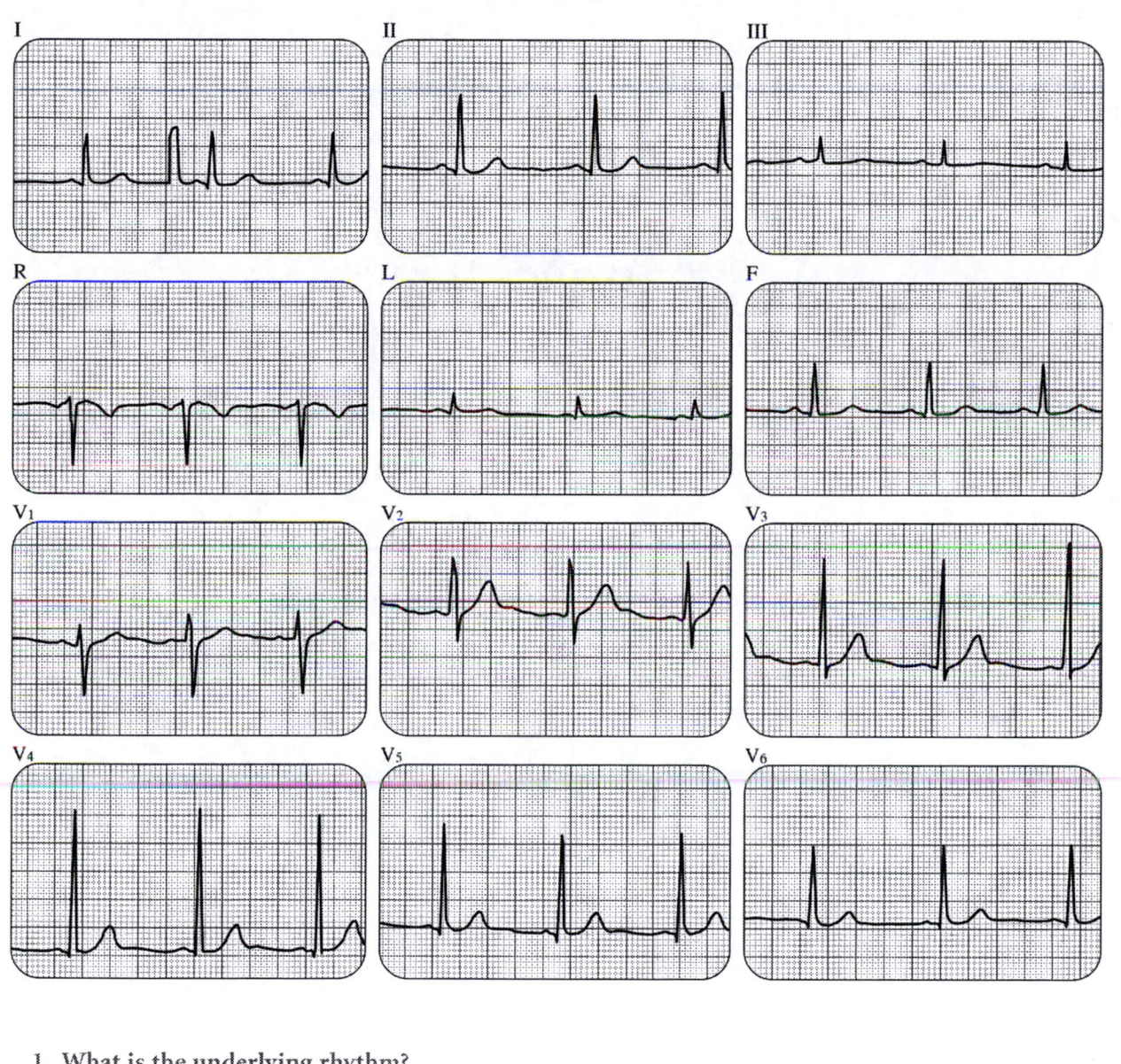

1. What is the underlying rhythm? _____

2. What are the acute changes? _____

3. What is your interpretation? _____

4. What can happen next? _____

Figure 6-17

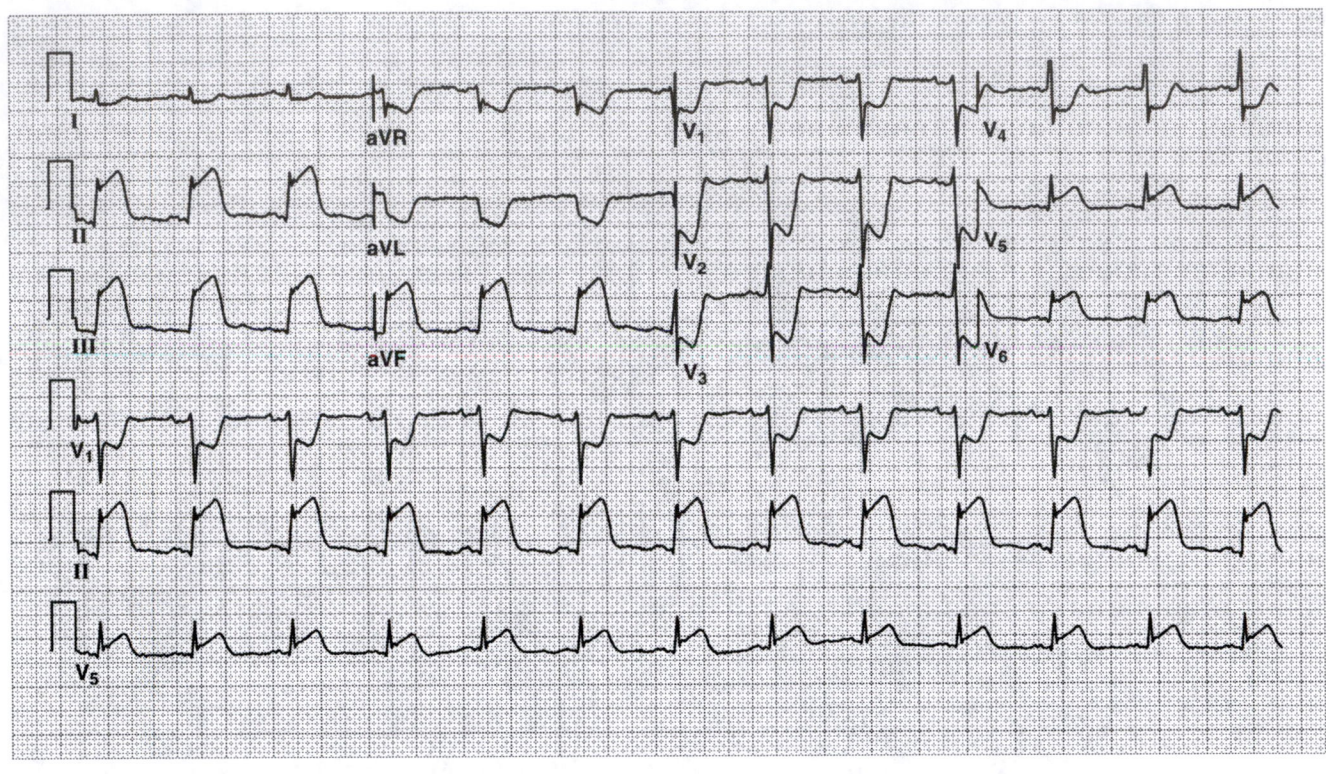

1. What is the underlying rhythm? _____
2. What are the acute changes? _____
3. What is your interpretation? _____
   _____
4. What can happen next? _____

Figure 6-18

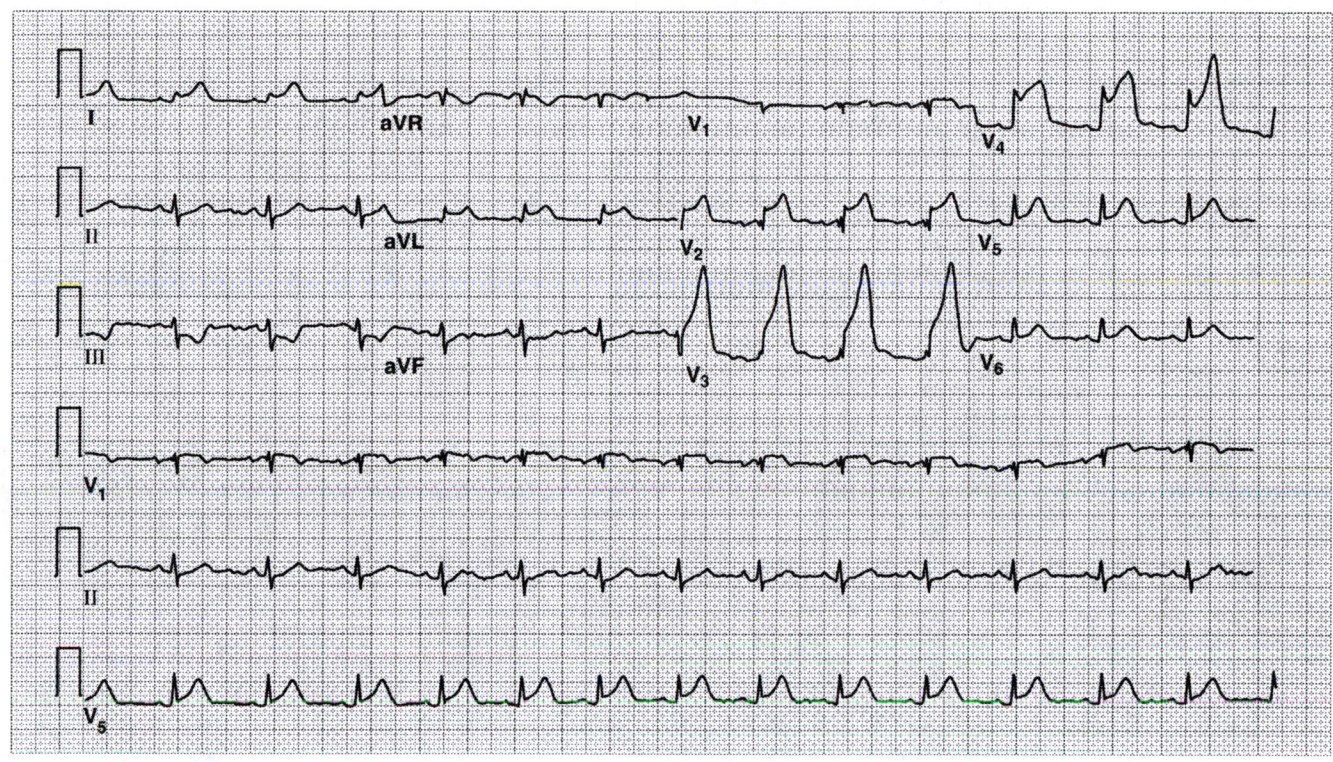

1. What is the underlying rhythm? _____

2. What are the acute changes? _____

3. What is your interpretation? _____

   _____

4. What can happen next? _____

Figure 6-19

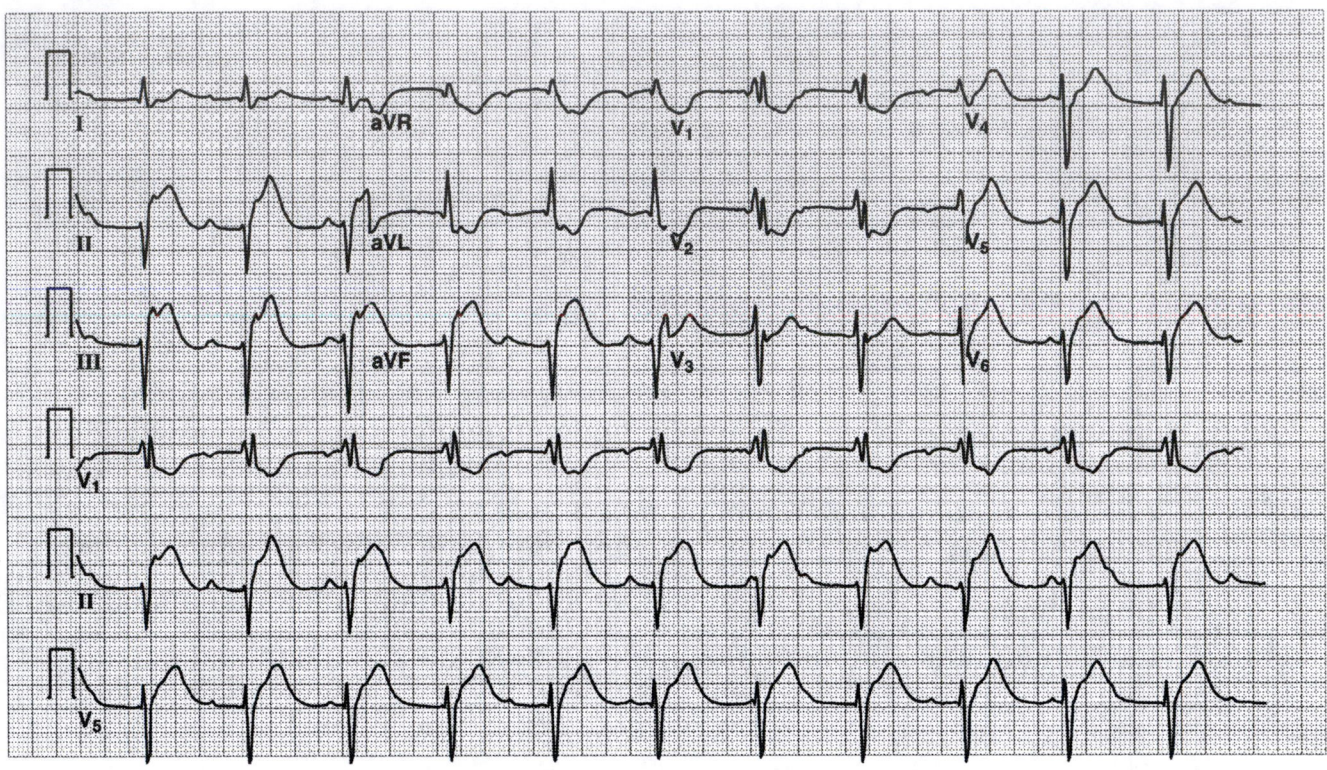

1. What is the underlying rhythm? _____

2. What are the acute changes? _____

3. What is your interpretation? _____

   _____

4. What can happen next? _____

Figure 6-20

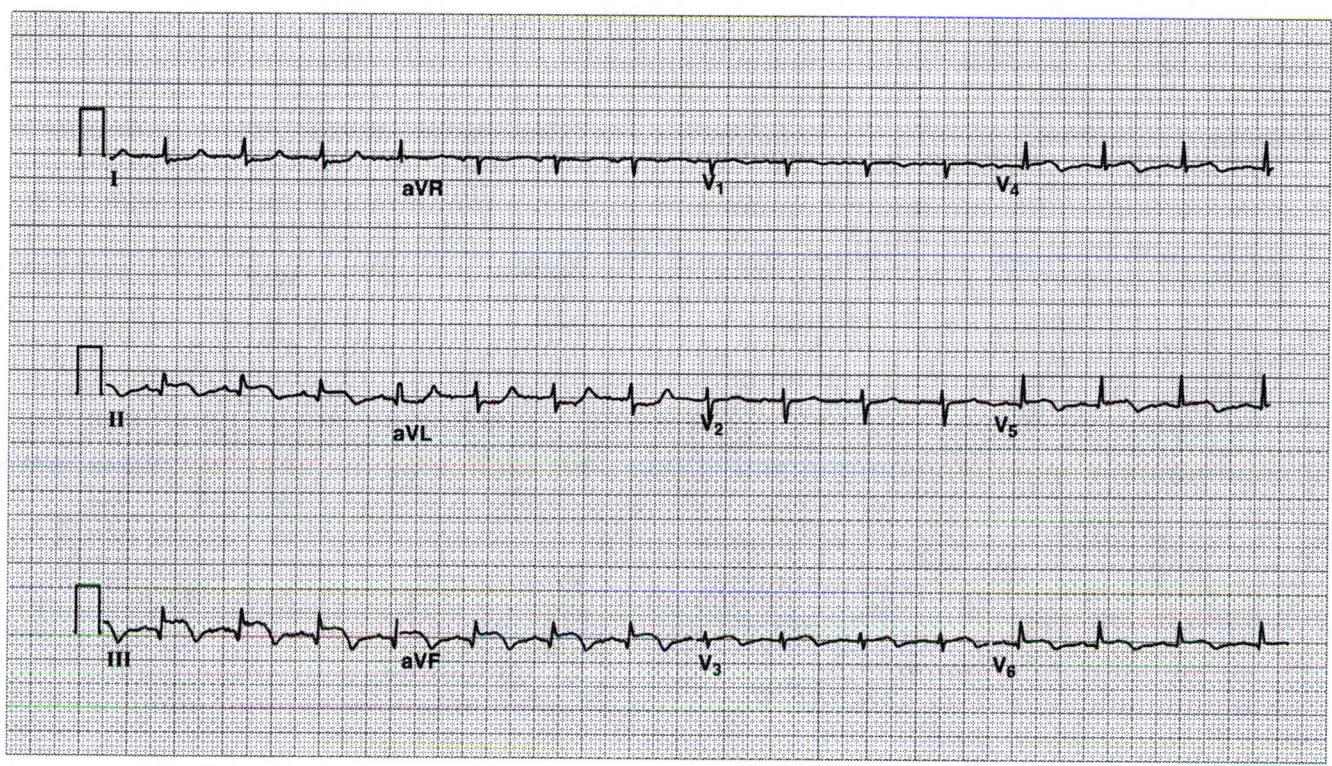

1. What is the underlying rhythm? _____

2. What are the acute changes? _____

3. What is your interpretation? _____

   _____

4. What can happen next? _____

Figure 6-21

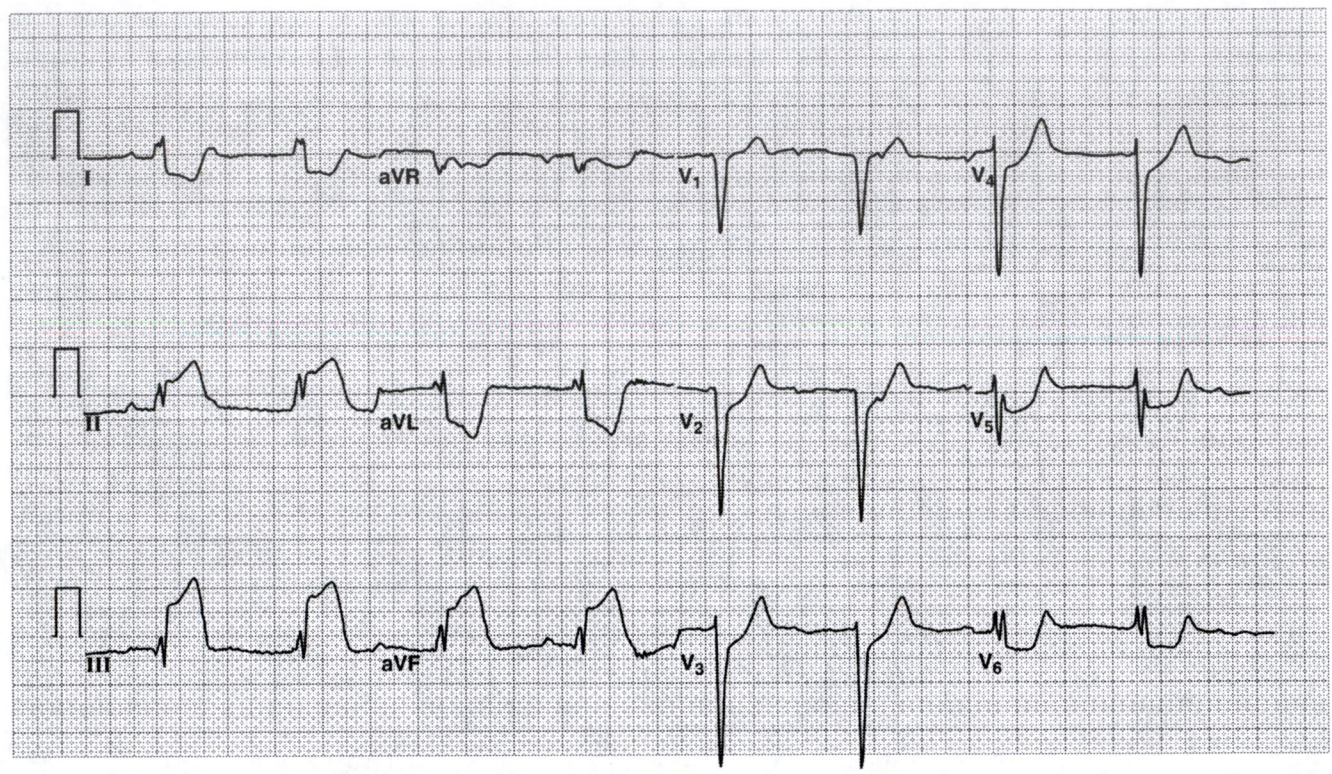

1. What is the underlying rhythm? _____

2. What are the acute changes? _____

3. What is your interpretation? _____

   _____

4. What can happen next? _____

Figure 6-22

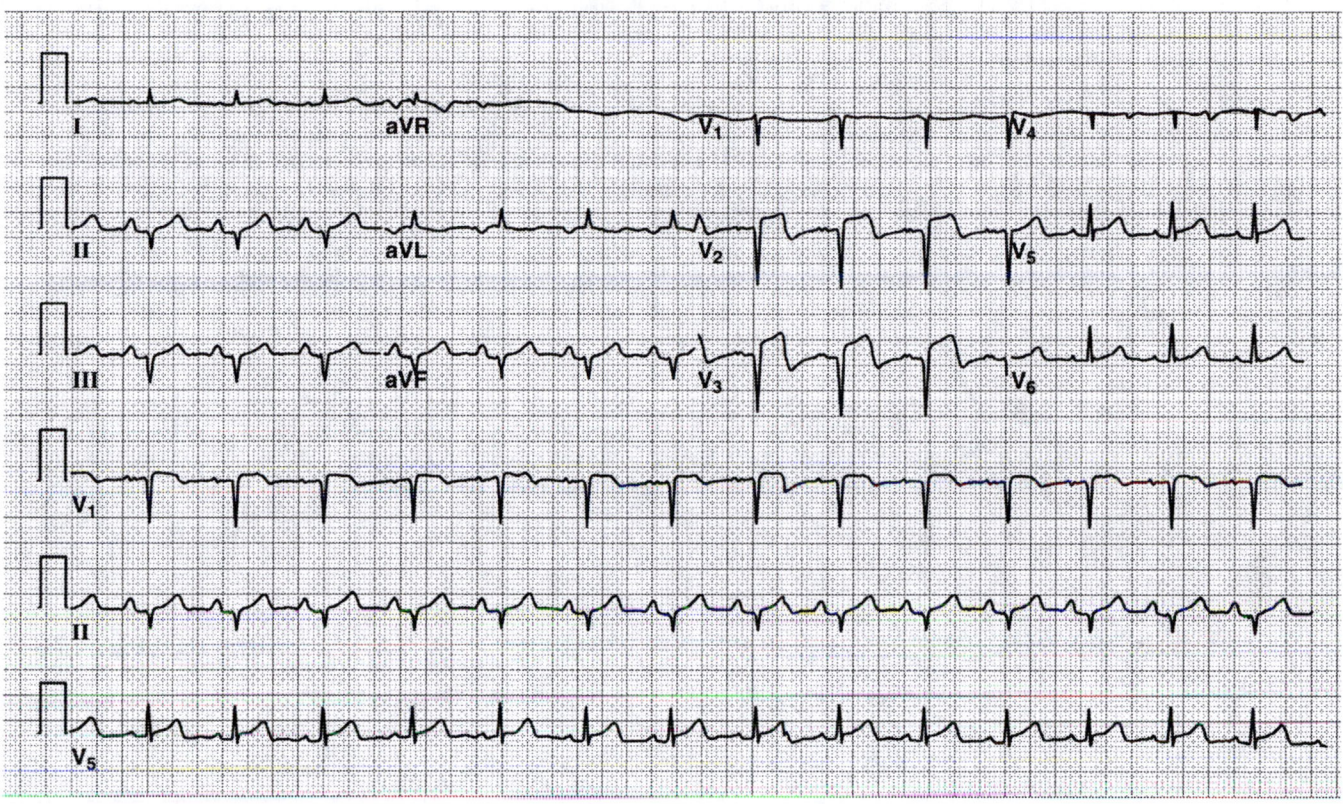

1. What is the underlying rhythm? _____

2. What are the acute changes? _____

3. What is your interpretation? _____

   _____

4. What can happen next? _____

References

Conover, M. B. (1996). *Understanding electrocardiography: Arrhythmias and the 12-lead ECG*. (7th ed.). St. Louis: Mosby-Year Book.

Conover, M. B. & Wellens, H. J. (1993). *The ECG in emergency decision making*. Philadelphia: W. B. Saunders.

Goldberger, E. (1982). *Textbook of clinical cardiology*. St. Louis: C. V. Mosby.

Marriott, H. J. & Conover, M. B. (1989). *Advanced concepts in arrhythmias*. (2nd ed.). St. Louis: C.V. Mosby.

Shlipak, M. G., Lyons W. L., & Go, A. S. (1999). Should the electrocardiogram be used to guide therapy for patients with left bundle branch block and suspected myocardial infarction? *Journal of the American Medical Association;* (24)281:714-719.

Surawicz, B. (1995). Abnormal depolarization: Intraventricular conduction disturbances. In *Electrophysiologic basis of ECG and cardiac arrhythmias*. Baltimore: Williams and Wilkins: 507-534.

Wagner, G. S. (Ed.). (1994). *Marriott's practical electrocardiography*. (9th ed.). Baltimore: Williams and Wilkins.

Wellens, J. L., Robles, De Medina, E. O., Bernard, R., et al. (1985). Criteria for intraventricular conduction disturbances. *Journal of the American College of Cardiology;* 5:1261-1275.

Zehender, M., et al. (1990). ECG variants and cardiac arrhythmias in athletes: Clinical relevance and prognostic importance. *American Heart Journal;* 119:1378.

CHAPTER 7

Intraventricular Conduction Defects

> **Premise** ○ The levels of the ventricular conduction system can be easily tracked using the 12-lead ECG.

Objectives

After reading the chapter and completing the Self-Assessment exercises, the student should be able to:

1. Identify the arterial perfusion of the bundle branches
2. Identify the ECG changes in right bundle branch block
3. Identify the ECG changes in left anterior and left posterior fascicular block
4. Identify the ECG changes in bifascicular block
5. List the clinical implications for each of the ventricular conduction defects.

Key Terms

bifascicular block	fascicular block	trifascicular block
bundle branch block	hemiblock	ventricular activation
fascicle	intrinsicoid deflection	time

Introduction

An *intraventricular conduction defect* is the result of impaired conduction of electrical impulses through 1 or more of the divisions of the intraventricular conduction system. The primary conduction pathways that make up the intraventricular conduction system are the right bundle branch and the left main branch. The left main bundle, also known as the common left bundle, divides into fascicles. The primary fascicles are the left anterior (LAF) and left posterior fascicle (LPF). The septal fibers that extend from the left main branch vary in length and breadth, and are not recognized as comprising a true fascicle. Figure 7-1 is an illustration of the intraventricular conduction system.

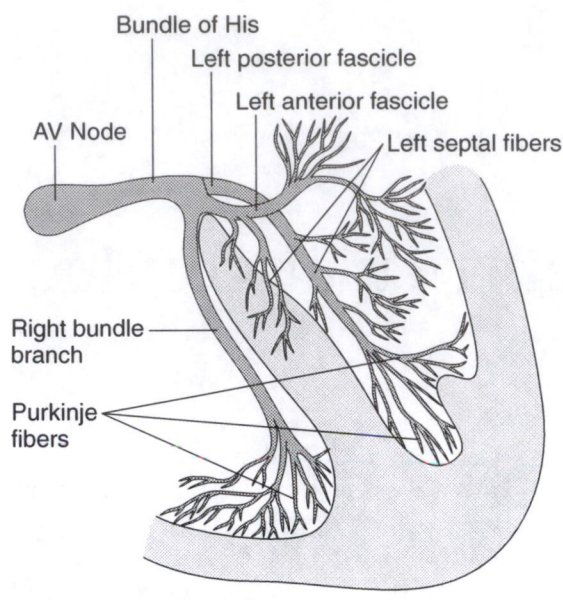

Bundle of His
Left posterior fascicle
Left anterior fascicle
AV Node
Left septal fibers
Right bundle branch
Purkinje fibers

Figure 7-1 Illustration of the conduction system from the AV node through to the His-Purkinje fibers. (Adapted with permission from *Principles of Clinical Electrocardiography*, 13th ed. by N. Goldschlager and M. Goldman, 1989, Appleton-Lange.)

When conduction through one or more of the bundle branches is impaired, there is a delay in the conduction pattern. One or parts of the ventricle can depolarize out of normal sequence, the ramifications of which include abnormal ventricular wall motion.

To understand the implications of **bundle branch block**, it is critical to know the anatomy of the intraventricular conduction system and the arterial supply to the right and left bundle branches. Bundle branch block of any kind can occur without infarction. However, if a patient presents with a myocardial infarction and the dominant blood vessel to the electrical conduction system is affected, the clinician should be able to anticipate the intraventricular conduction defects, predict the implications, and prepare accordingly.

THE BUNDLE BRANCHES AND ARTERIAL PERFUSION

Recall that the right bundle branch is a long fiber that begins at the level of the bundle of His and threads through the intraventricular septum to the base of the anterior papillary muscle of the right ventricle. The left anterior descending coronary artery perfuses the anterior myocardium and the anterior two-thirds of the septum. Its septal branch perfuses the proximal right bundle branch and the anterior division of the left bundle branch.

The left bundle branch divides into two primary fascicles; anterior and posterior. The more distal anterior fascicle has its origin in the bundle of His and threads through to the anterior superior endocardial surface and to the papillary muscle of the mitral valve. The anterior fascicle receives blood from the LAD and the right coronary artery (RCA). The posterior fascicle also has its origin in the bundle of His

⬤ **bundle branch block**

A conduction disorder in one or more of the bundle branches

⬤ **fascicles**

Bundles of fibers

and runs from the bundle to the posterior papillary muscle of the left ventricle. Perfusion to the posterior fascicle is by the RCA. The perforating arteries of the LAD also perfuse the posterior fascicle.

The RCA is responsible for perfusion to the posterior one-third of the septum. The AV nodal branch of the RCA perfuses the AV node and the bundle of His. As a result, occlusion in anterior wall myocardial infarction is a common cause of right bundle branch block (RBBB) while the left bundle branch block (LBBB) is seen with inferior wall myocardial infarction.

Arterial occlusion is one cause of a conduction disorder occurring in the bundle branch system. If the occlusion is not complete, the resulting ECG may show signs and symptoms of intermittent conduction defects. However, one of the more common causes of left bundle branch block is longstanding left ventricular hypertrophy with resulting thickening of heart muscle. Common causes of left ventricular hypertrophy include hypertensive heart disease, valvular heart disease, and as a sequela to open-heart surgery.

The presence of axis deviation on the ECG is recognized by many investigators as associated with delayed activation of tissue surrounding or near the infarcted area. The clinical significance of this phenomenon is the risk of sustained ventricular tachycardia (Flowers, 1990).

NORMAL SEQUENCE OF VENTRICULAR DEPOLARIZATION AND THE QRS VECTOR

Impulse propagation, usually from the sinus node, results in depolarization of the ventricular muscle and is responsible for the various components of the QRS vector—the wave form of depolarization. The first portion of the ventricular muscle to be activated is the junction of the middle and lower segments of the interventricular septum on the endocardial surface of the left ventricle. This depolarization wave causes vectorial forces that are oriented anteriorly, to the right, and superiorly or inferiorly. There is a counterclockwise rotation in the horizontal and left sagittal planes and a variable rotation in the frontal plane. From this point, the activation front proceeds rapidly toward the apex of the heart, speaking to both the right and left ventricular surfaces.

Because the left ventricle has greater muscle mass than the right, the depolarization forces responsible for activation of the left ventricle dominate the electrical field of the heart. As a result, the activation process is oriented primarily posteriorly, inferiorly, and to the left, corresponding to the anatomical position of the left ventricle. Simultaneous depolarization of the right and left free walls occurs well into the inscription of the QRS complex.

It is important to reemphasize that activation of the left ventricle is the result of impulse transmission through the two main branches of the left bundle, which has a short main trunk and bifurcates early into the anterior and posterior divisions or fascicles. The anterior branch provides conduction fibers to the anterior-superior aspects of the left ventricle and the posterior branch provides conduction fibers to the posterior-inferior aspects of the left ventricle. As the activation wave spreads inferiorly and posteriorly through the branches of the left bundle it causes a simultaneous depolarization of the inferior and lateral aspects of the left ventricle.

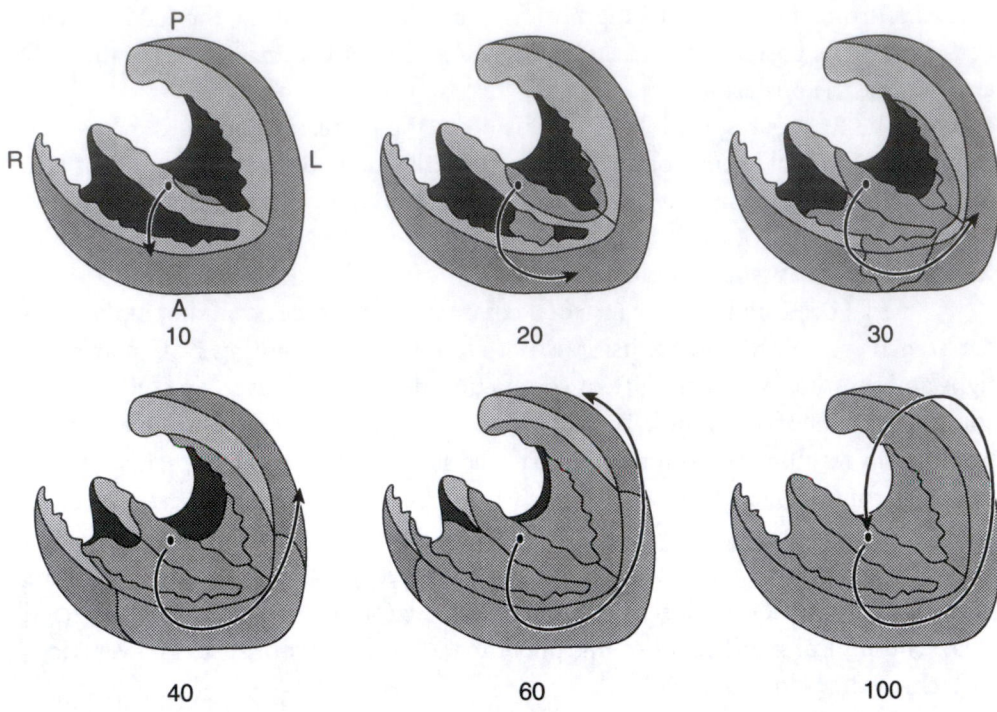

Figure 7-2 Sequence of ventricular activation as seen in the horizontal plane with QRS vectors superimposed at 10, 20, 30, 40, 60, and 100 milliseconds. From the point of view of lead II, the Q wave occurs over 10 to 20 milliseconds; the R wave over the next 30 to 40 milliseconds; and the S wave over the remaining 60 to 100 milliseconds. From the point of view of lead V_1, the small initial R wave occurs over 10 to 20 milliseconds and a negative S wave over the next 30 to 100 milliseconds. The progressive clearing in each model corresponds to the segments of myocardium that are being depolarized. (A = anterior; P = posterior; R = right; and L = left.)

Anatomically, the right bundle is a single trunk that bifurcates late into the Purkinje fibers. Occasionally, the time for completion of the left and right ventricular activation is not identical; in the majority of cases this is due to late activation of the outflow tract of the right ventricle or of the upper third of the interventricular septum. This disparity in the activation process may cause some vectorial forces that are oriented anteriorly and to the right. This is reflected on the ECG by the presence of an R′ in lead V_1 and a small S wave in leads V_5 or V_6. However, this pattern should not be interpreted as representative of a conduction abnormality of the right bundle or incomplete right bundle branch block as it is a normal event.

The entire ventricular activation process takes about 100 milliseconds or 0.10 second. Figure 7-2 illustrates the sequence of ventricular activation with QRS vectors superimposed from 10 to 100 milliseconds.

ECG CHANGES IN BUNDLE BRANCH BLOCK

In bundle branch block, the ST segment and T wave are usually in the opposite direction from the terminal portion of the QRS complex, primarily because repolarization of the ventricles is severely disturbed by this conduction defect. When bundle branch block is confirmed, these changes are called *secondary T waves*. On the other hand, segments and T waves that are the same polarity as the terminal portion of the QRS are called *primary ST-T wave changes*, and may be a sign of myocardial ischemia.

Right Bundle Branch Block

Significant alterations in the sequence of right ventricular depolarization occur when impulse propagation through the right main bundle is interrupted. The initial spread of activation, however, is normal during the first 40 milliseconds. The initial 10 to 20 milliseconds of ventricular depolarization represent septal depolarization which is normally oriented to the right and anteriorly, because this area is supplied by the conduction fibers from the left bundle. Therefore, in right bundle branch block, the beginning of the QRS complex is usually unchanged. What this means is there is a small R wave present in V_1 as the wave front crosses the septum. There is a small Q wave in V_6; normal activation of the left ventricle follows, producing an S wave in V_1 and an R wave in V_6. When the wave of electrical activity reaches the right bundle, the normal rapid conduction is halted. To depolarize the right ventricle, the impulse must travel through myocardial tissue rather than specialized conduction pathways. This takes time. Consequently, the QRS represents terminal conduction delay in the form of a late, broad R wave (R') in V_6 and a broad S wave in leads I, III, V_5 and V_6. The triphasic rsR' is seen in leads V_1 and V_6. Figure 7-3 is a graphic illustration of right bundle branch block and its associated ECG changes.

Causes of RBBB are:

- acute heart failure;
- anterior myocardial infarction;
- cardiomyopathy;
- Chagas' disease;
- congenital lesions;
- ischemic RCA disease;
- Legnegre's disease;
- Lev's disease;
- normal variant;
- rheumatic heart disease;
- surgical correction of Tetrology of Fallot;
- surgical correction of a ventricular septal defect;
- syphilis;
- trauma; and
- tumors

Rate-Related Right Bundle Branch Block. Occasionally, when heart rate increases as with stress testing, bundle branch block will occur at a particular rate. In this case, the bundle branch may still be in a refractory period and unable to

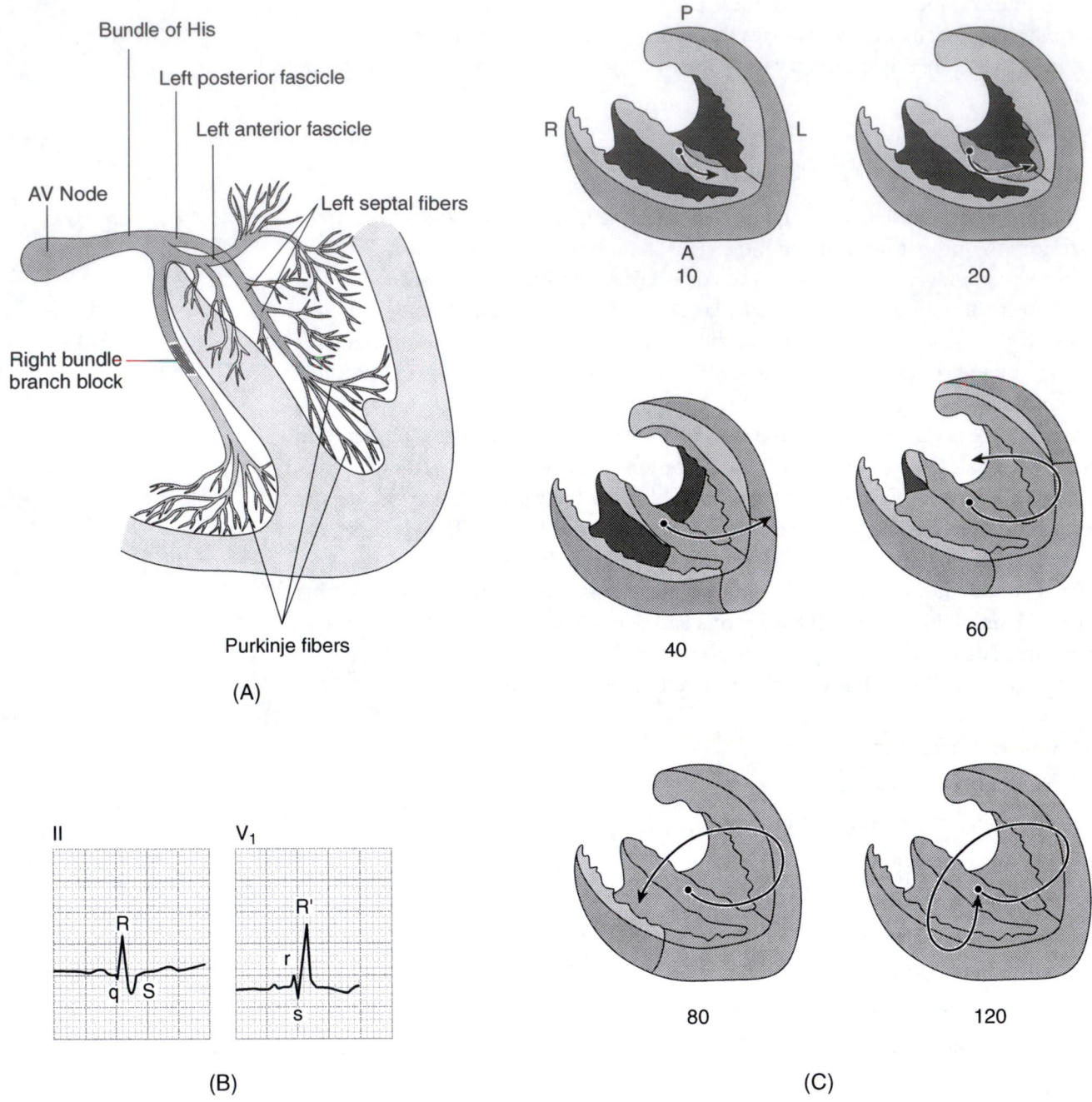

Figure 7-3 (A) Right bundle branch block; (B) shows the QRS complexes reflective of right bundle branch block; (C) shows the sequence of ventricular activation from 10-120 milliseconds. The QRS vector is superimposed on the heart with the corresponding cleared areas of the ventricles as they are being depolarized. Note the counterclockwise rotation of the QRS with delayed terminal appendage oriented anterior and to the right, occurring during between 80 and 120 milliseconds. Also notice that completion of depolarization takes 120 milliseconds or 0.12 second; *(continues)*

conduct the increased rate of incoming impulses normally. Rate-related bundle branch block is transient and once the heart rate returns to a normal, slower pace, the QRS will appear normal at 0.10 second.

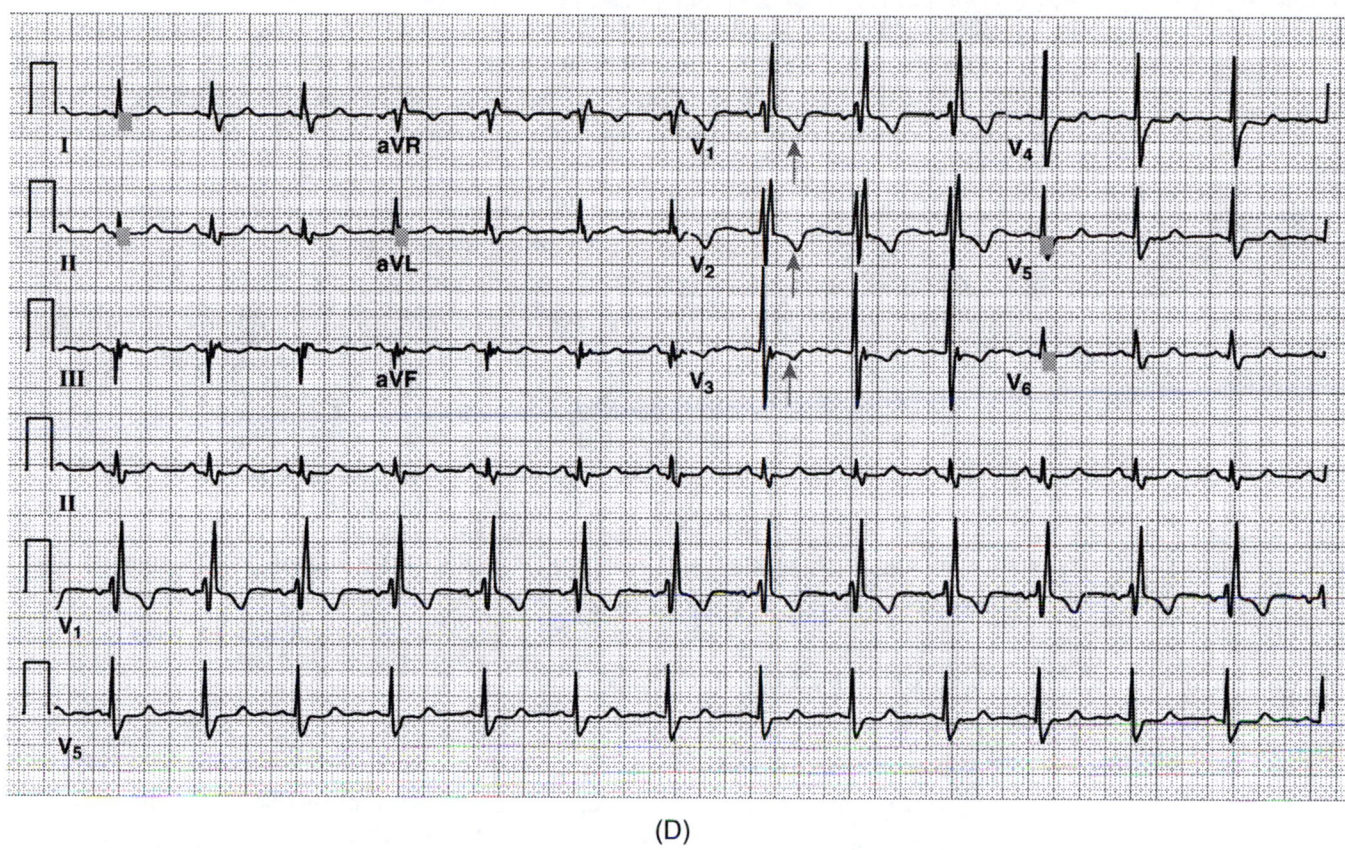

(D)

Figure 7-3 Continued (D) is a 12-lead ECG of right bundle branch block, showing the changes in the QRS complex in leads V_1 and V_2. The QRS complex is prolonged, greater than 0.10 second. There is a broad terminal S wave (shaded) in leads I, II, aVL, V_5, and V_6. The inverted T waves (arrow) seen in right precordial leads V_1 to V_3 are secondary T wave inversions.

Incomplete Right Bundle Branch Block. The term *complete* bundle branch block does not imply an irreversible condition. As we have seen, RBBB can occur when related to an increase in activity and heart rate. Premature atrial complexes followed by pauses, significant enough to support ventricular rest and recovery. When this happens, the morphology of RBBB remains but the QRS will be less than 0.12 second.

The clinical significance of incomplete right bundle branch block (IRBBB) remains controversial. ECG changes representative of incomplete right bundle branch block include:

- QRS complex less than 0.12 second; and
- rsR′ complex in V_1

Incomplete right bundle branch block in conditioned athletes may be related to an increase in muscle mass at the tip of the right ventricle. Once the activity is discontinued, the ECG signs of IRBBB disappear. Of the reported 14 percent of athletes affected with this phenomenon, 10 percent are between 20 and 35 years old.

Right Bundle Branch Block and Acute Myocardial Infarction. RBBB ECG patterns do not conflict with the patterns of infarction. The initial forces of left-to-right septal activation are intact, so when an infarction occurs, the resulting Q waves and ST segment elevation are visible.

RBBB that occurs within days of anterior wall myocardial infarction has a high risk of progressing to involve left anterior fascicular block and complete AV block. If MCL_1 or V_1 are the monitoring leads, the progressive involvement of the left bundle will be missed, since fascicular block is only diagnosed in the limb leads. In the case of anterior wall infarction, it is difficult to determine if the RBBB is new or pre-existing without obtaining previous records and 12-lead ECGs.

To summarize, ECG changes representative of right bundle branch block include:

- QRS complex greater than 0.10 second, 0.12 second, or more;
- Triphasic complex, rSR′ in V_1 and qRS in V_6;
- Small q and broad S waves in leads I, aVL, and V_6; and
- ST-T wave changes.

These changes in the terminal part of the QRS are all due to the late depolarization over right ventricular tissue.

Left Bundle Branch Block

Complete left bundle branch block (CLBBB) results when there is total interruption of transmission of the electrical impulse through the left main bundle or of the 2 main branches of the left bundle. Left bundle branch block is usually caused by occlusion in the left main branch or a simultaneous block in both anterior and posterior fascicles. It is usually the result of left anterior descending coronary artery disease. In left bundle branch block, the normal wave of depolarization is altered.

The sequence of left ventricular activation is markedly altered. Transmission of the impulse to the left ventricle occurs through excitation of the right septal mass, which is supplied by branches of the right bundle. Thus, the activation wave crosses the interventricular septum in a right-to-left direction. It follows, then, that the right ventricle depolarizes before the left. It is generally accepted that most of the conduction abnormalities of this type happen due to a delay in transmission across the interventricular septum, as with anteroseptal myocardial infarction.

The normal septal Q wave is not recorded in leads I, V_5, and V_6 with the abnormal septal depolarization. If Q waves are recorded in the presence of LBBB, the possibility of concurrent problems such as infarction should be considered.

Recall the left bundle is thick and broad and has a blood supply from both right and left coronary arteries. Consequently, left bundle branch block in a patient with diagnosed myocardial infarction usually reflects underlying heart disease because a very large lesion is required to block the left bundle branch. LBBB without underlying heart disease is very rare. Figure 7-4 illustrates left bundle branch block and its associated ECG changes.

Causes of left bundle branch block include:

- acute heart failure;
- acute myocardial infarction;
- cardiomyopathy;
- congenital lesions;
- ischemic LCA disease;

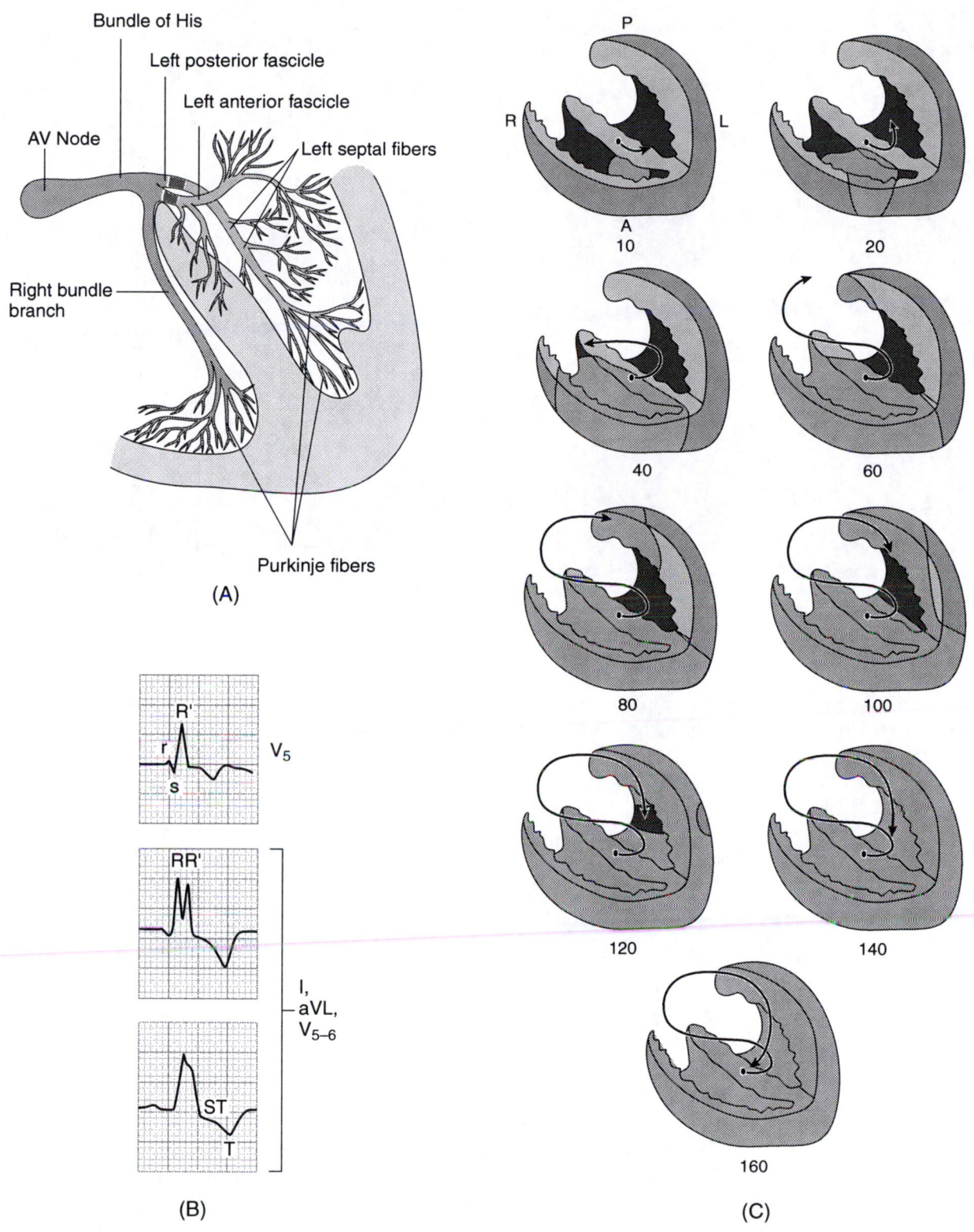

Figure 7-4 (A) Left bundle branch block. (B) The QRS complex that reflects the ECG changes associated with left bundle branch block is slurred and prolonged, greater than 0.12 second. (C) The sequence of ventricular activation from 10 to 160 milliseconds. The QRS vector is superimposed on the heart with the corresponding cleared areas of the ventricles as they are being depolarized. Note the near figure eight pattern reflecting the abnormal depolarization. Also note that completion of depolarization is 160 milliseconds or 0.16 second. *(continues)*

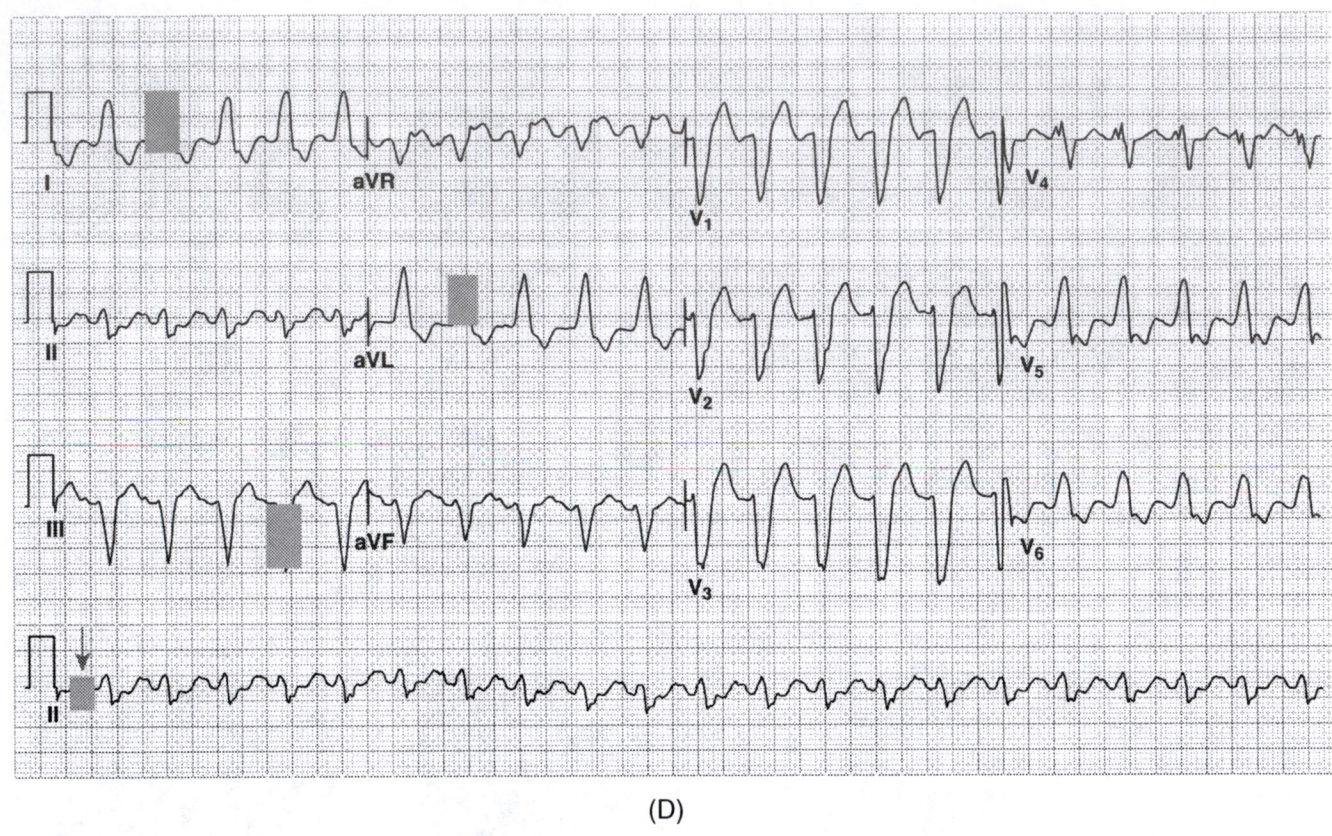

(D)

Figure 7-4 Continued (D) The broad, positive QRS complex in leads I, II, and aVL and the broad negative deflection in lead III reflect the direction of septal depolarization from right to left. There is first degree AV block (arrow).

- Legnegre's disease;
- Lev's disease;
- rheumatic heart disease;
- syphilis;
- trauma; and
- tumors

Rate-Related Left Bundle Branch Block. Occasionally, when heart rate increases as with stress testing, bundle branch block will occur. One explanation is that the bundle branch may still be in a refractory period and unable to conduct the increased rate of incoming impulses normally. Rate-related bundle branch block is transient and once the heart rate returns to a normal, slower pace, the QRS appears normal at 0.10 second.

ECG criteria for diagnosing left bundle branch block are:

- QRS greater than 0.12 second;
- QS or rS complexes in V_1;
- monophasic R wave in V_5 and V_6;

- notched or slurred QRS;
- No Q or S waves in leads I, aVL, or V_6;
- VAT time exceeds 0.02 second in V_1 and 0.04 second in V_6; and
- secondary ST-T wave changes in the left precordial leads V_5 and V_6.

Incomplete Left Bundle Branch Block. An ECG showing the pattern of left bundle branch block with a QRS of less than 0.12 second may indicate an incomplete left bundle branch block (ILBBB). However, cause for this type of conduction defect remains controversial. It has been suggested that left bundle branch block occurs when transmission of the electrical impulse through the left main bundle is partially interrupted. This produces an abnormal sequence of ventricular activation, with the right ventricle activating slightly earlier than the left through the intact right bundle branch. This blockage causes various degrees of delay through the left bundle, resulting in degrees of abnormalities in the QRS vector. These are particularly evident during the initial 30 milliseconds, meaning that ventricular activation time is delayed.

The time from the beginning of the initial inscription of the QRS to the point where the impulse arrives under a particular electrode of a lead measure is called the **ventricular activation time (VAT)**. The corresponding deflection produced is called the **intrinsicoid deflection**. V_1 measures VAT for the right ventricle, which is normally 0.02 second because the right ventricle is thin-walled. It is measured from the beginning of the small R wave to the peak of that small R wave.

V_6 measures VAT for the left ventricle, which is usually 0.04 second. It is calculated from the beginning of the QRS to the peak of the R wave. Recall that the left ventricle is thicker than the right and it takes longer for the impulse to arrive under the V_6 electrode. In left bundle branch block, the VAT exceeds 0.02 second in V_1 and 0.04 second in V_6. Figure 7-5 shows the measurement of the ventricular activation time in V_1 and V_6.

- **ventricular activation time (VAT)**

The time from the beginning of the initial inscription of the QRS, to the point where the impulse arrives under a particular electrode of a lead

- **intrinsicoid deflection**

The deflection made during the time from the beginning of the initial inscription of the QRS, to the point where the impulse arrives under a particular electrode of a lead; used to measure ventricular activation time

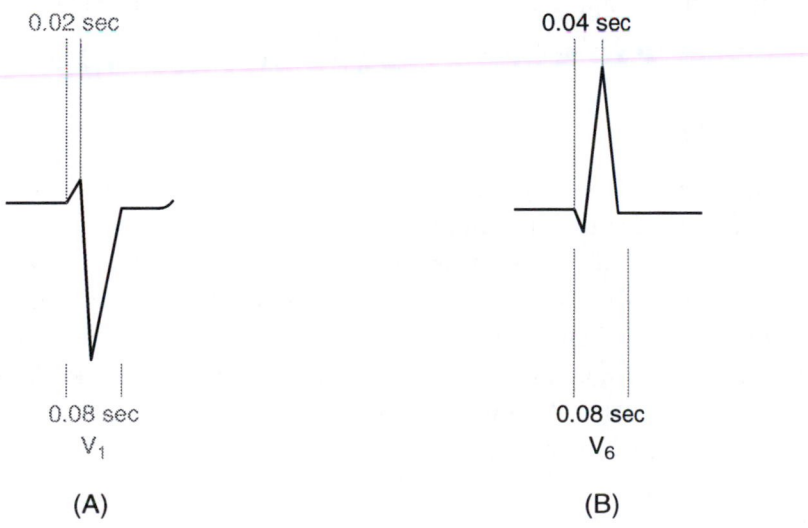

Figure 7-5 (A) VAT time for the right ventricle measured from the beginning of the QRS to the peak of the small R wave in V_1; (B) VAT time for the left ventricle measured from the beginning of the QRS to the peak of the R wave in V_6.

Left Bundle Branch Block Resulting from Myocardial Infarction. Left bundle branch block can result from arterial occlusion and concomitant with a myocardial infarction. Though left bundle branch block can be a preexisting disease, it most commonly occurs after anterior wall myocardial infarction.

In left bundle branch block, septal activation has to be reversed. Recall that the left bundle branches are incapable of conduction, therefore, depolarization of the right ventricle appears first, followed by the left. Consequently, any Q waves that originate because of left ventricular problems are obscured. Without clear Q waves, it's really difficult to confirm the diagnosis of myocardial infarction.

Many clinicians believe that the ECG is not helpful in diagnosing an MI in the presence of left bundle branch block. When left bundle branch block is present, an upright T wave in V_5 and V_6 may indicate ischemia in that area. This is because the ST segment and T wave in left bundle branch block are usually opposite in polarity from the terminal portion of the QRS (a secondary T wave). When the ST segment and T wave are of the same polarity of the terminal portion of the QRS, (a primary T wave), this is an acute sign of a possible ischemia. Therefore, with ECG changes of left bundle branch block and positive T waves are present in a lead with a negative terminal QRS, the clinician must suspect an acute MI is in progress. Other ECG findings with left bundle branch block and myocardial infarction are:

- decrease in R wave amplitude over left ventricular leads;
- Q waves in I, aVL, or V_6 greater than 0.04 second, which may indicate anteroseptal or lateral wall myocardial infarction; and
- ST segment and T wave displacement, affecting the normal ST segment convex appearance

While these changes may be useful indicators, there is no way to diagnose an acute myocardial infarction in the presence of left bundle branch block using the ECG. Nevertheless, the presence of left bundle branch block should alert the clinician to the possibility of an MI. The patient who presents with acute chest pain, shortness of breath, diaphoresis, pallor, and all the clinical findings of an acute MI should be treated appropriately. In these circumstances, the ECG is a valuable tool that must be supported with clinical correlation.

FASCICULAR BLOCKS

The main left bundle divides early into the anterior-superior and the posterior-inferior branches. Conduction abnormalities through the left anterior branch result in a marked degree of frontal plane left axis deviation called left anterior **fascicular block** (LAFB) or left anterior **hemiblock** (LAH). Similarly, a conduction abnormality through the left posterior branch results in a marked degree of frontal plane right axis deviation and is called *left posterior fascicular block* (LPHB) or *left posterior hemiblock* (LPH). The anatomic distribution of this branch makes isolated left posterior fascicular block rare.

Left Anterior Fascicular Block

Blood to the left anterior fascicle is supplied from the septal branch of the left anterior descending coronary artery. In some instances, there is an additional blood sup-

● fascicular block

Disruption in conduction within one or more of the extensions of the bundle branches

● hemiblock

Also known as fascicular block; disruption in conduction within one or more of the extensions of the bundle branches

ply from the AV nodal branch of the right coronary artery. LAH can be congenital or can occur with hypertensive heart disease, aortic valve disease and cardiomyopathy. LAH can also be intermittent, rate-related or transient. Clinically, the most common cause is arterial occlusion involving the ventricular septum, with acute anterior myocardial infraction, but it can also occur with inferior wall myocardial infarction.

The sequence of ventricular activation in left anterior fascicular block causes delayed activation of the superior aspect of the left ventricular wall. The abnormal ventricular activation process causes large, late ventricular forces oriented superiorly and to the left. The activation process begins in the inferior-posterior aspects of the left ventricle, which depolarizes first through the intact left posterior-inferior branch.

Patients with fascicular block must be closely monitored for **bifascicular block** (RBBB and LAH), also known as *complete heart block*. The QRS is usually 0.10 second and presents with a rS in leads II, III, and aVF. The negative amplitude of the QRS is most prominent in lead III and the axis is shifted to the far left. There may be small Q waves in leads I and aVL. Figure 7-6 is an illustration of ECG changes with left anterior fascicular block.

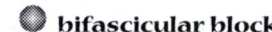

bifascicular block

The term that describes right bundle branch block occurring concomitantly with left anterior fascicular block

The ECG characteristics of left anterior fascicular block include:

- QRS complex usually at 0.10 second;
- left axis deviation of −40 degrees or more;
- rS in leads II, III, and aVF, with no terminal R wave;
- small Q waves in leads I and aVL due to the shift of initial forces inferiorly and to the right; and
- a terminal r or R in aVR

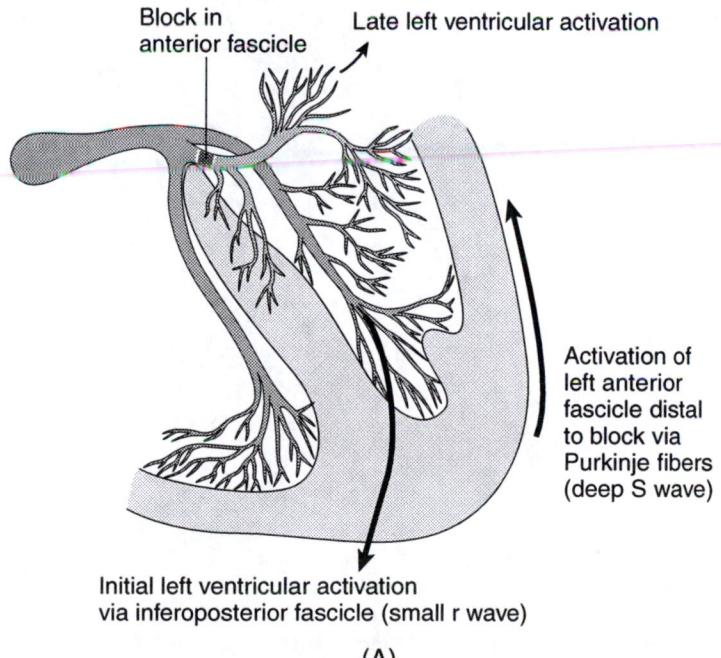

Block in anterior fascicle

Late left ventricular activation

Activation of left anterior fascicle distal to block via Purkinje fibers (deep S wave)

Initial left ventricular activation via inferoposterior fascicle (small r wave)

(A)

Figure 7-6   (A) Left anterior fascicular block. *(continues)*

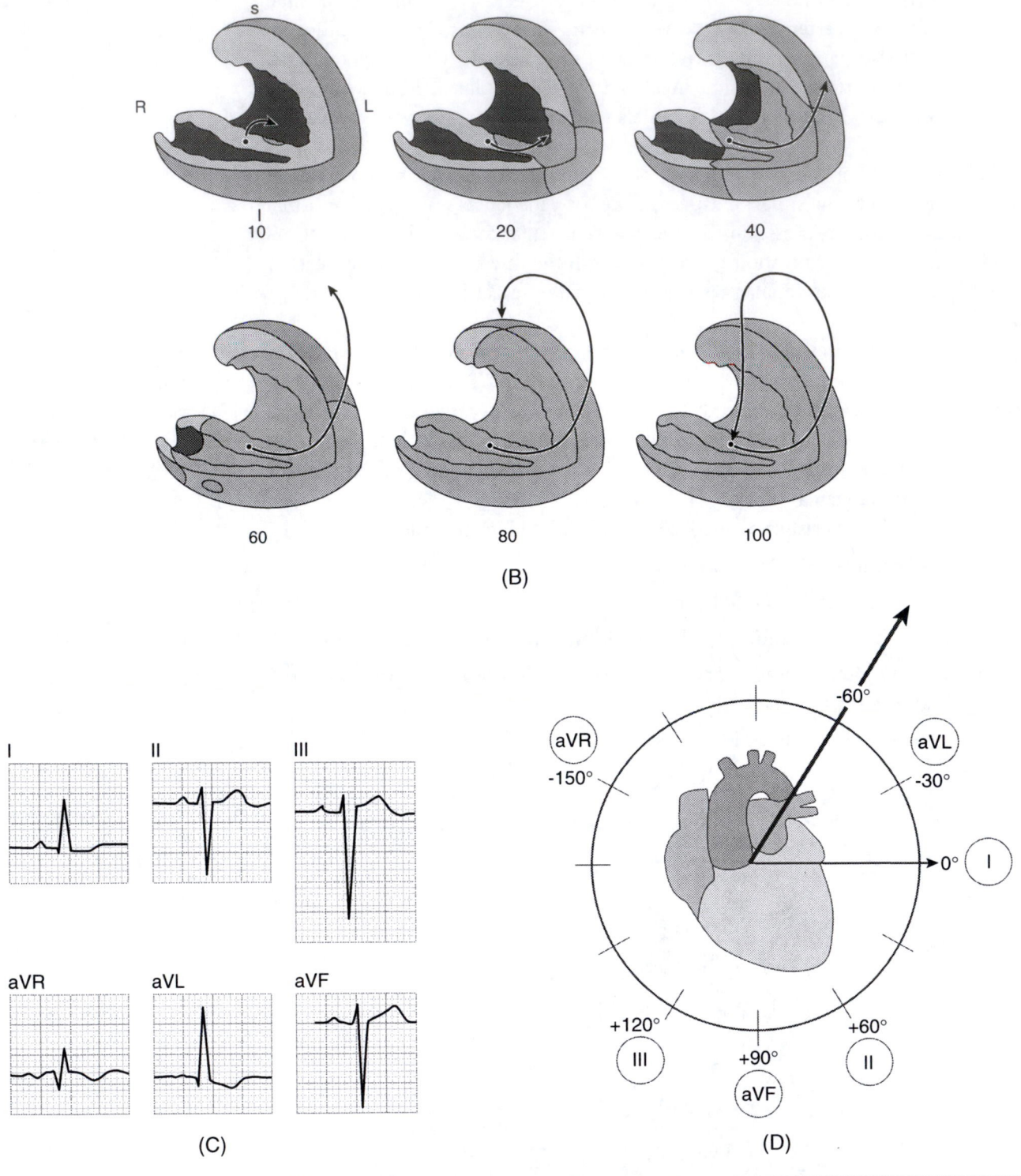

(B)

(C)

(D)

Figure 7-6 (Continued) (B) The sequence of activation from 10 to 100 milliseconds. QRS vectors in the frontal plane with the corresponding areas of the ventricles being depolarized in patients with left anterior hemiblock. The QRS vector is superimposed on the heart with the corresponding darkened areas of the ventricles as they are being depolarized. Note the normal inferior orientation of the QRS during the first 10 to 20 milliseconds. The QRS vectors continue with counterclockwise rotation causing a marked superior displacement of the maximum forces of the QRS; left axis deviation. (C) Associated ECG changes. Note that the QRS complex is an rS configuration in leads II, III, and aVF; the Rs configuration in leads I and aVL. (D) The Lewis circle plotting the mean flow of current as affected by LAFB. The two arrows directed superior and to the left indicate a superior, leftward shift. The QRS in lead III is most negative of the limb leads and leads I and aVL are positive, with lead I the most positive.

Left Anterior Fascicular Block and RBBB

Left anterior fascicular block (LAH) can occur with right bundle branch block, because the structures involved are similar and share much of the same blood supply. On the ECG right bundle branch block is recognized in V1; if the S wave is greater than the R wave, then left axis deviation is present. When right bundle branch block is concomitant with a left anterior fascicular block it is called bifascicular block. Often the LAH obscures the RBBB.

ECG characteristics of bifascicular block are:

- QRS complex usually at 0.10 second;
- RBBB pattern with left axis deviation (RBBB + LAH); and
- RBBB pattern with right axis deviation (RBBB + LPH)

Left Anterior Fascicular Block and Myocardial Infarction

If some portion of the anterior wall is involved with inferior wall myocardial infarction (IWMI), or if the AV nodal artery is affected as with proximal right coronary artery disease, LAH may obscure the ECG signs of MI. The Q wave one would anticipate will be missing from leads II, III, and aVF. In addition, IWMI and LAH can each cause left axis deviation. With IWMI an axis shift is usually leftward to about 30 degrees. This is due to the loss of inferior forces. If the axis is 60 degrees, concomitant LAH is probably the cause.

An analytical assessment can still be made. Recall, LAH with or without IWMI will produce deep S waves in lead II but no terminal r wave. In aVR a terminal r or R will occur with LAH.

Left Posterior Fascicular Block

Left posterior fascicular block (LPFB), also called left posterior hemiblock (LPH), is caused by an obstruction of the posterior-inferior division of the left bundle branch block. Isolated LPFB is rare since it is shorter and thicker than the anterior fascicle and has a dual blood supply. LPFB has more serious clinical implications since it implies compromise to both the right and left coronary arteries as well as damage to large areas of myocardial muscle and to the electrical conduction system in the left ventricle. In patients with posterior or lateral wall myocardial infarction LAFB is often associated with RBBB.

When left posterior fascicular block is present, the sequence of activation is characterized by initial depolarization of the anterior-superior aspect of the left ventricle. This causes the QRS forces to be oriented superiorly and to the right or left. Late activation of the posterior-inferior walls of the left ventricle results in large forces oriented inferiorly and to the right. The left ventricle is depolarized by a left anterior fascicle and right axis deviation is obvious. There are tall R waves in lead III, and an rS wave in leads I and aVL. Right axis deviation can be caused by other conditions; for instance, right ventricular hypertrophy, chronic obstructive lung disease, and lateral wall myocardial infarction. Each of these has to be ruled out clinically before making the diagnosis of left posterior fascicular block. Figure 7-7 is a illustration of ECG changes with left posterior fascicular block.

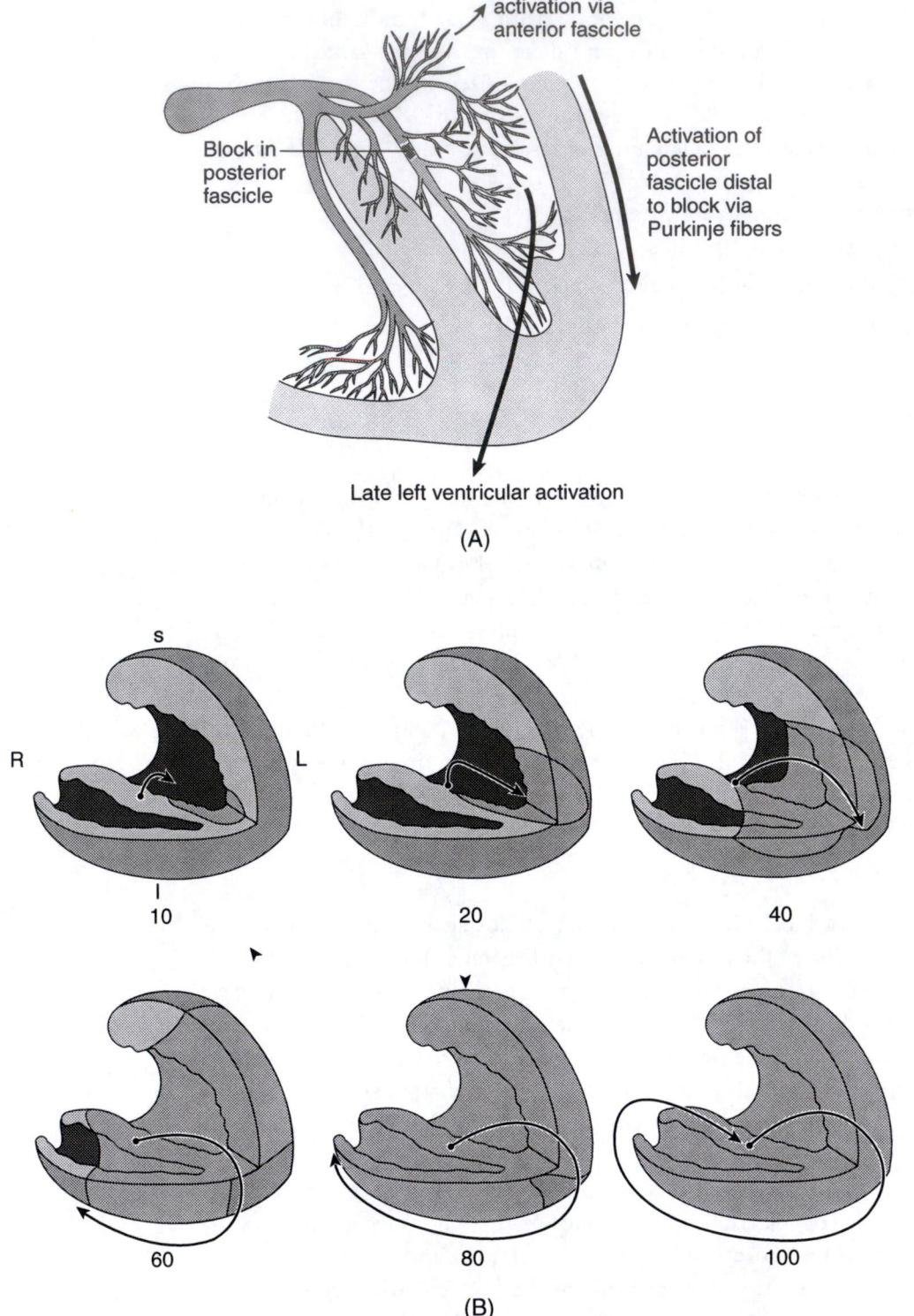

Figure 7-7 (A) Left posterior fascicular block; (B) The sequence of activation from 10 to 100 milliseconds. QRS vectors are shown with the corresponding area of the ventricles being depolarized in patients with left posterior hemiblock. The QRS vector is superimposed on the heart with corresponding darkened areas of the ventricles as they are being depolarized. Note the superior orientation of the QRS during the first 10 to 20 milliseconds. The QRS vectors continue and the result is the anterior and rightward orientation of the maximum QRS forces. *(continues)*

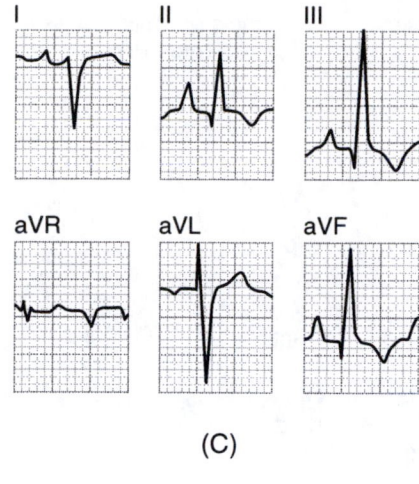

(C)

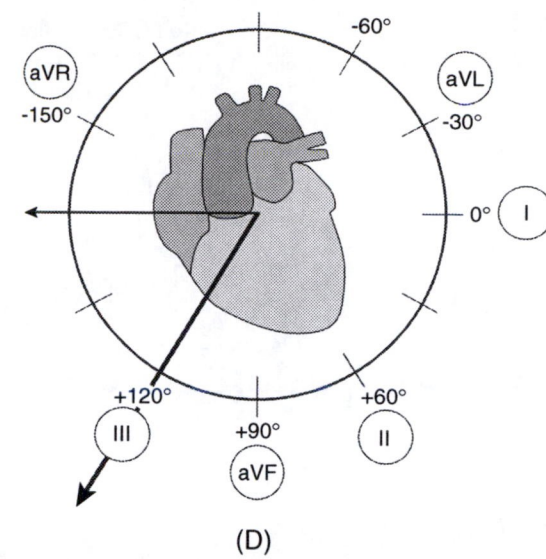

(D)

Figure 7-7 Continued (C) The associated ECG changes. The QRS complex is prolonged, greater than 0.10 second; note the rS configuration in leads I and aVL and the Rs configuration in leads II, III, and aVF. (D) The Lewis circle plotting the mean flow of current as affected by LPFB. The longer arrow is directed inferior and to the right indicating a rightward shift. The QRS in lead III is most positive of the limb leads; leads I and aVL are negative, with lead I the most negative.

COMPLETE LEFT BUNDLE BRANCH BLOCK

With complete left bundle branch block (CLBBB), the QRS axis is usually within normal limits or a mild degree of left axis deviation (LAD). Complete left bundle branch block with marked degree of LAD could represent the result of complete block of the anterior division of the left bundle, with partial block of the posterior division. Complete left bundle branch block and a marked degree of right axis deviation (RAD) probably represents a complete block of the posterior division with a partial block of the anterior division. In isolated complete left anterior hemiblock, there is a marked degree of left axis deviation, usually secondary to complete block of the anterior division of the left bundle. Isolated left posterior hemiblock usually shows a marked degree of right axis deviation that is due to complete block of the posterior division of the left bundle.

Figure 7-8 summarizes the implications of various levels of conduction defects within the left bundle branch.

Table 7-1 provides an overview of conduction abnormalities of the left bundle, indicating the site of the conduction defect, the direction of the QRS axis, and the duration of the QRS complex.

TRIFASCICULAR BLOCK

A block located in each of the three main fascicles on the bundle branch system is called a **trifascicular block**. If the block is complete, the patient will be left with an escape ventricular pacemaker below the lesions. Assessment of the ECG involves

● **trifascicular block**

A block is located in each of the three main fascicles on the bundle branch system

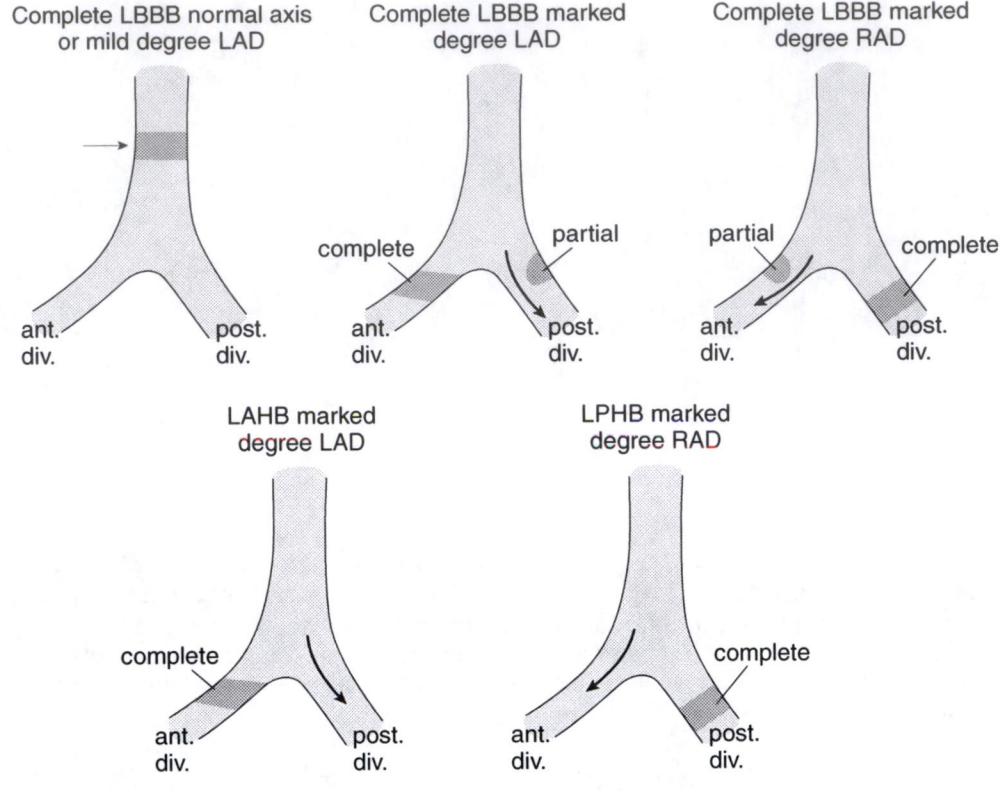

Figure 7-8 Types of left bundle branch conduction defects and associated axis deviations

Table 7-1 Summary of conduction abnormalities of the left bundle, indicating the site of the conduction defect, the direction of the QRS axis, and the duration of the QRS complex.

Conduction Defect	Site of the Defect	Axis	QRS duration
Left anterior hemiblock	anterior-superior branch	above -45°	0.12 second or less
Left posterior hemiblock	posterior-inferior branch	greater than +100°	0.12 second or less
Complete left bundle branch block	left main	below -30°	0.14 second or more
Complete left bundle branch block with left axis deviation	complete anterior-superior branch	above -45°	0.14 second or more
Complete left bundle branch block with right axis deviation	complete posterior-inferior branch partial superior-inferior branch	greater than +110°	0.14 second or more

reviewing leads II, III, and aVF for axis shift with LAH as well as assessment of the PR interval for signs of complete AV block. Lead V_1 should be assessed for RBBB. In addition, the clinician should look for the following:

- rS in leads II, III, and aVF, with no terminal R wave;
- small Q waves in leads I and aVL due to the shift of initial forces inferiorly and to the right; and
- a terminal r or R will occur in aVR

Summary

Structure and function are related throughout the human body. The heart is especially revealing when there is the slightest alteration in its electrical system. Without the flow of electric impulses the muscular pump fails to be effective. The 12-lead ECG reveals in its entirety the framework of the heart's critical action potential. Nutrition via arterial blood flow is as important to the bundle branch system as it is to the myocardium.

Self-Assessment Exercises

● ECG Rhythm Identification Practice

Identify the ECG criterion listed below each ECG. Use the Lewis circle to help with calculation of axis. Compare your answers with those in the back of the book.

Figure 7-9

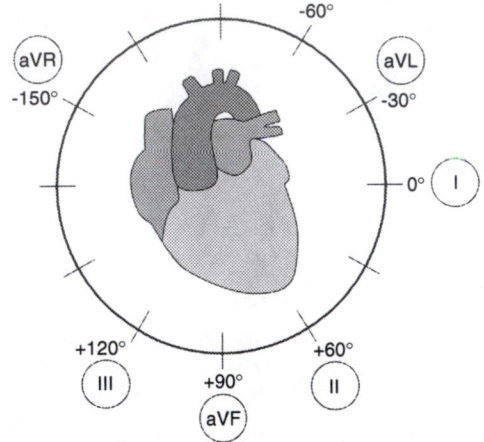

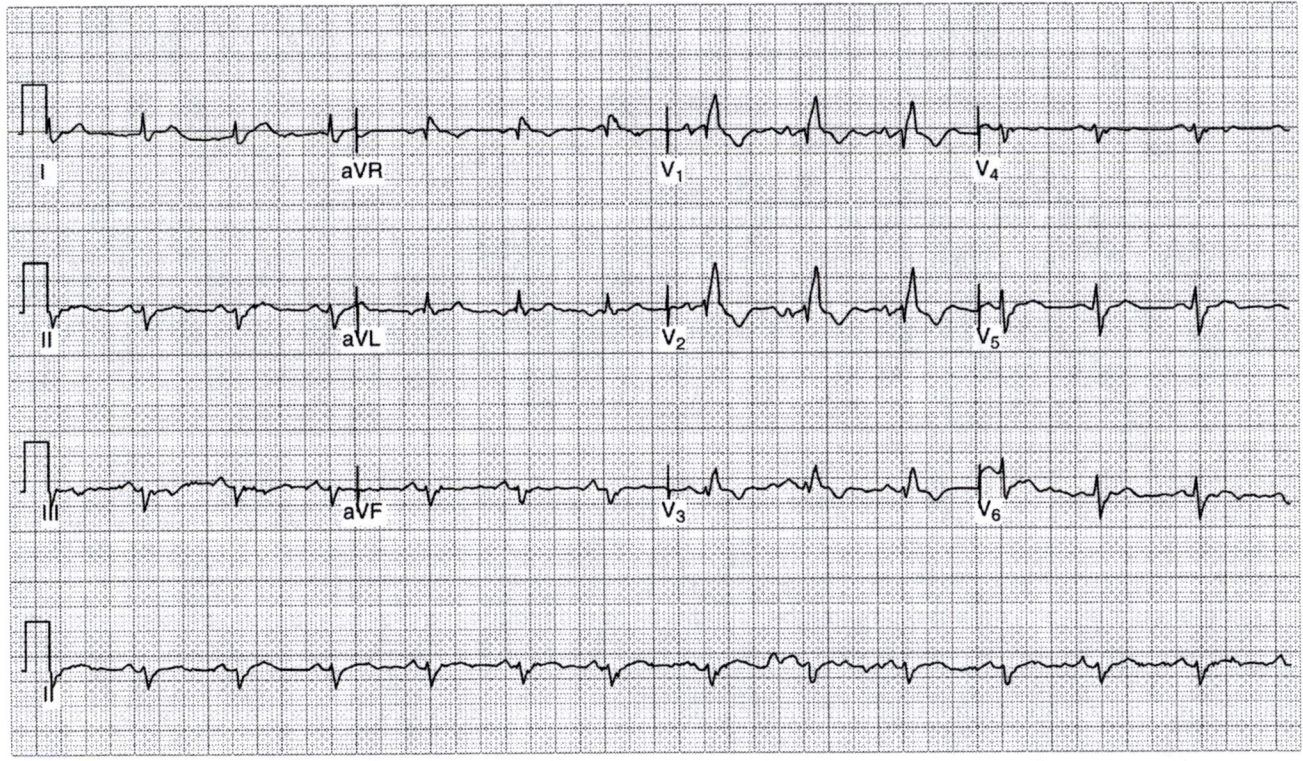

1. What is the underlying rhythm? _____

2. What are the acute changes? _____

3. What is your interpretation? _____

    _____

4. What can happen next? _____

    _____

Figure 7-10

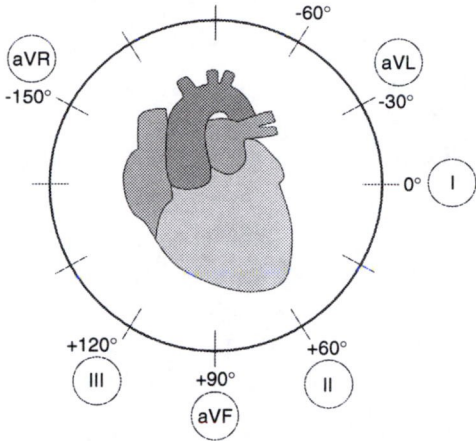

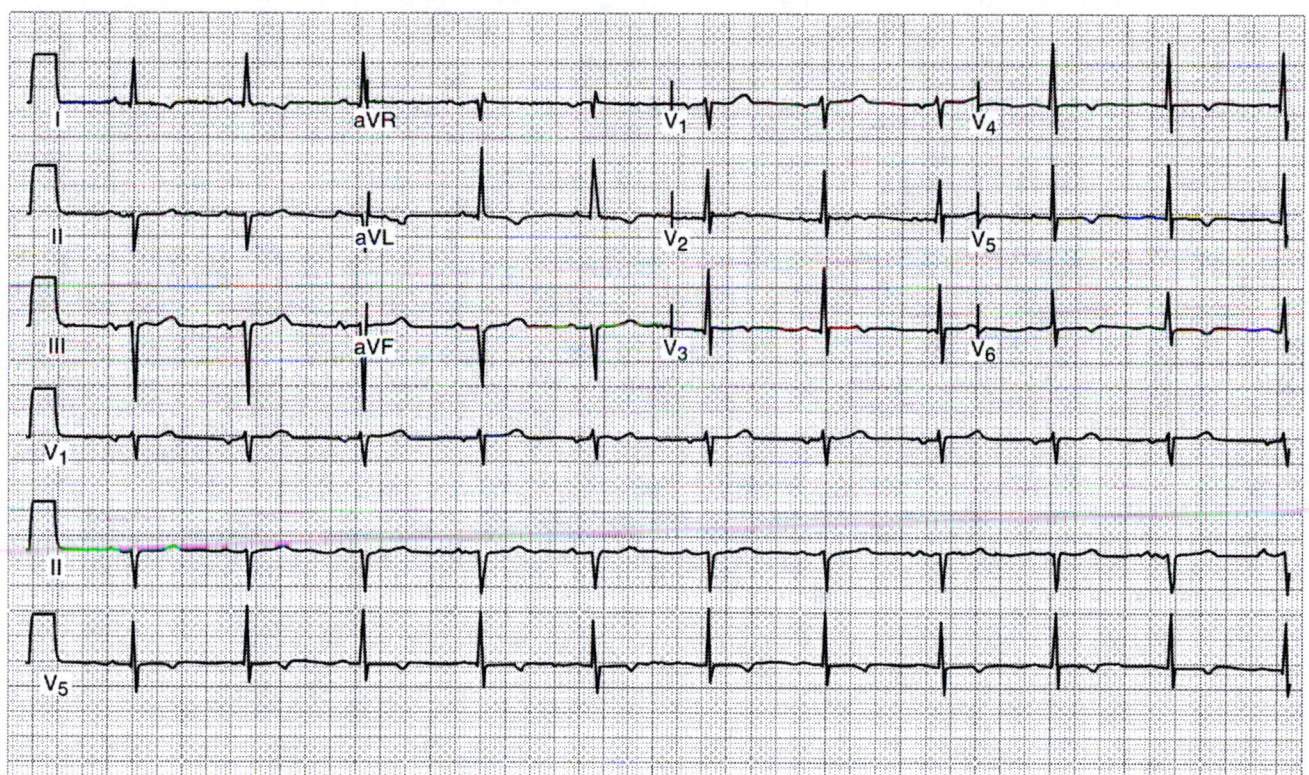

1. What is the underlying rhythm? _____

2. What are the acute changes? _____

3. What is your interpretation? _____

_____

4. What can happen next? _____

_____

Figure 7-11

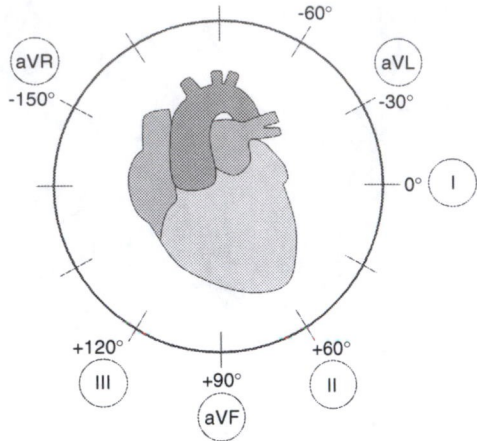

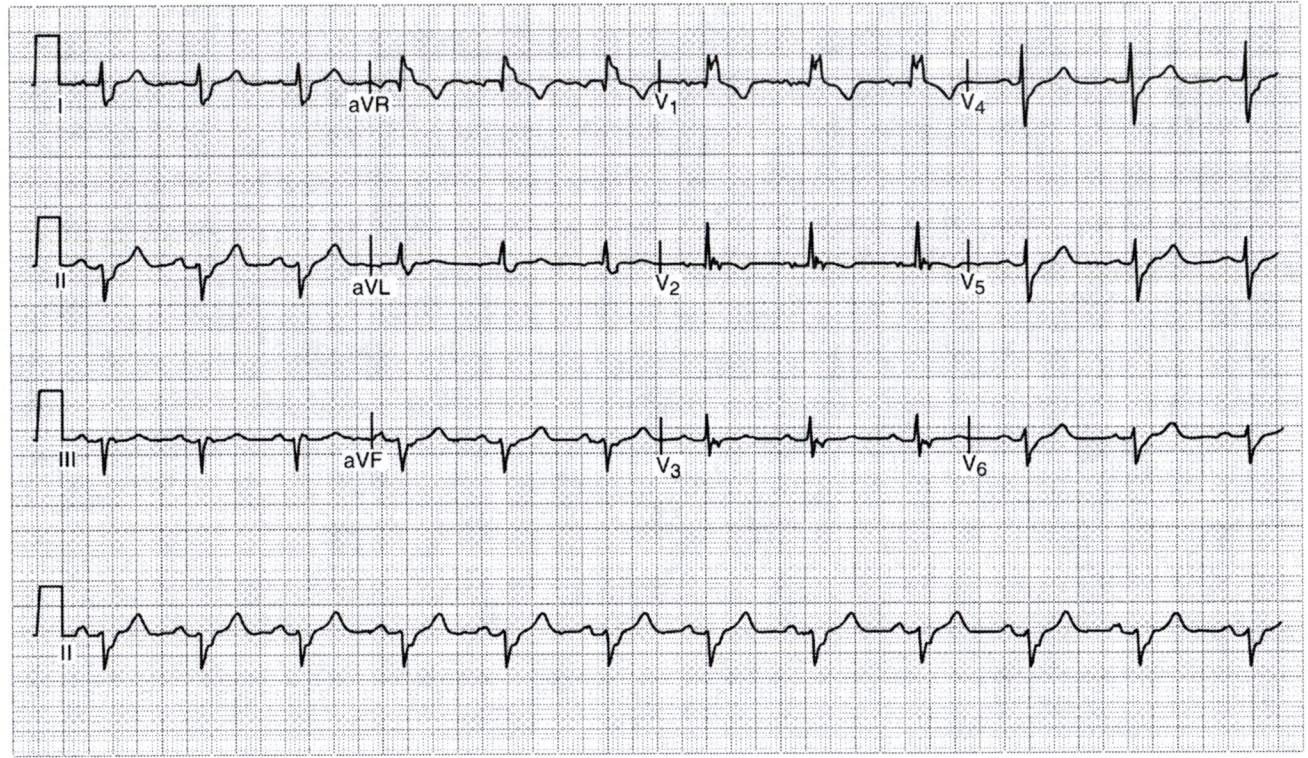

1. What is the underlying rhythm? _____

2. What are the acute changes? _____

3. What is your interpretation? _____

_____

4. What can happen next? _____

_____

Figure 7-12

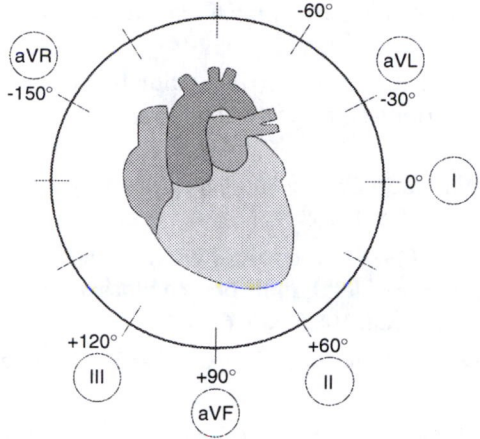

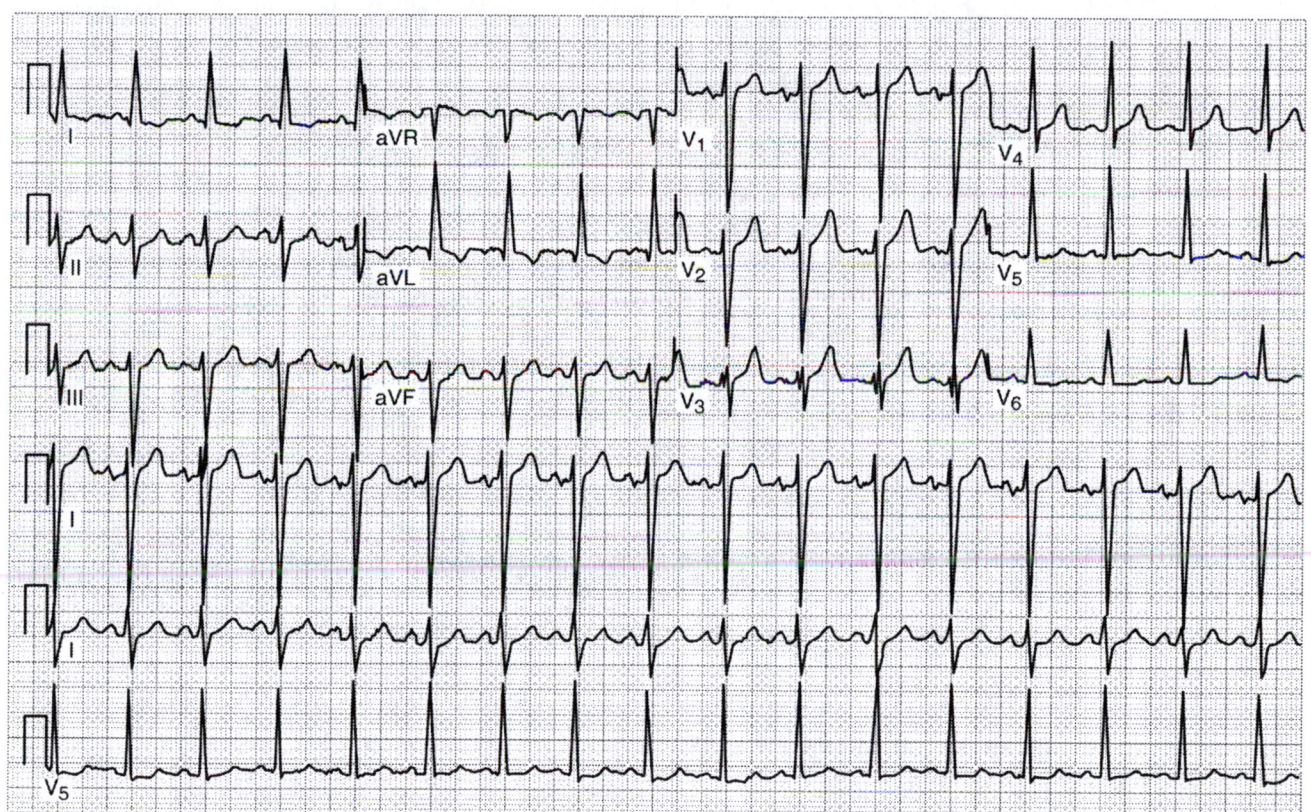

1. What is the underlying rhythm? _____
2. What are the acute changes? _____
3. What is your interpretation? _____
   _____
4. What can happen next? _____
   _____

References

Chou T. C. (1996). *Left ventricular hypertrophy in electrocardiography in clinical practice: Adult and pediatric.* Philadelphia: WB Saunders; 37-53.

Conover, M. B. (1996). *Understanding electrocardiography: Arrhythmias and the 12-lead ECG.* (7th ed.). St. Louis: Mosby-Year Book.

Flowers, N. S., Horan, L. F. & Wylds, A. C. (1990). Relations of peri-infarction block to ventricular late potentials in patients with inferior wall myocardial infarction. *American Journal of Cardiology*; 66:568.

Futterman, L. G. & Lemberg, L. (July 1999). Commotio Cordis: Sudden cardiac death in athletes. *American Journal of Critical Care.* Vol. 8. No. 4.

Klein, R. C., Vera, Z., DeMaria, A. N., Mason, D. T. (1984). Electrocardiographic diagnosis of left ventricular hypertrophy in the presence of left bundle branch block: An echocardiographic study. *American Heart Journal*; 108:502-506.

Mandel, W. J. (Ed.). (1987). *Cardiac arrhythmias: Their mechanisms, diagnoses and management.* (2nd ed). Philadelphia: Lippincott.

Marriott, H. J., & Conover, Mary, B. (1989). *Advanced concepts in arrhythmias* (2nd ed.). St. Louis: C.V. Mosby.

Okin, P. M., Roman, M. J., Devereux, R. B., & Kligfield, P. (1995). Electrocardiographic identification of left ventricular mass by simple voltage-duration products. *Journal of the American College of Cardiology*; 25:417-423.

Sgarbossa, E.B. & Wagner, G. (1998). Electrocardiography. In Topol, E. J., (Ed.). *Textbook of cardiovascular medicine.* Lippincott-Raven; 1545-1589.

Surawicz, B. (1998). Electrocardiographic diagnosis of chamber enlargement. *Journal of the American College of Cardiology*; 8:711-724.

Wellens, H. J. J. (1995). Atrioventricular nodal and subnodal conduction disturbances. In Willerson, J. R. & Cohn, J. N. (Eds.). *Cardiovascular medicine.* New York: Churchill Livingstone.

Zelender, M. et al. (1990). ECG variants and cardiac arrhythmias in athletes: Clinical relevance and prognostic importance. *American Heart Journal*; 119:1378.

Chamber Enlargement and Hypertrophy

Premise ⊙	Increased amplitude of ECG wave forms does not equal the diagnosis of hypertrophy or chamber enlargement.

Objectives

After reading the chapter and completing the Self-Assessment exercises, the student should be able to:

1. Identify the ECG characteristics of left and right atrial enlargement
2. Identify the ECG patterns seen in ventricular hypertrophy
3. Identify the ECG signs of ventricular strain pattern

Key Terms

hypertrophy   P mitrale   P pulmonale

Introduction

Patients who have atrial or ventricular hypertrophy or atrial or ventricular enlargement can have otherwise normal ECGs. ECG changes can be masked in patients who are obese and those patients who have chronic obstructive lung disease. This is because air and fat are very poor electrical conductors, so these changes may be masked or lost to the clinician using the ECG as a diagnostic tool. Patients with normal hearts may show ECG changes indicative of enlargement of atria and the ventricles or even hypertrophy, because they have a very thin chest wall or simply as a normal variant.

RIGHT ATRIAL ENLARGEMENT

Recall that P waves represent atrial depolarization. In right atrial enlargement, the P wave in lead II is 3 mm or greater in amplitude and may have a normal duration. Such P waves are referred to as **P pulmonale**. Right atrial enlargement (RAE) is frequently accompanied by right ventricular hypertrophy. Figure 8-1 is an illustration of the increased amplitude of a P wave.

⊙ **P pulmonale**

Peaked abnormal P waves

P pulmonale

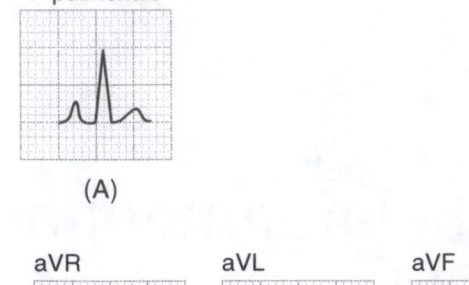

(A)

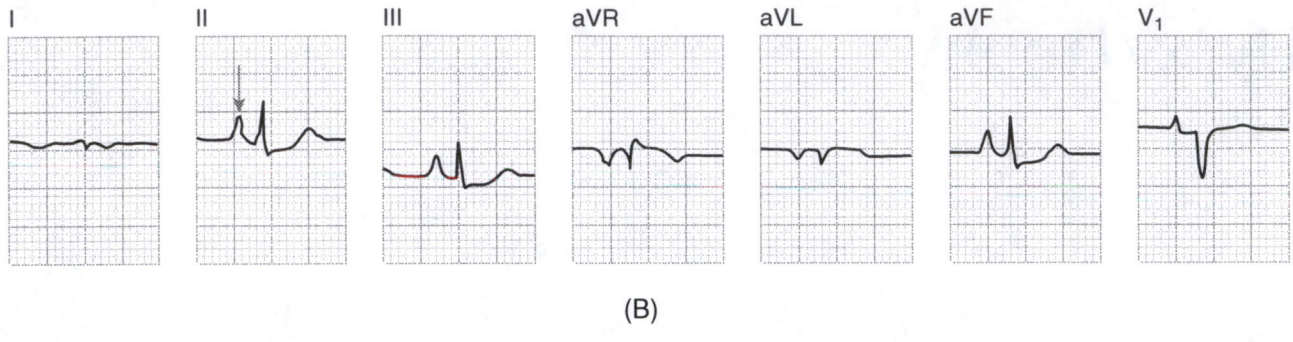

(B)

Figure 8-1 (A) PQRST complex with a P wave of 3 mm and 0.08 second; (B) frontal plane ECG tracing showing increased P wave amplitude significant for P pulmonale

The most frequent causes for right atrial enlargement are:
- pulmonary hypertension;
- pulmonary emboli;
- chronic pulmonary disease;
- pulmonary valve disease; and
- tricuspid valve disease

LEFT ATRIAL ENLARGEMENT

The presence of left atrial enlargement (LAE) is revealed on the terminal configuration of the P wave. First of all, the P wave is increased to about 0.12 second or more and may have a notched or diphasic appearance in lead II. This is called **P mitrale** and suggests LAE. Figure 8-2 contains ECG tracings showing the increased duration and change in morphology of a P mitrale.

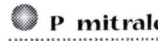 **P mitrale**

Notched abnormal P waves

The most frequent causes for left atrial enlargement are:
- systemic hypertension;
- aortic valve disease;
- mitral valve disease; and
- left ventricular failure

VENTRICULAR HYPERTROPHY

In ventricular hypertrophy the increase in muscle mass, secondary to hemodynamic effects of pressure or volume load, exaggerates the vectorial forces generated by the left ventricle. For instance, mitral valve disease causing insufficiency can pro-

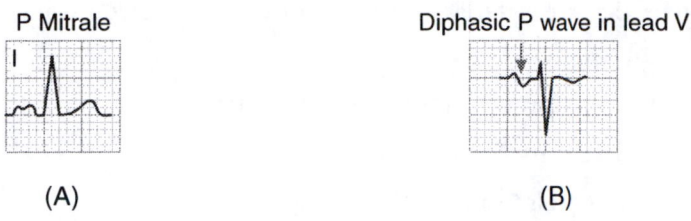

P Mitrale

Diphasic P wave in lead V$_1$

(A)

(B)

Figure 8-2 ECG tracings showing changes in P wave morphology associated with P mitrale. (A) a notched P wave is visible in lead I; (B) a diphasic P wave is seen in lead V$_1$.

mote retrograde blood flow and chamber enlargement. As a result, the increased workload will cause an increase in left ventricular mass called hypertrophy. Figure 8-3 is an illustration of the relative size of the ventricle with hypertrophy.

Right Ventricular Hypertrophy

Because left ventricular activity overshadows the right, when right ventricular hypertrophy is visible on the ECG the condition is extremely severe. The most useful clue to right ventricular hypertrophy is right axis deviation and abnormalities in V$_1$ (recall that V$_1$ faces the right ventricle). The most frequent causes for right ventricular hypertrophy are:

- congenital heart disease such as pulmonary stenosis, tetralogy of Fallot, and Eisenmenger's Syndrome;
- congenital defects with ventricular overload;
- mitral insufficiency with pulmonary hypertension, mitral stenosis;
- primary pulmonary disease;
- pulmonary vascular hypertension;
- pulmonary emboli; and
- pulmonary stenosis

hypertrophy

A condition in which there is an increase in left ventricular muscle mass as a result of increased workload on the heart

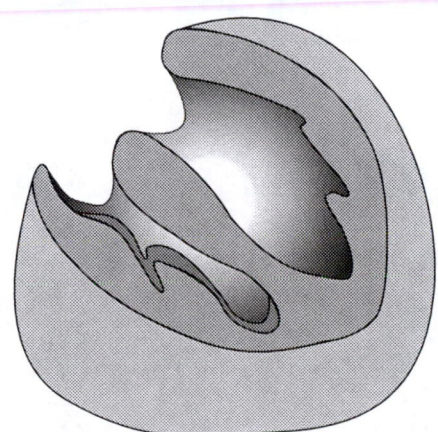

Figure 8-3 An illustration of the change in the relative size of the right ventricular wall with hypertrophy. Note the thickness in the myocardial layer, as well as the affected septum and the papillary muscles. Also note the change in volume capacity of the affected ventricle.

ECG changes that are criteria for right ventricular hypertrophy include:

- right axis deviation;
- R wave height to S wave depth ratio greater than 1 in V_1;
- R wave equals 7 mm in V_1;
- S wave equals 7 mm in V_5 and V_6;
- R wave in V_1 plus the S wave in V_5 or V_6 is greater than 10 mm;
- rSr with R wave greater than 10 mm or qRS pattern in V_1;
- right ventricular strain pattern; and
- associated right atrial enlargement .

Figure 8-3 illustrates change in the relative size of the ventricular wall and the change in volume capacity of the affected ventricle, while Figure 8-4 illustrates the sequence of activation in right ventricular hypertrophy.

Left Ventricular Hypertrophy

Left ventricular muscle mass in the normal human heart is roughly 2 to 3 times thicker than right ventricular muscle mass. This is due to the force with which blood

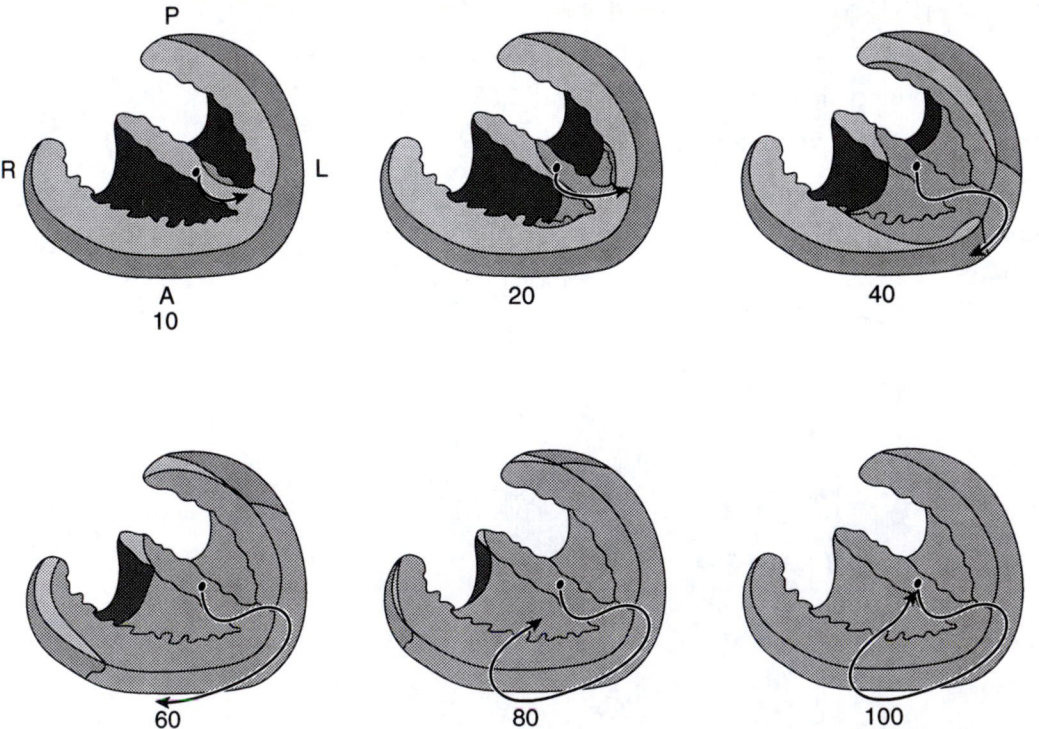

Figure 8-4 Sequence of ventricular activation from 10 to 100 milliseconds as displayed in the horizontal plane in **right** ventricular hypertrophy. The QRS vector is superimposed on the heart with the corresponding cleared areas of the ventricles as they are being depolarized.

is pumped into systemic circulation, which can be 10 times greater than blood flow to the pulmonic circulation. The QRS complex depicted on a normal ECG represents depolarization of the ventricles and reflects left ventricular muscle mass. It follows, then, that left ventricular enlargement will be represented on the ECG by changes in the duration of the QRS complex in some of the leads.

Common causes of left ventricular hypertrophy include:

- systemic arterial hypertension;
- aortic stenosis or insufficiency;
- coarctation of the aorta;
- hypertrophic cardiomyopathy;
- primary pulmonary disease; and
- mitral insufficiency

There are major criteria for assessment of the ECG and determinants of left ventricular hypertrophy:

1. Direction of the QRS vector

2. QRS duration

3. QRS morphology

4. Voltage criteria

5. Axis

Changes in the QRS. In left ventricular hypertrophy (LVH), the QRS vector is directed somewhat more leftward and more posterior, greater than 30 degrees. Figure 8-5 illustrates the change in the relative size of the left ventricular wall. The ECG leads show changes reflecting the hypertrophy. Figure 8-6 illustrates the sequence of activation in left ventricular hypertrophy. Measurement and shape of the QRS (0.10 or less) is rarely changed as a result of the sequence of depolarization remaining the same.

Voltage Criteria. There are several ways to determine the presence of left ventricular hypertrophy using the 12-lead ECG, and many point systems for more elaborate identification. It is best to work with a method that uses 2 levels of certainty: voltage criteria and secondary ST-T changes. The clinician should not favor any one criteria, but adapt to the patient circumstance by taking into consideration individual variables. In fact, using voltage criteria alone can result in a false negative identification.

The most common change in the ECG is the increased voltage of the mean QRS vector, reflected in the tall R waves in leads I and/or aVL, V_3, or V_6. Deep S waves in V_1 may also be seen.

The amplitude of the R wave is greater than 27 mm in V_5 or greater than 25 mm in V_6. (This application has merit for those patients older than 35 years).

There are many methods that can be used to determine voltage. The methods outlined here are the Index of Lewis, R wave height, Sokolow-Lyon criteria, R/S voltage criteria, and the Cornell voltage test.

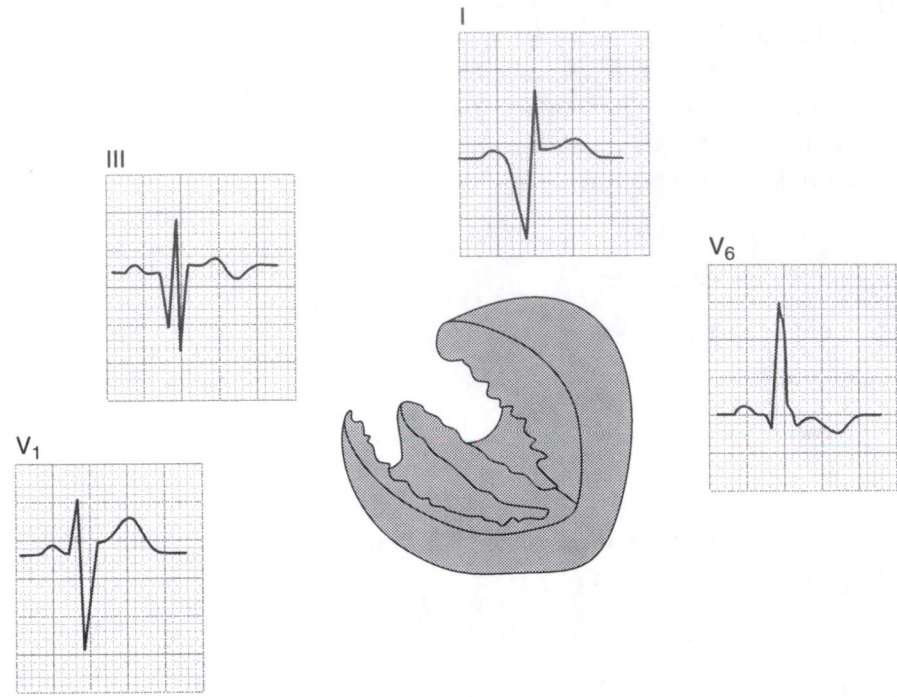

Figure 8-5 Illustration of the heart showing excessive thickness of the left ventricle and the septum. The ECG leads demonstrate evidence of LVH by R/S voltage criteria; $SV_1 + RV_6 = {>}35$ mm.

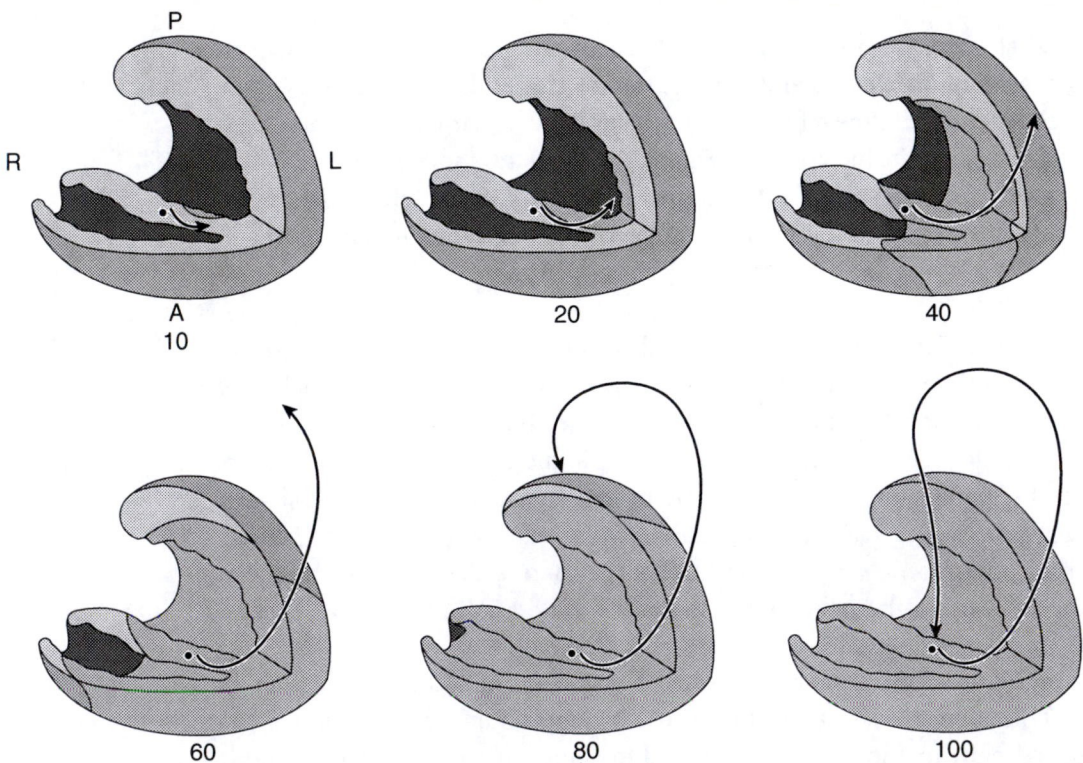

Figure 8-6 Sequence of ventricular activation from 10 to 100 milliseconds as displayed in the horizontal plane in **left** ventricular hypertrophy. The QRS vector is superimposed on the heart with the corresponding cleared areas of the ventricles as they are being depolarized.

There are natural instances of increased amplitude in the QRS complexes of young persons with slight builds who tend to have a higher voltage. The Lewis criteria can differentiate in such cases, with fewer false positives. Also, if left anterior fascicular block is present, the increased voltage criteria will correct for this factor. (See LVH with LBBB and LVH with RBBB in Chapter 7.) The Index of Lewis criteria is outlined below.

Add:

the net positive deflection in lead I in mm

+ the net negative deflection in lead III in mm

= > 21 mm = left ventricular hypertrophy

The Height of the R Wave. The height of the R wave in aVL should measure greater than 13 mm. Although this system is straightforward, there are frequent false positives. Most authorities recommend use of the Index of Lewis or Sokolow-Lyon to confirm the interpretation using R wave height as a sole measure.

Sokolow-Lyon Criteria. This method is very popular, but is not recommended for patients *under* the age of 35 years:
1. Look at leads V_1, V_5, and V_6
2. When the S wave in V_1 plus the R wave in V_5 or V_6 is 35 mm or greater, it is positive for LVH ($SV_1 + RV_5$ or $RV_6 = >35$ mm is indicative of LVH).

Figure 8-7 shows a 12-lead ECG illustrating the relative size of QRS complexes consistent with left ventricular hypertrophy.

R/S Voltage Criteria.
- The R wave in aVL is greater than 11 mm; or
- The S wave in V_1 (SV_1) plus the R wave in V_5 (RV_5) or the R wave in V_6 (RV_6) is greater than 35 mm; or
- The R wave in V_5 or V_6 is greater than 25 mm.

The specificity is greater than 95 percent using this criteria, but the sensitivity is low, less than 30 percent.

Cornell Voltage Test. Add the height of the R wave in aVL and the depth of the S wave in V_3. If the result is greater than 28 mm in males or greater than 20 mm in females, left ventricular hypertrophy is present. This test has a sensitivity, or true positive rate, of 42 percent and a specificity, or true negative rate, of 96 percent.

Axis. In left ventricular hypertrophy there is a leftward, posterior shift and poor R wave progression across the precordium. Occasionally, there is loss of terminal rightward forces manifested by the presence of secondary ST and T wave abnormalities.

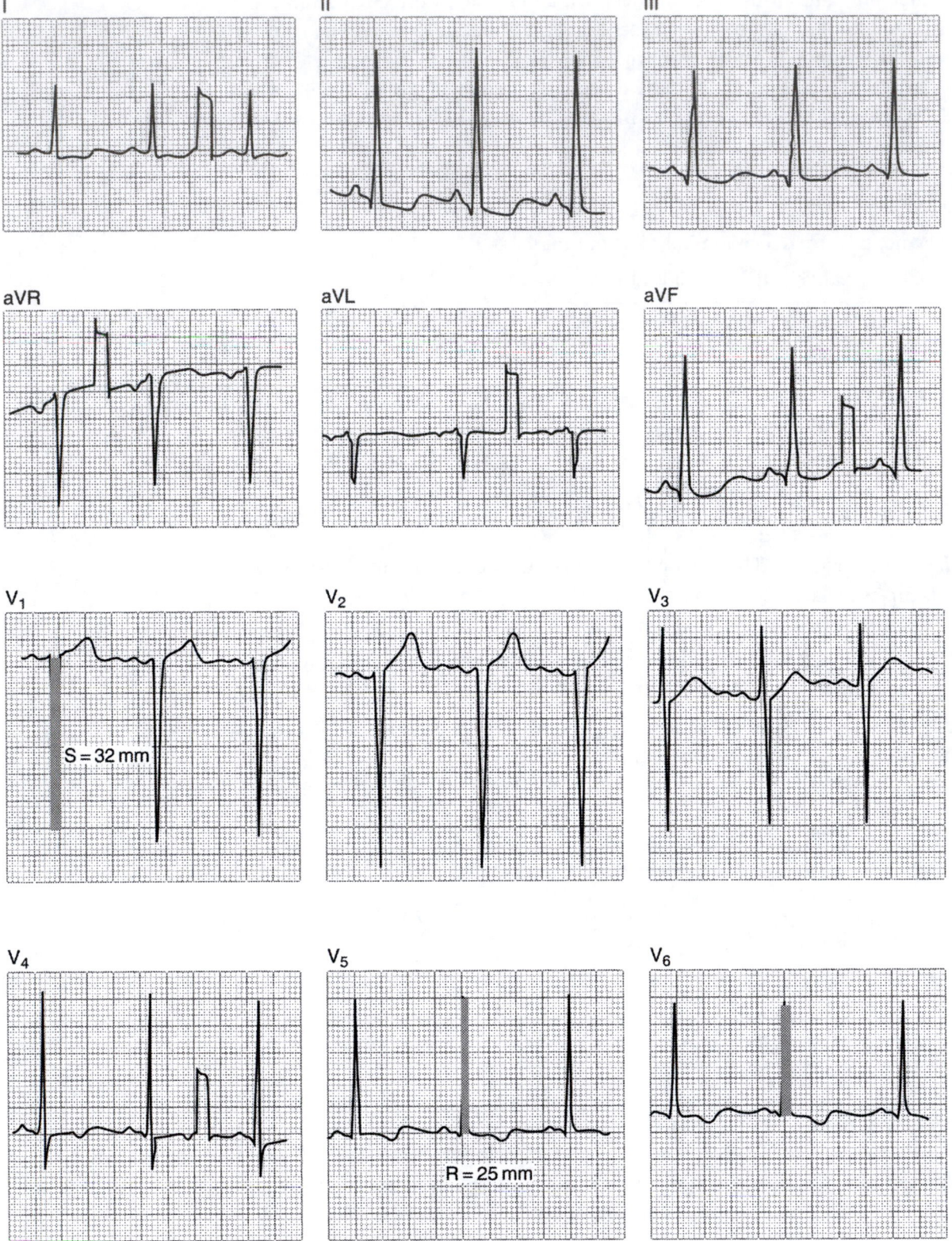

Figure 8-7 A 12-lead ECG illustrating QRS complexes (shaded) with left ventricular hypertrophy. Look at leads V_1, V_5, or V_6. Add the values of the S wave in V_1 plus the value of the R wave in V_5 or RV_6. Note the value is greater than 35 mm and, therefore, is indicative of LVH.

Left Ventricular Hypertrophy (LVH) with Left Bundle Branch block (LBBB). Most patients with LBBB also have anatomic left ventricular hypertrophy, making the increased duration of the QRS difficult to determine. Klein and colleagues found that the sum of the S wave amplitude in V_2 and the R wave amplitude in V_6 of 4.5 mV or more had an 86 percent sensitivity and a 100 percent specificity to detect left ventricular hypertrophy in patients with LBBB.

Left Ventricular Hypertrophy (LVH) with Right Bundle Branch Block (RBBB). The sensitivity of ECG criteria for LVH decreases in the presence of RBBB. A useful sign when these two exist is the presence of left atrial enlargement. The presence of a P wave terminal force in V_1 increases the sensitivity for LVH to over 70 percent with an approximate specificity of 80 percent. A Sokolow index of greater than or equal to 3.5 mV is 100 percent specific for LVH in patients who are not obese.

Ventricular Strain Pattern

Ventricular strain is denoted by ST segment and T wave changes that are frequently seen with ventricular hypertrophy. The reason for these changes is not altogether clear. It is thought that conduction delays through the thickened walls certainly play an important role as does ischemia due to the increase in muscle fiber diameter. Left ventricular strain manifests on the ECG with ST segment depression and asymmetrical T wave inversion in leads that face the affected ventricle, I, aVL, V_5, and V_6. The affected ST segments have a downsloped appearance, frequently referred to as hockey stick in shape.

Reciprocal ST elevation in upright T waves is seen in V_1 and V_2 which face the right ventricle; therefore, left ventricular hypertrophy with a strain pattern will cause 1 mm to 2 mm of ST elevation in V_1 and V_2 and may be mistaken for an acute injury pattern. Right ventricular strain shows the same kind of ST segment changes in left ventricular strain, but in different leads. In right ventricular strain, leads V_1, V_2, II, III, and aVF show ST segment depression with asymmetrical T wave inversion. Figure 8-8 shows two 12-lead ECGs illustrating ventricular hypertrophy and strain.

There are several ECG changes with ventricular strain. Secondary ST-T wave changes, sometimes referred to as left *ventricular strain pattern*, are the most suggestive criteria. The spatial changes can be approximated by identifying:

- sagging ST segments and inverted T waves in every lead with a tall R wave; and

- a rising ST and upright T in every lead with a deep S wave.

The ECG diagnosis of hypertrophy and strain is not realistic without a 12-lead ECG. However, clinical presentation and medical history are vital in validating changes with the 12-lead in the clinical setting.

Left ventricular strain pattern

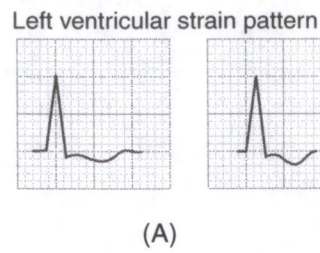

(A)

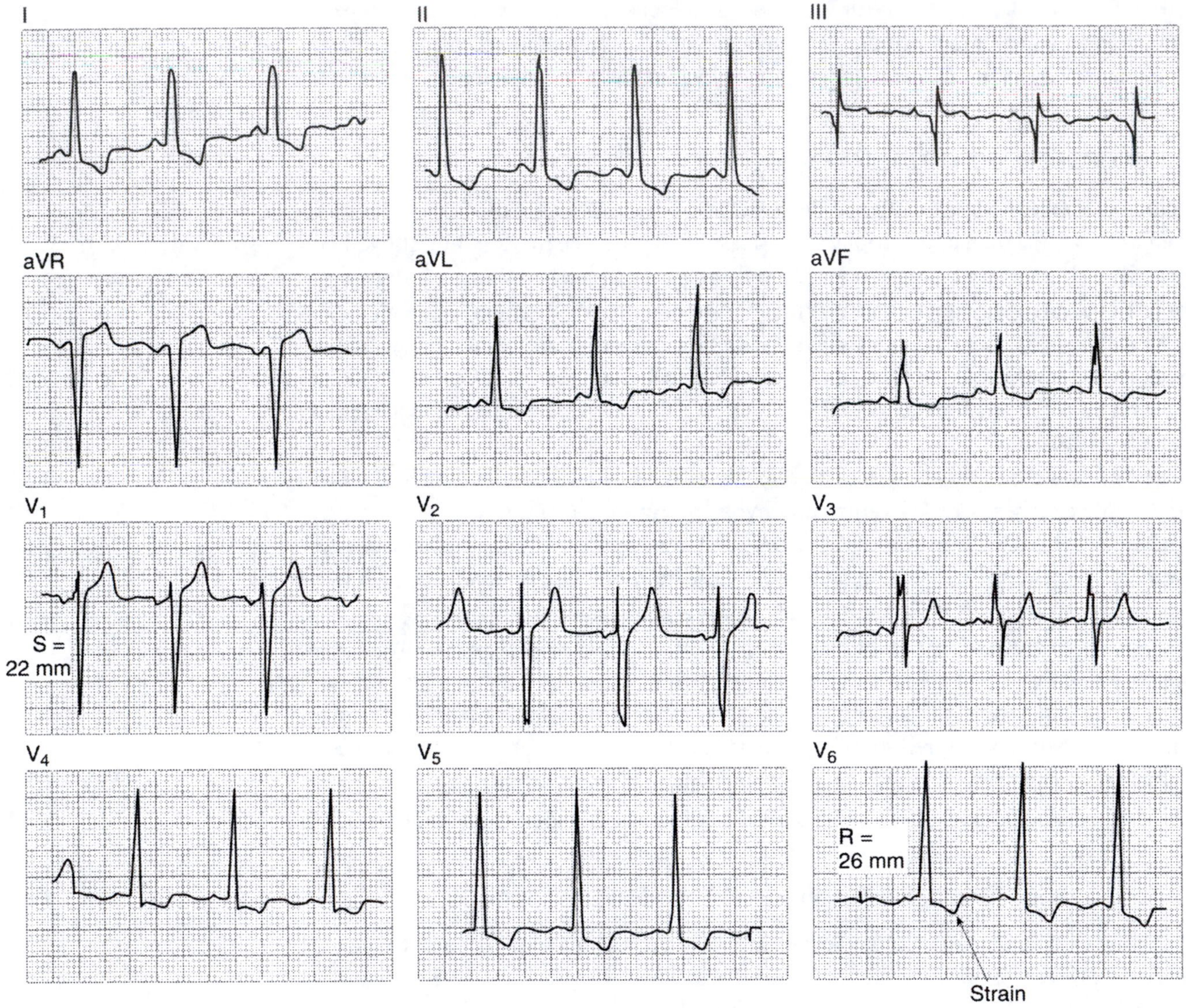

I   II   III

aVR   aVL   aVF

V_1 V_2 V_3

S = 22 mm

V_4 V_5 V_6

R = 26 mm

Strain

(B)

Figure 8-8   (A) ECG complexes illustrating the ST-T wave changes seen in a strain pattern; (B) a 12-lead ECG in left ventricular hypertrophy. Note the deep S waves in V_1, increased R wave amplitude in V_5 and V_6, with ST-T wave changes reflecting strain in V_6. (Adapted with permission from *Principles of Clinical Electrocardiography*, 13th ed., by N. Goldschlager and M. Goldman, 1989, Appleton-Lange.) *(continues)*

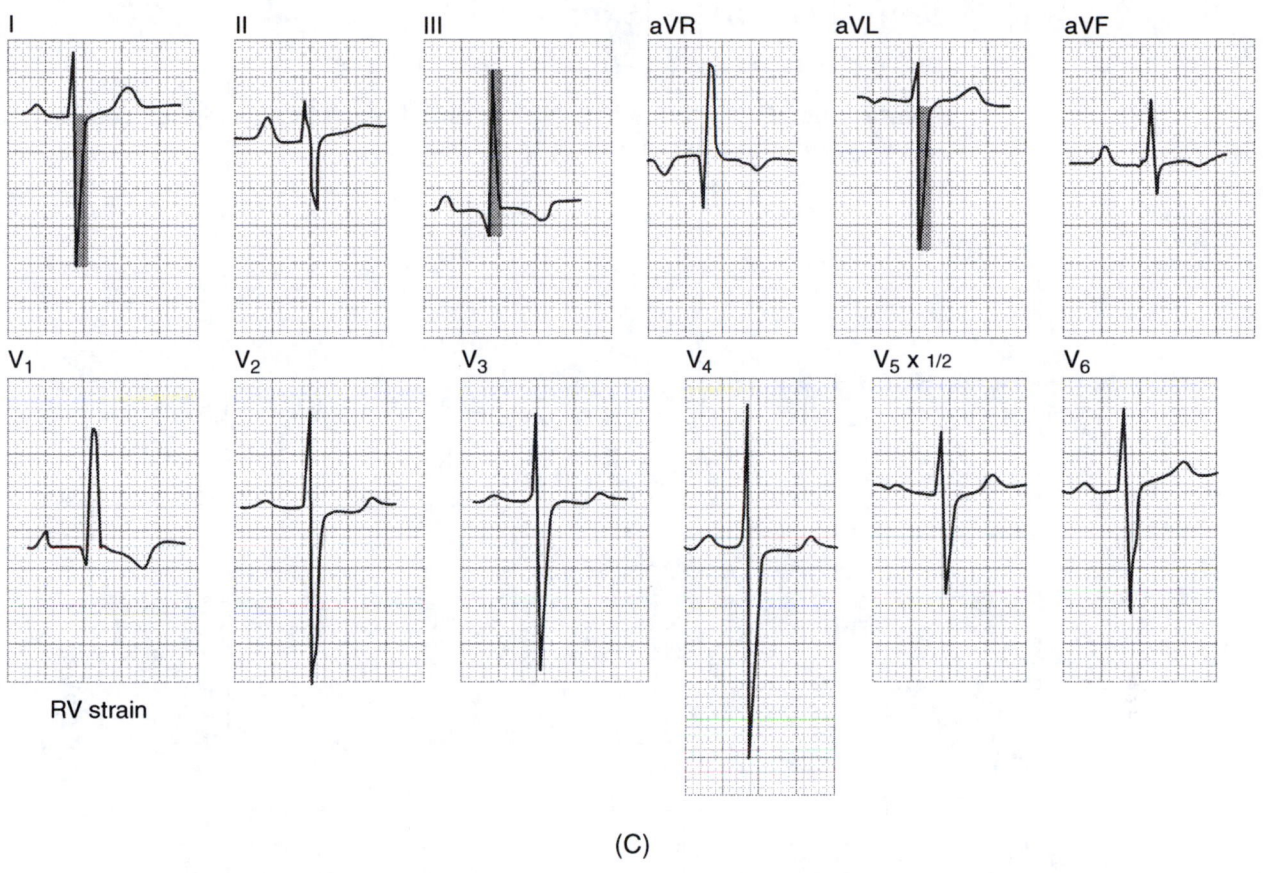

(C)

Figure 8-8 Continued (C) a 12-lead ECG in right ventricular hypertrophy. Note the increased amplitude (shaded) of R waves in lead III and deep S waves in I and aVL. Lead V₅ has been minimized to "make it fit" for mounting purposes. Note that the QRS in V₅ is half the true illustration of that lead, while V₁ shows the characteristic ST-T wave strain pattern. (Adapted with permission from *Principles of Clinical Electrocardiography*, 13th ed., by N. Goldschlager and M. Goldman, 1989, Appleton-Lange.)

Summary

The 12-lead ECG is very revealing in regard to all four of the heart's chambers and affords the clinician the ability to interpret nonacute conditions. The assessment of increased amplitude can support the diagnosis of chamber enlargement due to chronic disease. Confirmation by use of 12-lead ECG is a valuable tool in diagnosing the existence of chamber hypertrophy. Awareness of the existence of chamber abnormality may alter choice of intervention and affect long-term outcome.

In this chapter we have discussed tools for assessing atrial and ventricular enlargement. Atrial enlargement is infrequently seen, and occurrence of right atrial enlargement is more common than left. Ventricular hypertrophy must be substantiated with clinical assessment and history. Ventricular changes are more commonly encountered and many measurement criteria exist. As with any other diagnosis, the use of the ECG as a tool requires a consistent approach, remembering that vigilance and verification with clinical assessment is critical.

Self-Assessment Exercises

● **ECG Rhythm Identification Practice**

Identify the ECG criterion listed below each 12-lead ECG, and then compare your answers with those in the back of the book.

Figure 8-9

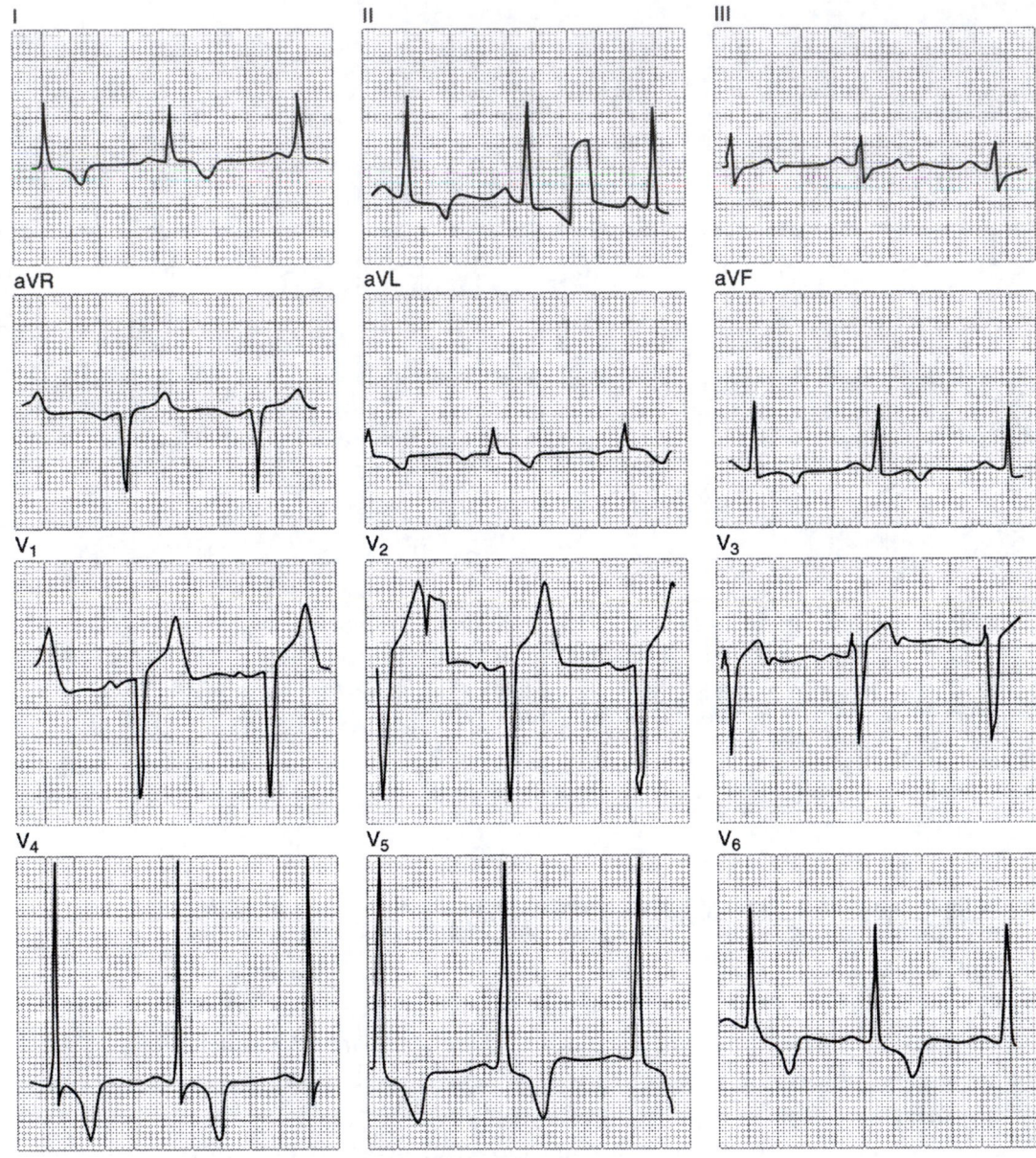

1. What is the underlying rhythm? _____

2. What are the acute changes? _____

3. What is your interpretation? _____

_____

4. What can happen next? _____

Figure 8-10

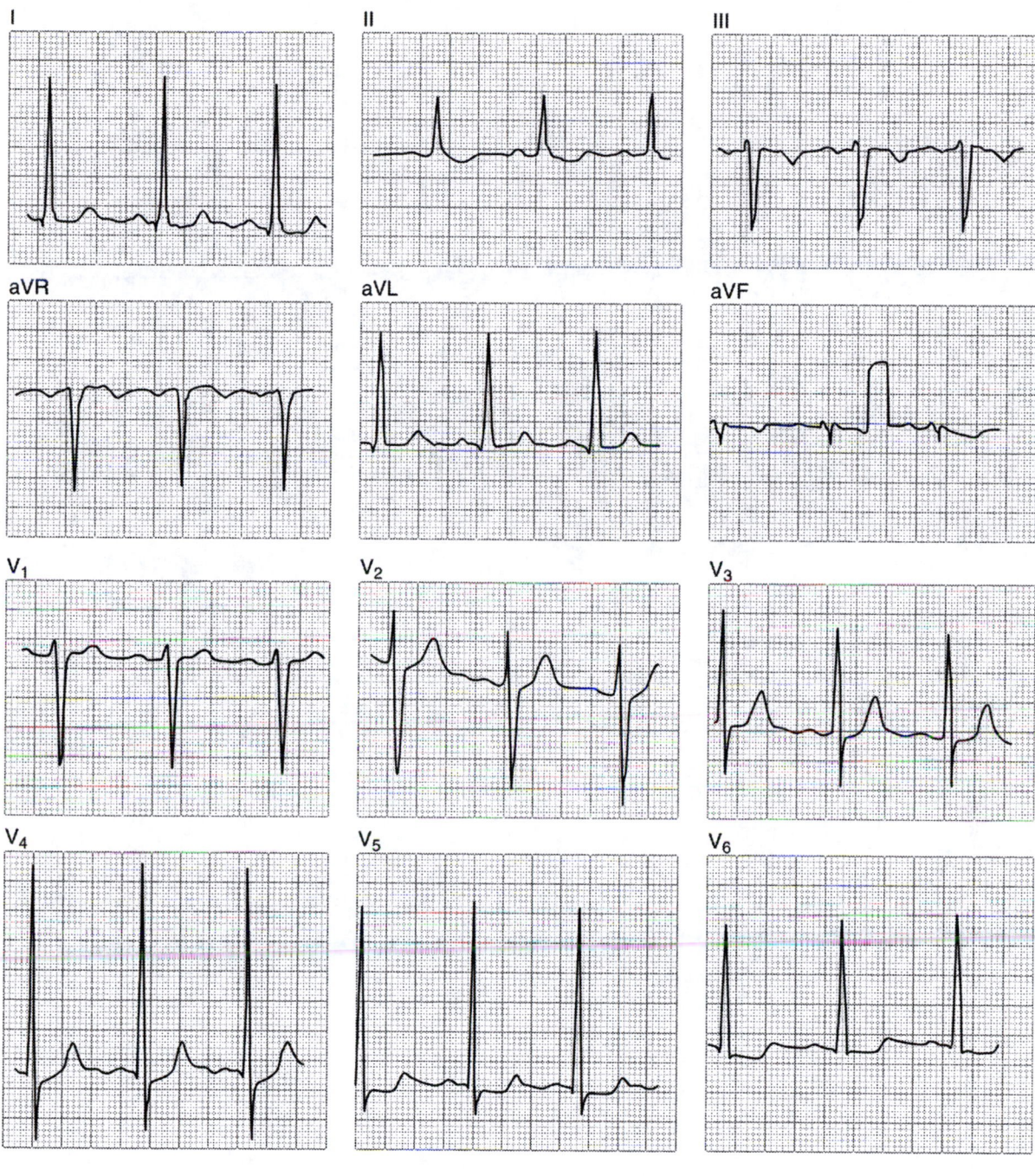

1. What is the underlying rhythm? _____
2. What are the acute changes? _____
3. What is your interpretation? _____
   _____
4. What can happen next? _____
   _____

Figure 8-11

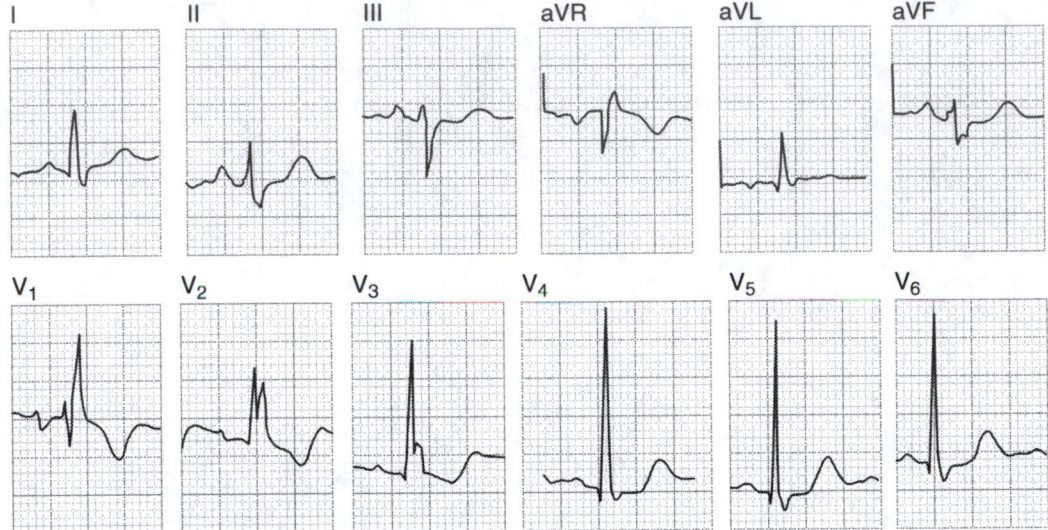

1. What is the underlying rhythm? _____
2. What are the acute changes? _____
3. What is your interpretation? _____
   _____
4. What can happen next? _____
   _____

Figure 8-12

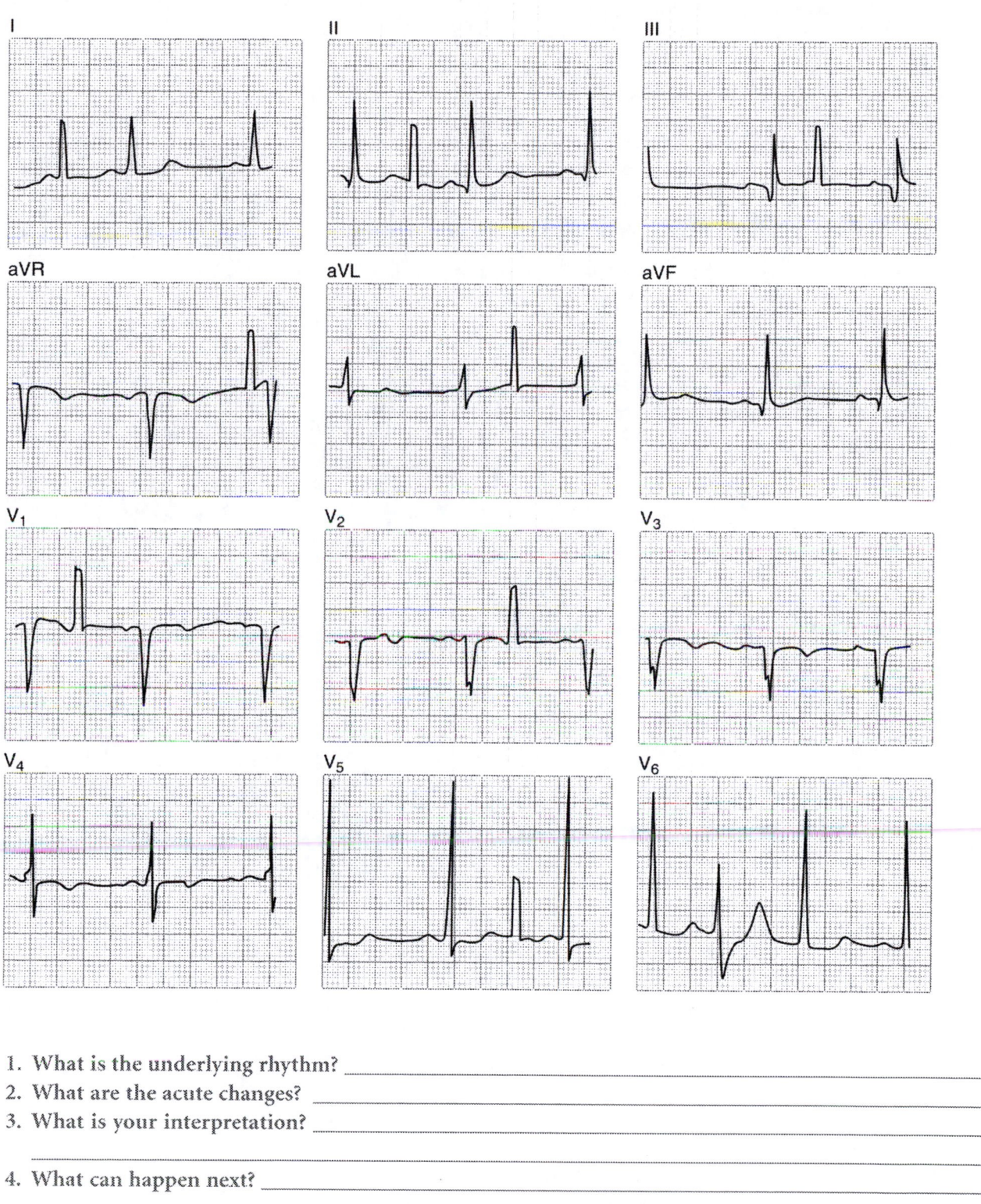

1. What is the underlying rhythm? _____
2. What are the acute changes? _____
3. What is your interpretation? _____

   _____

4. What can happen next? _____

   _____

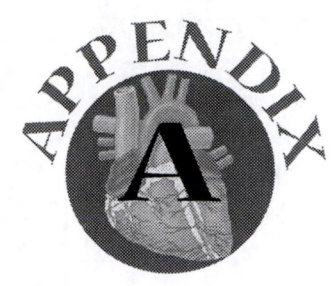

Answers to Self-Assessment Exercises

CHAPTER 1 THE HEART'S CONDUCTION SYSTEM

Matching

1. F
2. A
3. G
4. H
5. I

6. B
7. C
8. D
9. E
10. J

CHAPTER 2 THE ECG AND THE 12-LEAD SYSTEM

Fill in the Blanks

1. left free wall
2. apical and inferior surface
3. right inferior surface
4. right bundle branch
5. right anterior surface

6. anterior septal surface
7. left anterior surface
8. left ventricle
9. left lateral surface

CHAPTER 3 RATE, RHYTHM, AND WAVE FORMS

ECG Rhythm Identification Practice

Figure 3-27

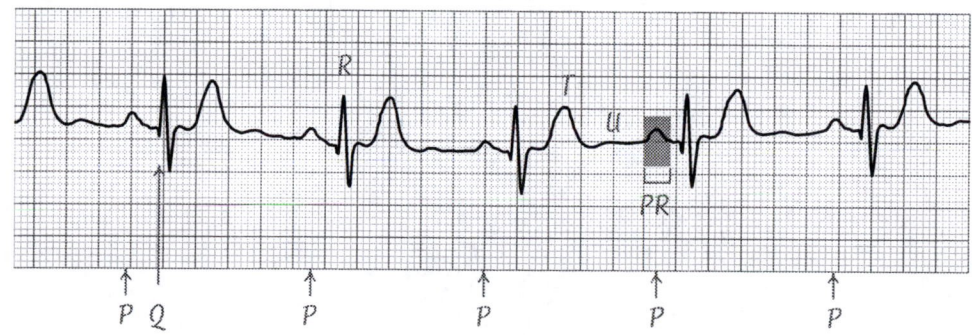

1. There are P, Q, R, S, T, and U waves. ST segment is on the line.
2. The P wave is positive (+).

3. QRS/ventricular rate/rhythm = 56/min/regular.
4. P (atrial) rate/rhythm = 55/minute/regular.
5. PR interval = 0.20 second and consistent.

Figure 3-28

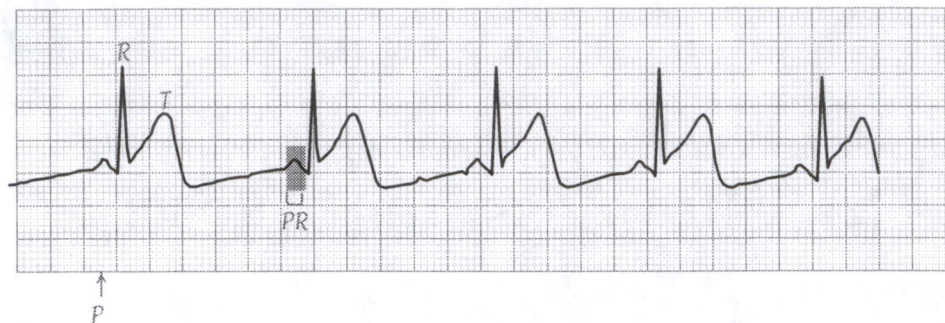

1. There are P, R, and T waves
2. The P waves are positive (+).

3. QRS (ventricular) rate = 55/minute/regular.
4. P (atrial) rate/rhythm = 55/minute/regular.
5. PR interval = 0.12-0.16 second. seconds and consistent.

CHAPTER 4 AXIS DETERMINATION AND IMPLICATIONS

Matching

1. A. E is not an option until voltage and axis are calculated
2. B. B is not an option until voltage and axis are calculated
3. E.

4. C.
5. D.

ECG Rhythm Identification Practice

Figure 4-11

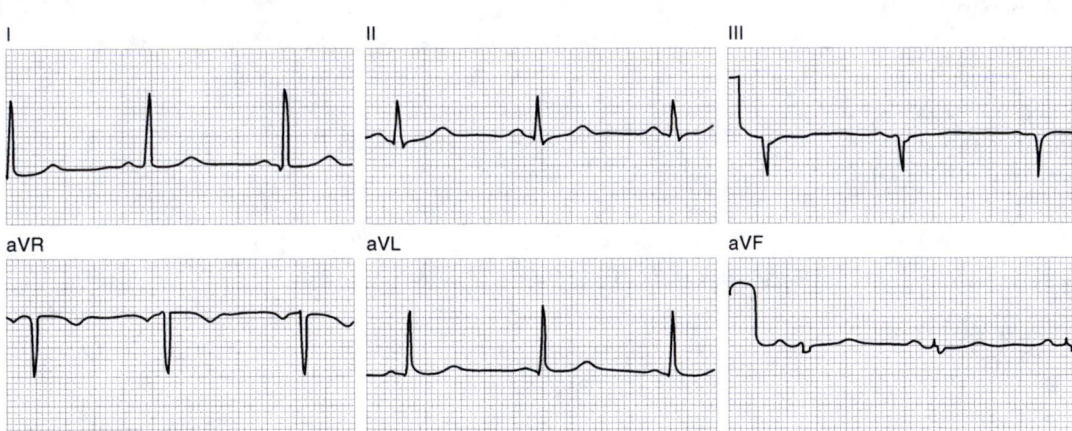

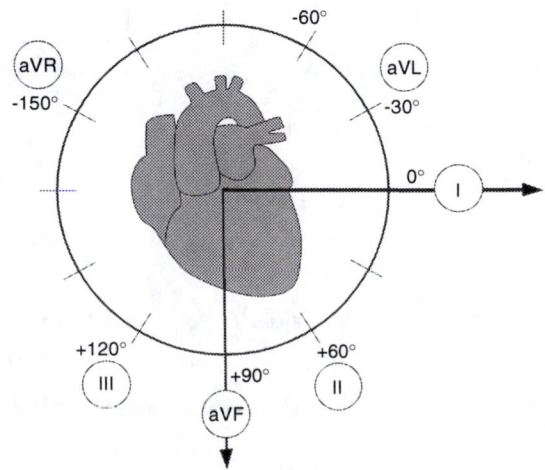

1. What is the underlying rhythm?

   Sinus at 67 beats per minute.

2. What is the axis?

   a. Look at leads I and II. Are leads I and II positive?

   Both leads I and II are positive. No other calculations are vital; axis is to the left at +0°.

   b. Are there equiphasic deflections?

   Yes, in aVF. Lead I is perpendicular to lead aVF and lead I is the greatest positive net area.

   c. See the arrows on the Lewis circle to verify your calculations.

3. What is your interpretation?

   Sinus at about 67 beats per minute.

Figure 4-12

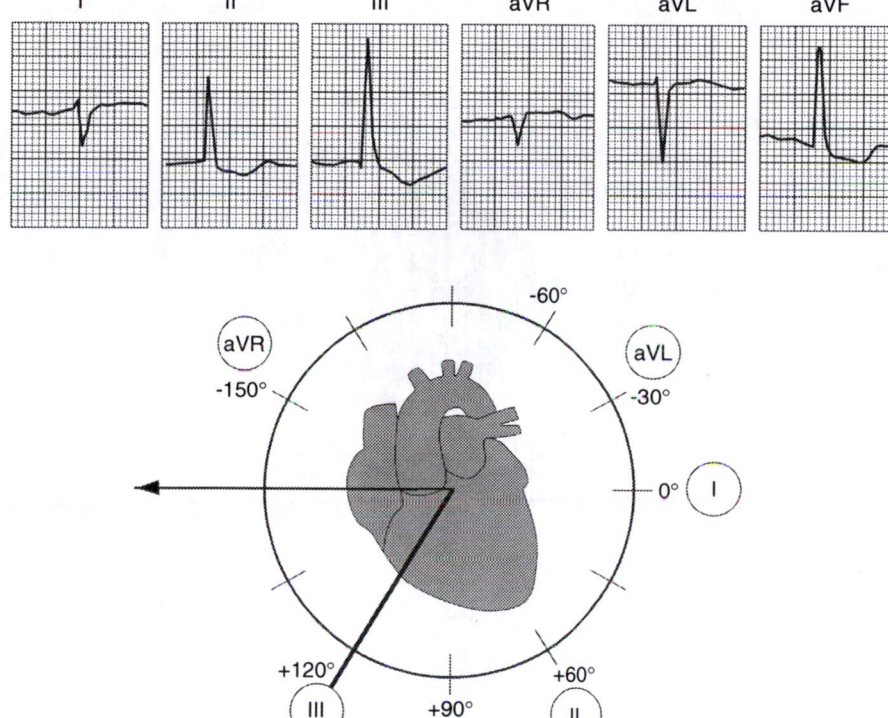

1. What is the underlying rhythm?

   Cannot tell, perhaps sinus.

2. What is the axis?

   a. Look at leads I and II. Are leads I and II positive?

   Lead I is negative and II is positive; therefore calculation is in order. There are no equiphasic deflections. Using the Lewis circle and the Handal-Lewis quadrant method, lead I is negative so the shift is away from lead I, to the right; lead III has the greatest positive net area; therefore axis is inferior and to the right at +120°.

   b. Are there equiphasic deflections?

   No, not really.

   c. See the arrows on the Lewis circle to verify your calculations.

3. What is your interpretation?

   Sinus with right axis deviation at +120°.

Figure 4-13

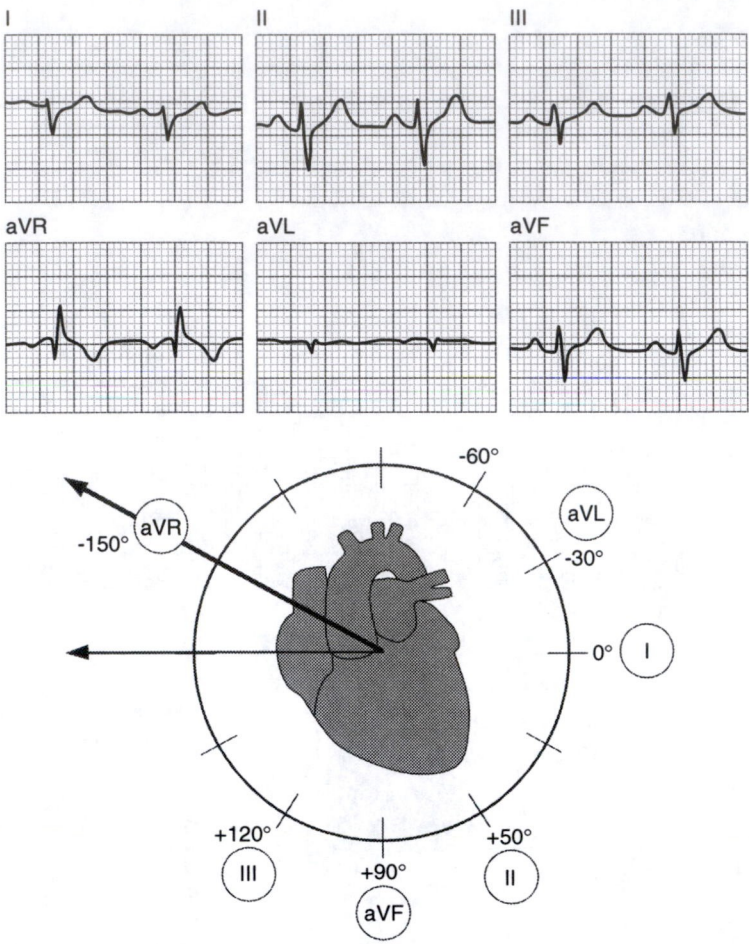

1. What is the underlying rhythm?

   Sinus at 86 beats per minute.

2. What is the axis?

   a. Look at leads I and II. Are leads I and II positive?

   Lead I is negative and leads II and III are equiphasic; therefore calculation is in order. Leads II, III and aVF are equiphasic. Lead I is negative so the flow of current is away from lead I, to the right; lead aVR has the greatest positive net area; axis is in no-mans' land, superior and to the right at about -150°.

   b. Are there equiphasic deflections?

   Yes, that is what was confusing; II, III and aVF are equiphasic.

   c. See the arrows on the Lewis circle to verify your calculations.

3. What is your interpretation?

   Sinus at 86 beats per minute with axis deviation at -150°.

Figure 4-14

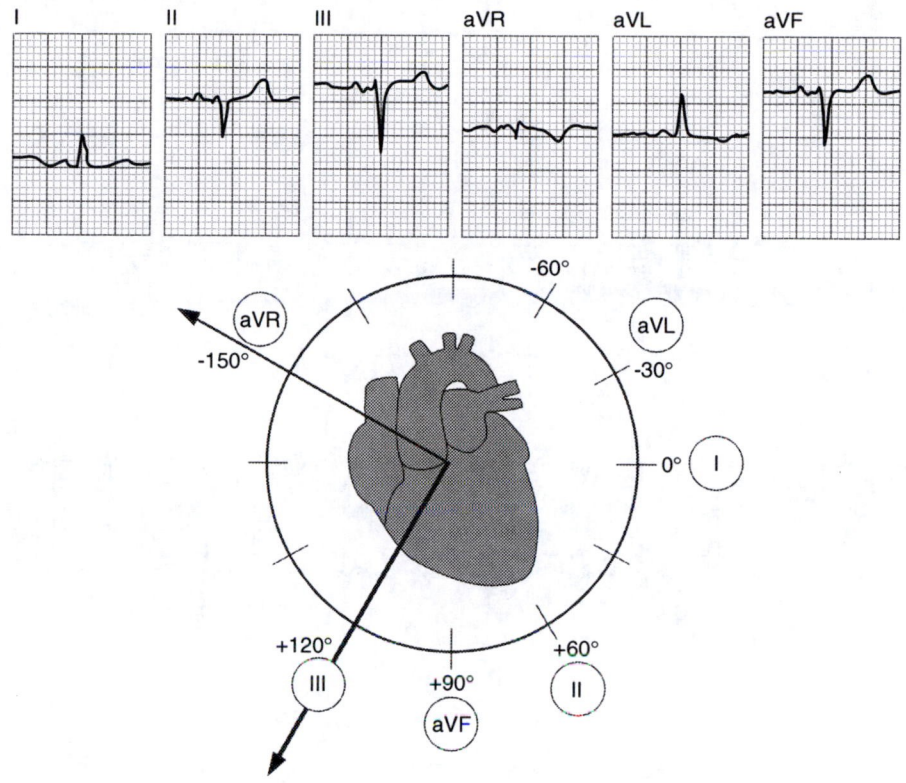

1. What is the underlying rhythm?

    Sinus.

2. What is the axis?

    a. Look at leads I and II. Are leads I and II positive?

    Lead I is positive and II is negative so calculation is in order. Lead aVR is equiphasic and lead III is perpendicular to aVR; lead III is negative and has the greatest net negative, so the axis is inferior and to the right at +120°.

    b. Are there equiphasic deflections?

    Yes, in aVR. The Q and R waves are very small, but on close inspection, the complex is equiphasic.

    c. See the arrows on the Lewis circle to verify your calculations.

3. What is your interpretation?

    Sinus with right axis deviation at +120°.

Figure 4-15

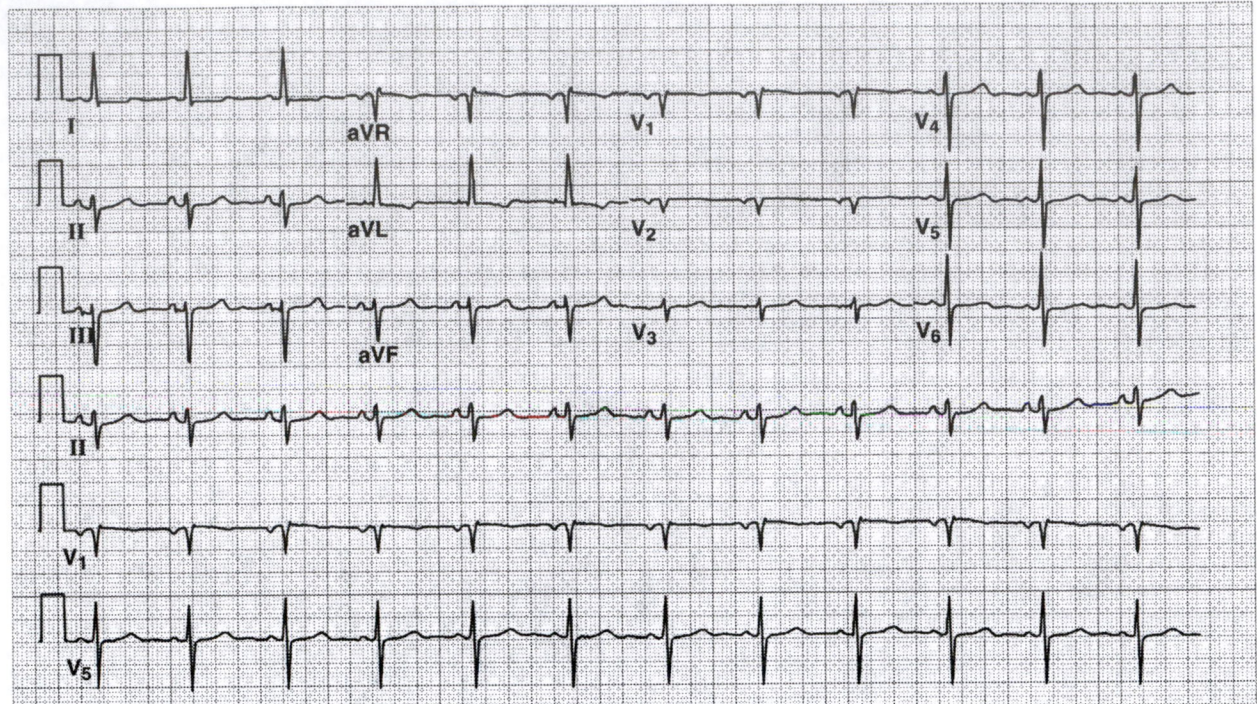

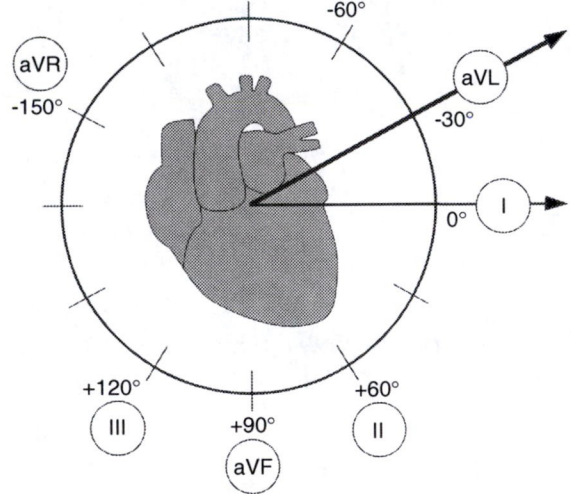

1. What is the underlying rhythm?

   Sinus at 75 beats per minute.

2. What is the axis?

   a. Look at leads I and II. Are leads I and II positive?

   Lead I is positive and II is equiphasic, therefore calculation is in order. Using the two-step method, lead II is equiphasic and lead aVL is perpendicular to lead II. Lead III is negative, and the net area of leads I, III, and aVL are similar so the average would be at aVL, or -30°.

   b. Are there diphasic deflections?

   Yes, lead II.

   c. See the arrows on the Lewis circle to verify your calculations.

3. What is your interpretation?

   Sinus at 75 beats per minute with axis at -30°.

CHAPTER 5 SINUS RHYTHM AND THE ARRYTHMIAS

ECG Rhythm Identification Practice

Figure 5-59

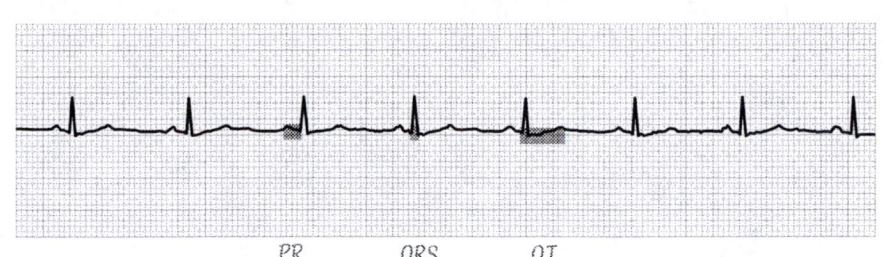

QRS duration _0.06 second_ QT _0.32 second_   Identification _sinus rhythm vent rate at 67/minute_

Ventricular rate/rhythm _67/minute/regular_

Atrial rate/rhythm _67/minute/regular_   Symptoms _probably none_

PR interval _0.16 second_   Treatment _be supportive_

Figure 5-60

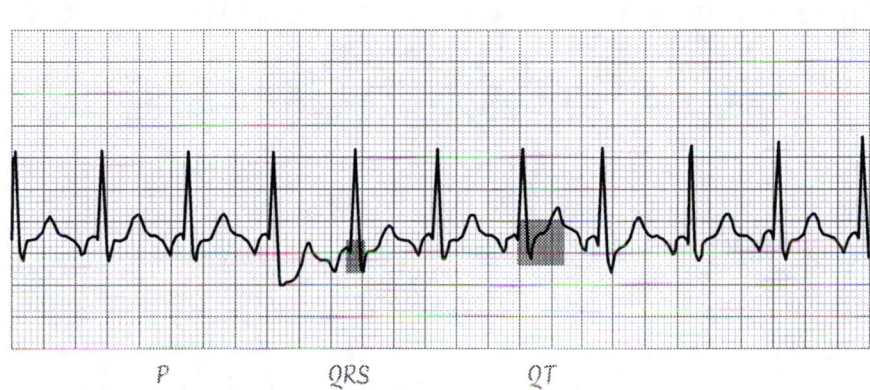

QRS duration _0.10 second_ QT _0.24-0.28 second_   Identification _junctional tachycardia vent rate 110/minute._

Ventricular rate/rhythm _110/minute/regular_

Atrial rate/rhythm _110/minute/regular_   Symptoms _? dizziness, postural hypotension_

PR interval _0.12 second_   Treatment _assess for s/s ↓ perfusion; ? why_

Figure 5-61

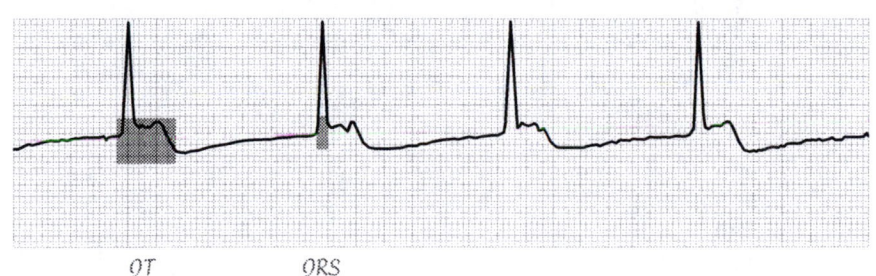

QRS duration _0.08-0.10 second_ QT _0.24-0.28 second_   Identification _junctional rhythm, vent rate 46/minute_

Ventricular rate/rhythm _46/minute/regular_   Symptoms _? dizziness, postural hypotension_

Atrial rate/rhythm _UTD_   _if hypotensive and hypoperfusing, ABCs, O₂, (P),_

PR interval _UTD_   Treatment _IV, ? meds/med Hx, V/S/ allergies; consider_
    atropine, fluids, dopamine, pace

Figure 5-62

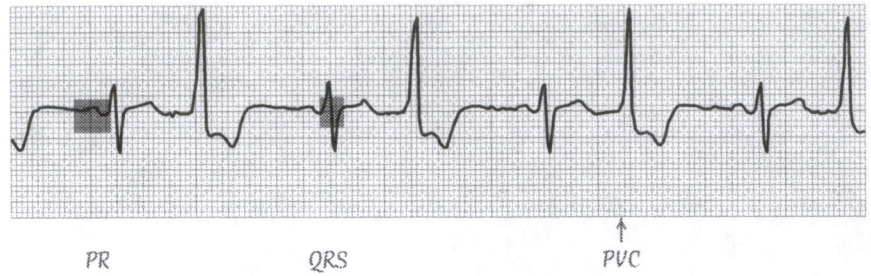

QRS duration _0.12 second_ QT _0.36 second_

Ventricular rate/rhythm _70/bigeminal_

Atrial rate/rhythm _35/minute_

PR interval _0.16 second_

Identification _sinus with ventricular bigeminy; overall rate is 70/minute (QRS = 0.12 second rS pattern)_

Symptoms _probably none_

Treatment _? meds/med Hx; be supportive_

Figure 5-63

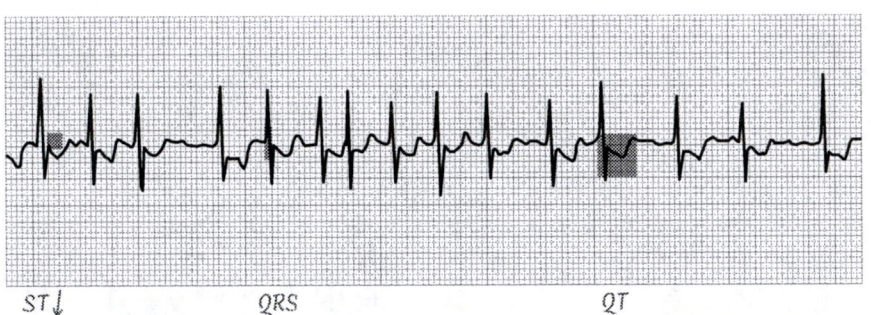

QRS duration _0.06 second_ QT _0.32 second_

Ventricular rate/rhythm _100-296/minute_

Atrial rate/rhythm _UTD_

PR interval _UTD_

Identification _atrial fib 100-296/minute with 2-3 mm ST ↓_

Symptoms _? meds/med Hx, vital signs, allergies_

Treatment _be supportive; if tachycardia persists and patient is symptomatic, may consider verpamil_

Figure 5-64

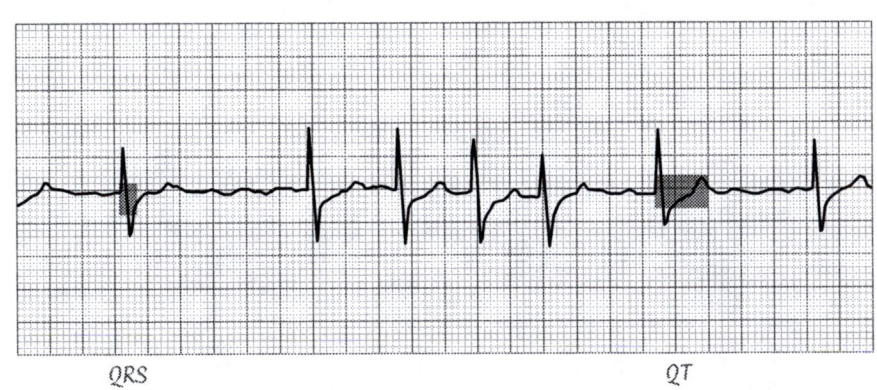

QRS duration _0.10 second_ QT _0.32-0.40 second_

Ventricular rate/rhythm _50-150/minute_

Atrial rate/rhythm _UTD_

PR interval _UTD_

Identification _atrial fib vent rate range is 50-150/minute 2 mm ST ↓_

Symptoms _probably none_

Treatment _? meds/med Hx, V/S/ allergies; be supportive_

Figure 5-65

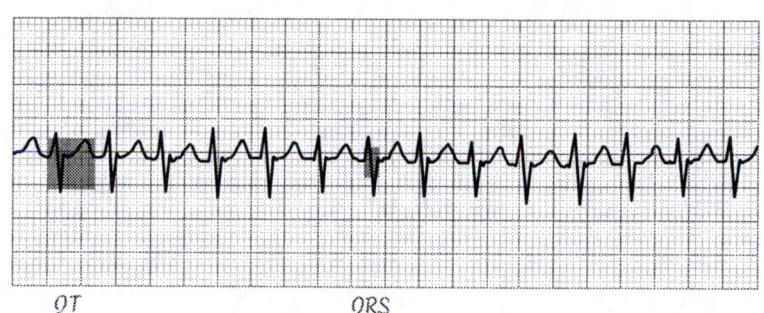

QT   QRS

QRS duration   *0.06 second*   QT *0.24-0.28 second*   Identification   *SVT at 188/minute*

Ventricular rate/rhythm   *188/minute/regular*

Atrial rate/rhythm   *UTD*   Symptoms   *? dizziness, hypotension, ALOC*

PR interval   *UTD*   Treatment   *ABCs, O₂, (P), IV, ? meds/med Hx, V/S/ allergies; consider vagal maneuvers, adenosine*

Figure 5-66

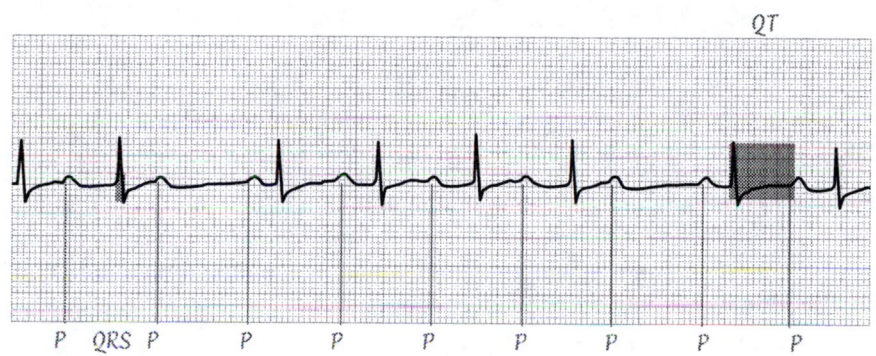

QT

P   QRS   P   P   P   P   P   P   P   P

QRS duration   *0.08 second*   QT *0.40-0.44 second*   Identification   *sinus at 100; 2° AV block probably Type 1*

Ventricular rate/rhythm   *55-100/minute*   *(QRS = 0.08), Wenkebach*

Atrial rate/rhythm   *100/minute/regular*   Symptoms   *probably none*

PR interval   *0.24, 0.32, 0.40 second*   Treatment   *ABCs, O₂, (P), IV, ? meds/med Hx, V/S/ allergies*

Figure 5-67

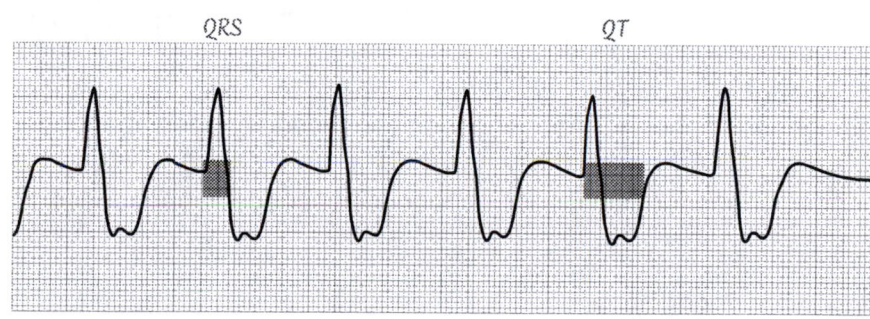

QRS   QT

QRS duration   *0.16-0.20 second*   QT   *0.44 second*   Identification   *accelerated ventricular rhythm vent rate of*

Ventricular rate/rhythm   *67/minute/regular*   *55/minute*

Atrial rate/rhythm   *UTD*   Symptoms   *? pulse; if pulse present, ALOC*

PR interval   *UTD*   Treatment   *If pulseless: CPR, intubate, epi/TCP; if pulse is present: consider fluids, TCP ASAP*

Figure 5-68

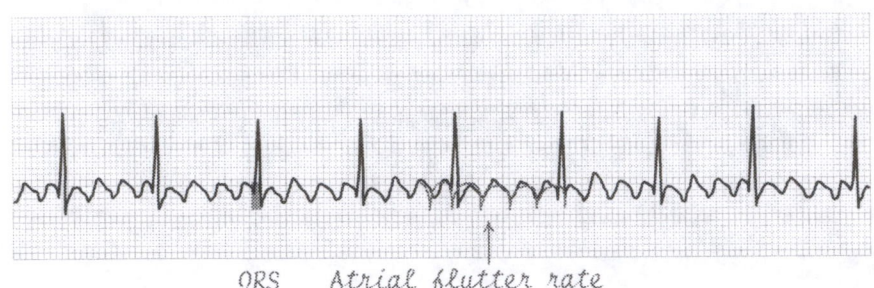

QRS   Atrial flutter rate

QRS duration   0.04-0.10 second   QT   UTD   Identification   atrial flutter vent rate 86-100/minute

Ventricular rate/rhythm   86-100/minute

Atrial rate/rhythm   300   Symptoms   none anticipated

PR interval   none   Treatment   ? meds, med Hx, be supportive

Figure 5-69

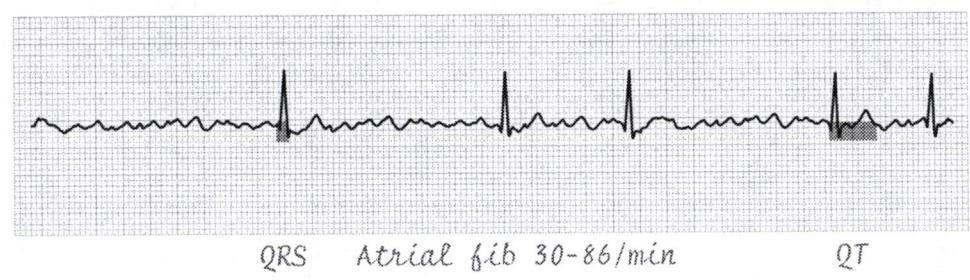

QRS   Atrial fib 30-86/min   QT

QRS duration   0.08-0.10 second   QT   0.38 second   Identification   atrial fibrillation vent rate 30-86/minute

Ventricular rate/rhythm   30-86/minute

Atrial rate/rhythm   UTD   Symptoms   may be related to slower rates; ? digitalis

PR interval   none   Treatment   ? meds, med Hx, be supportive; consider
fluids/dopamine/pace if s/s hypotension, hypoperfusion

Figure 5-70

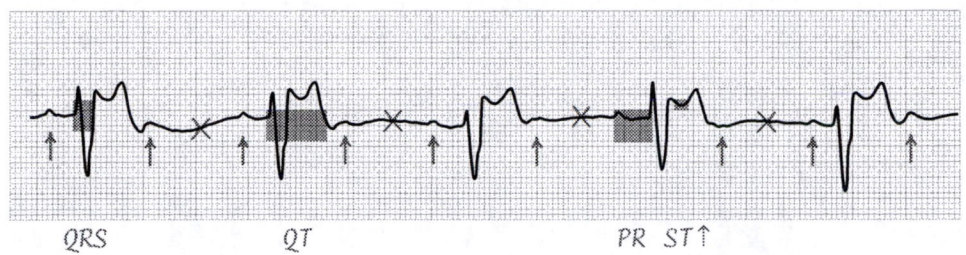

QRS   QT   PR ST↑

QRS duration 0.12 second   QT 0.42 second

Ventricular rate/rhythm 41/minute

Atrial rate/rhythm 41/minute

PR interval 0.28 second

Identification *sinus bradycardia, 1° AV block, 2 mm ST↑*
QRS 0.12 second

Symptoms *associated with bradycardia; dizziness,*
postural hypotension

Treatment *? meds/med Hx, be supportive; consider*
Atropine, fluids, dopamine, TCP

Figure 5-71

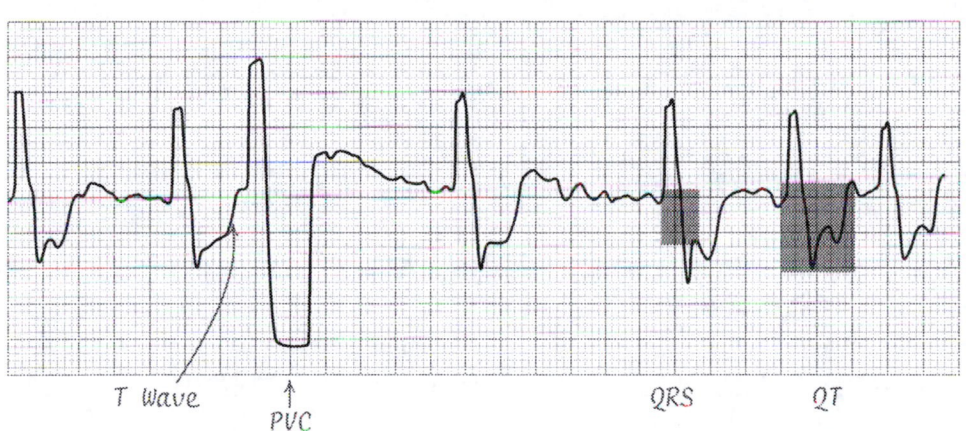

T Wave   ↑   QRS   QT
PVC

QRS duration 0.16 second   QT n/a

Ventricular rate/rhythm 55-100/irregular

Atrial rate/rhythm n/a

PR interval n/a

Identification *atrial fibrillation vent rate at 55-100/minute*
6 mm ST ↓ and an R on T PVC

Symptoms *none noted*

Treatment *? meds/med Hx/vitals*

Figure 5-72

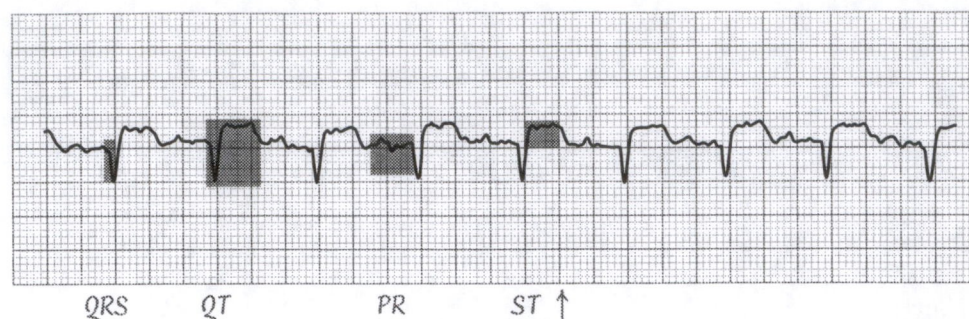

QRS duration _0.04-0.06 second_   QT _0.28 second_
Ventricular rate/rhythm _100/minute_
Atrial rate/rhythm _100/minute_
PR interval _0.24 second_

Identification _sinus at 100/minute with 1° AV block with 3 mm ST segment; Q waves 4-5 mm._
Symptoms _may have pain_
Treatment _? meds/med Hx, be supportive, if pain, Rx the pain_

Figure 5-73

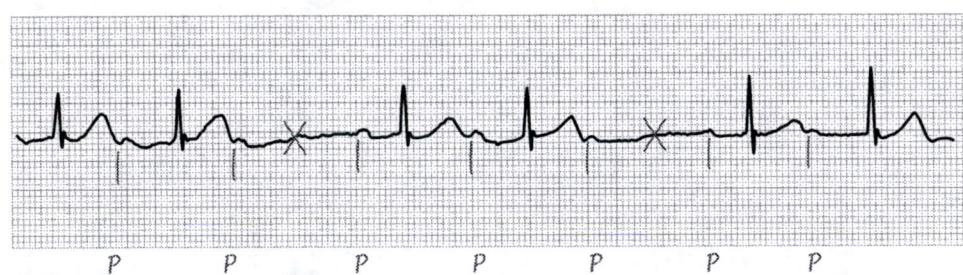

QRS duration _0.08 second_   QT _0.40 second_
Ventricular rate/rhythm _40-75/minute_
Atrial rate/rhythm _75/minute_
PR interval _0.32, 0.38_

Identification _sinus at 75 with vent rate 40-75/minute, 2° AV block probably Type 1 (QRS=0.08)_
Symptoms _none noted_
Treatment _? meds/med Hx/vitals_

Figure 5-74

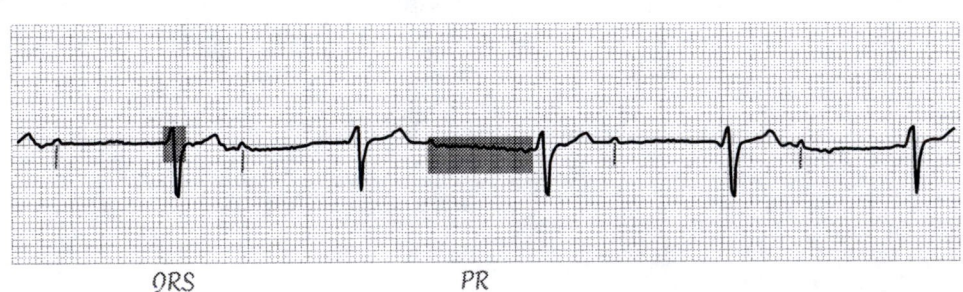

QRS duration _0.10 second_   QT _0.38 second_
Ventricular rate/rhythm _50/minute_
Atrial rate/rhythm _50/minute_
PR interval _0.78 second_

Identification _sinus brady at 50/minute with 1° AV block ? isorhythmic AV dissociation_
Symptoms _associated with bradycardia, i.e., dizziness, postural hypotension_
Treatment _if symptomatic with bradycardia, consider Atropine, fluids, dopamine, TCP_

CHAPTER 6 MYOCARDIAL PERFUSION DEFICITS AND ECG CHANGES

Matching

1. D
2. B
3. C
4. E
5. A

ECG Rhythm Identification Practice

Figure 6-16

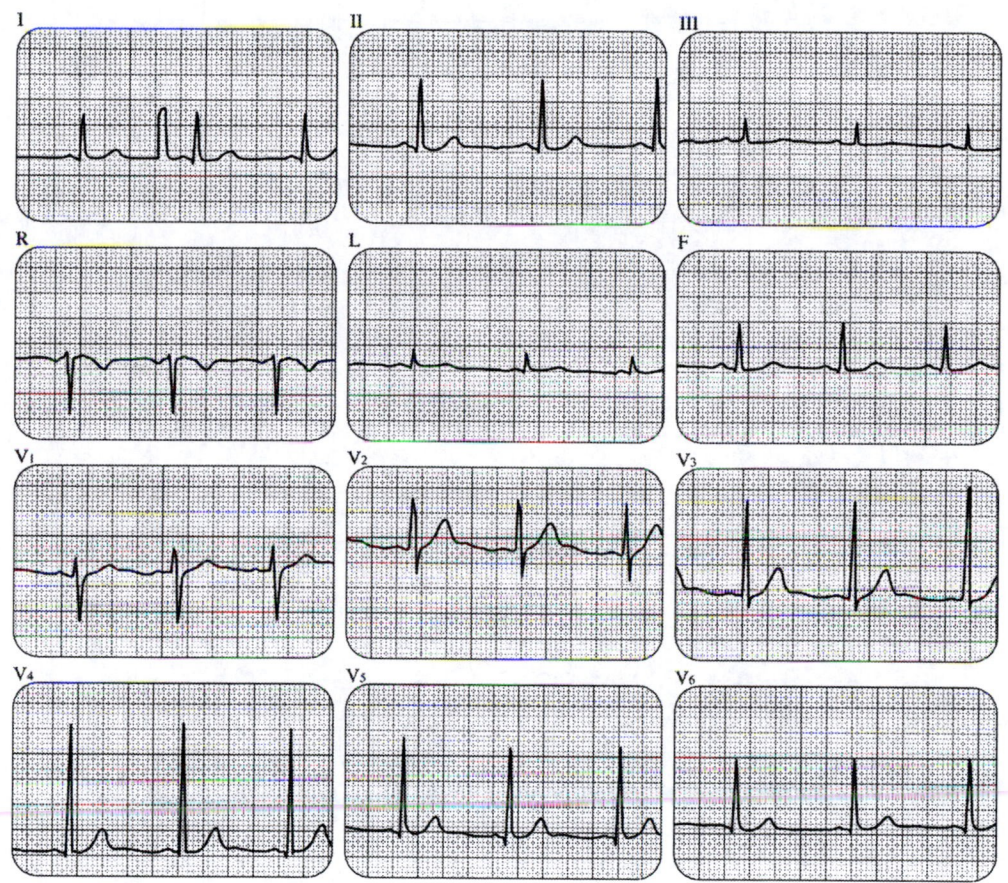

1. What is the underlying rhythm?
   Underlying rhythm is sinus at 60/minute.

2. What are the acute changes?
   None noted.

3. What is your interpretation?
   Interpretation is sinus at 60/minute.

4. What can happen next?
   Be supportive.

Figure 6-17

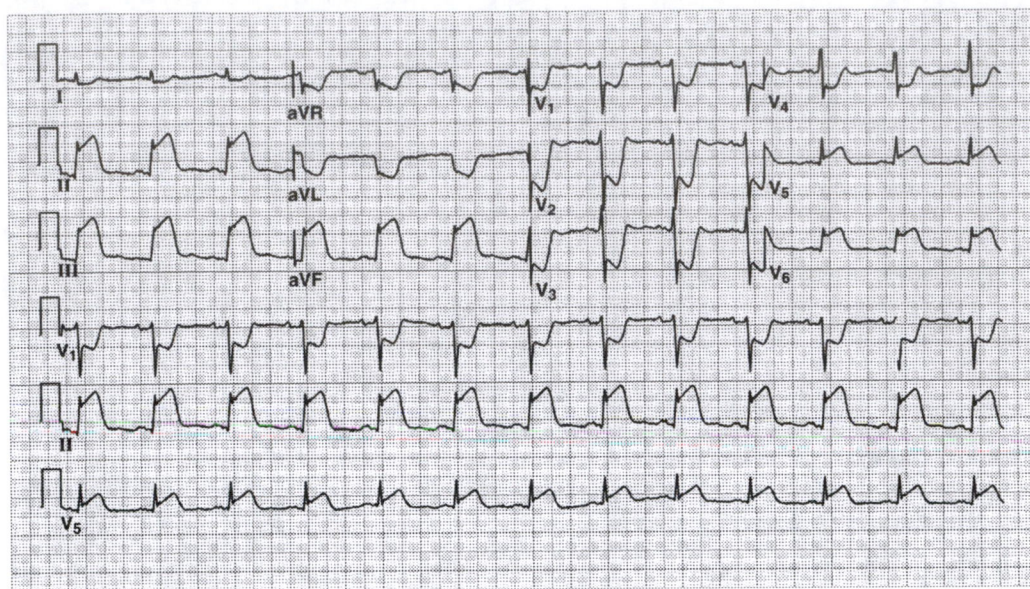

1. **What is the underlying rhythm?**
   Underlying rhythm is sinus at 75/minute.

2. **What are the acute changes?**
   Acute changes are 7 mm ST seg ↑ in II, III, and with reciprocal changes in aVL (ST ↓). There are R waves in $V_2 \rightarrow V_4$ with ST ↓ in V_2, V_3, V_4; ST ↑ in V_5 and V_6.

3. **What is your interpretation?**
   Interpretation is acute infero-posterior wall MI

   ? Extension to the LL surface?

4. **What can happen next?**
   Observe for SA and AV conduction problems, s/s failure.

Figure 6-18

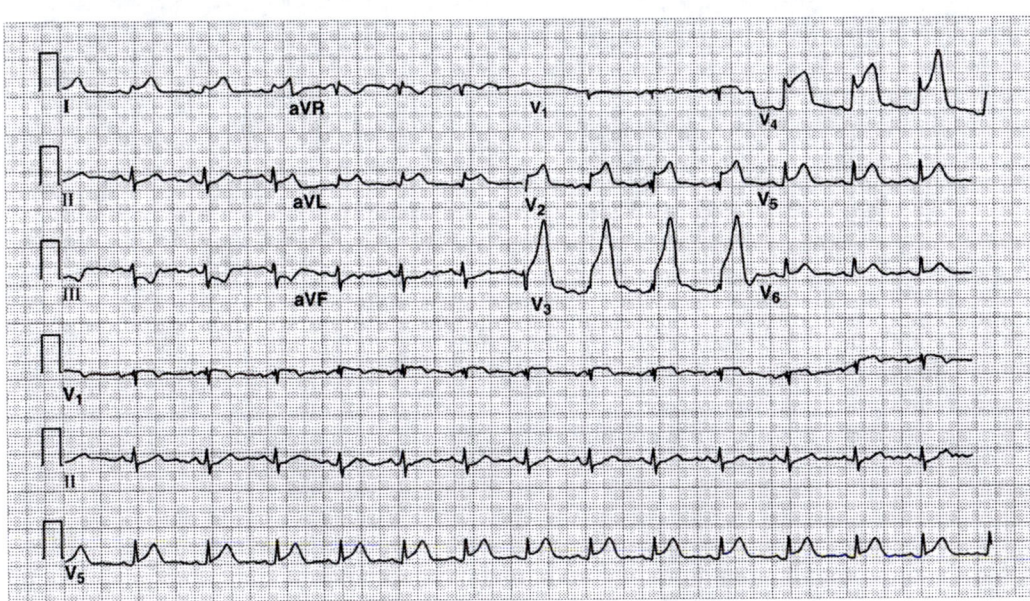

1. **What is the underlying rhythm?**
   Underlying rhythm is sinus at 85/minute.

2. **What are the acute changes?**
   Acute changes are 2mm ST seg ↑ in I, aVL and with reciprocal ST ↓ in II, III, and aVF. There are Q waves in V_1 and V_2. There is progressive ST ↑ in V_2, V_3, and V_4, 2-3 mm ST ↑ in V_5 and V_6.

3. **What is your interpretation?**
   Interpretation is sinus at 85/minute with acute anteroseptal myocardial infarction, extension of injury and ischemia to the antero-lateral surface.

4. **What can happen next?**
   Observe for AV and BB conduction problems, s/s failure.

Figure 6-19

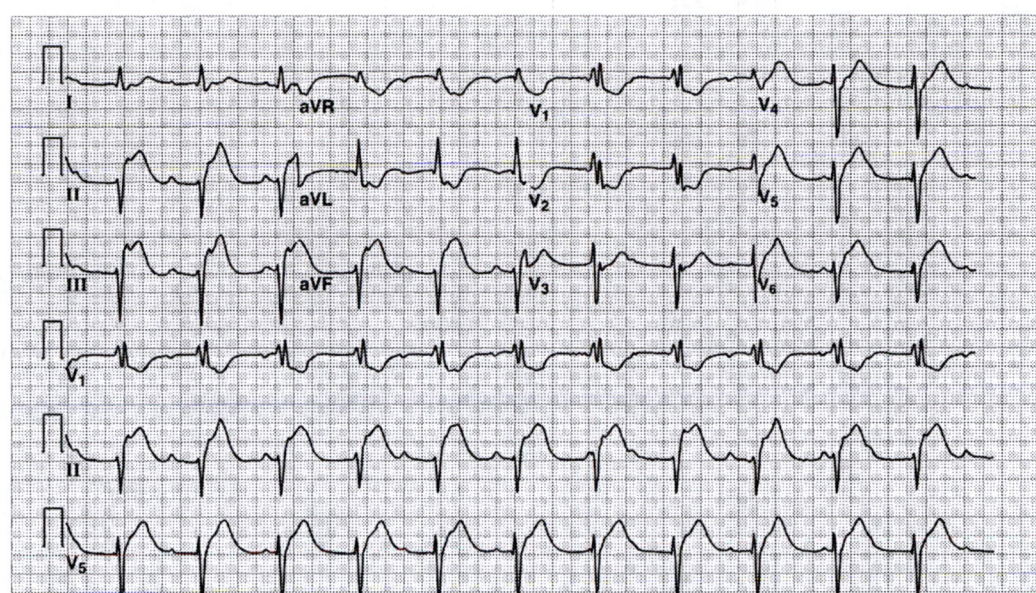

1. What is the underlying rhythm?
   Underlying rhythm is sinus at 60 with complete AV block, accelerated junctional rhythm at 67/minute

2. What are the acute changes?
   Acute changes are broad S wave in I, aVL; ST ↑ in II, III, and aVF; rS configuration in II, III, and aVF. The QRS in V₁, V₂ and V₃ shows an RSR'. There is ST ↓ in V₂, V₃ with ST ↑ in V₄, V₅ and V₆.

3. What is your interpretation?
   Interpretation is sinus at 60/minute with acute inferior, possible posterior MI, RBB which may mask the posterior injury pattern.

4. What can happen next?
   Observe for BB conduction problems, s/s failure. Consider standby for TCP.

Figure 6-20

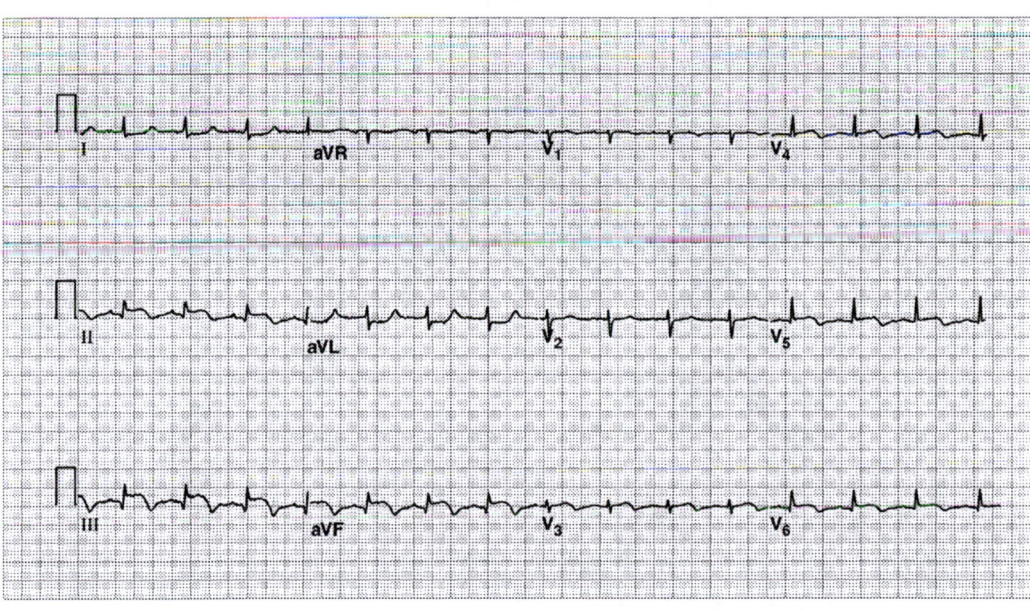

1. What is the underlying rhythm?
   Underlying rhythm is sinus at 86/minute; QT 0.40 second.

2. What are the acute changes?
   Acute changes are small Qs and ST ↑ in leads II, III, and aVF reciprocal ST ↓ in leads I and aVL. T waves in V₄, V₅, and V₆.

3. What is your interpretation?
   Interpretation is sinus at 86/minute with inferior myocardial infarction.

4. What can happen next?
   Observe for SA and AV conduction problems.

Figure 6-21

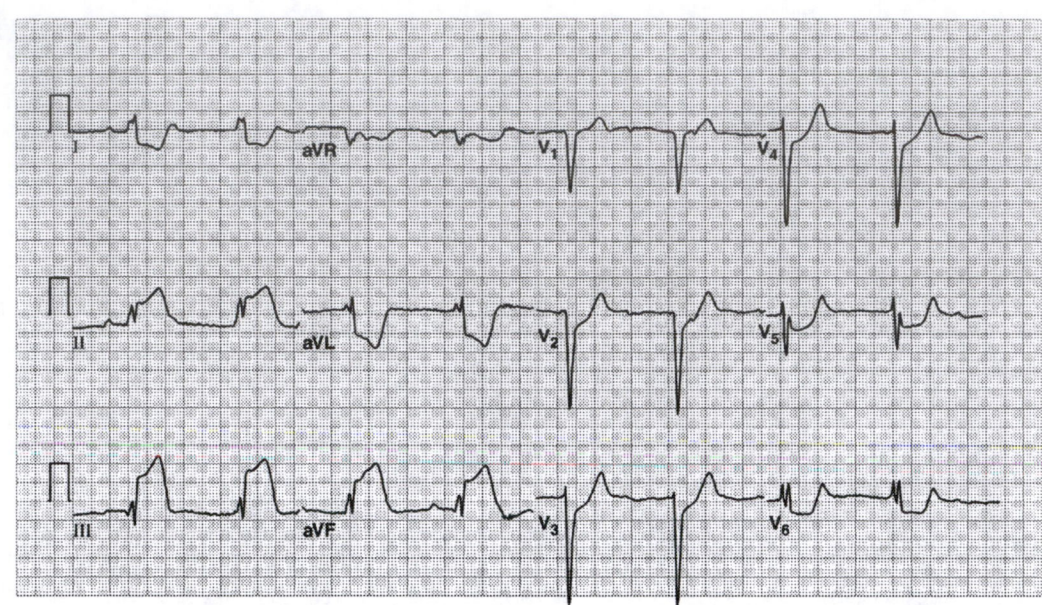

1. **What is the underlying rhythm?**
   Underlying rhythm is sinus at 86 complete AV block with ventricular rate at 50/minute.
2. **What are the acute changes?**
   Acute changes are broad QRS, notched, 0.14 second in leads I, II, III, and V_6. ST ↑ in leads II, III, and aVF; reciprocal ST ↓ in I and aVL. There are deep Qs; ST ↓ in V_2, V_4, V_5, and V_6. There is a broad, notched R wave in leads I, aVL, and V_6.

3. **What is your interpretation?**
   Interpretation is sinus at 86/minute with complete AV block; idiojunctional rhythm at 50/minute. Acute anteroseptal MI. Current of injury pattern in II, III, and aVF showing inferior involvement. There is left bundle branch block.
4. **What can happen next?**
   Observe for AV s/s failure; stand by for TCP.

Figure 6-2?

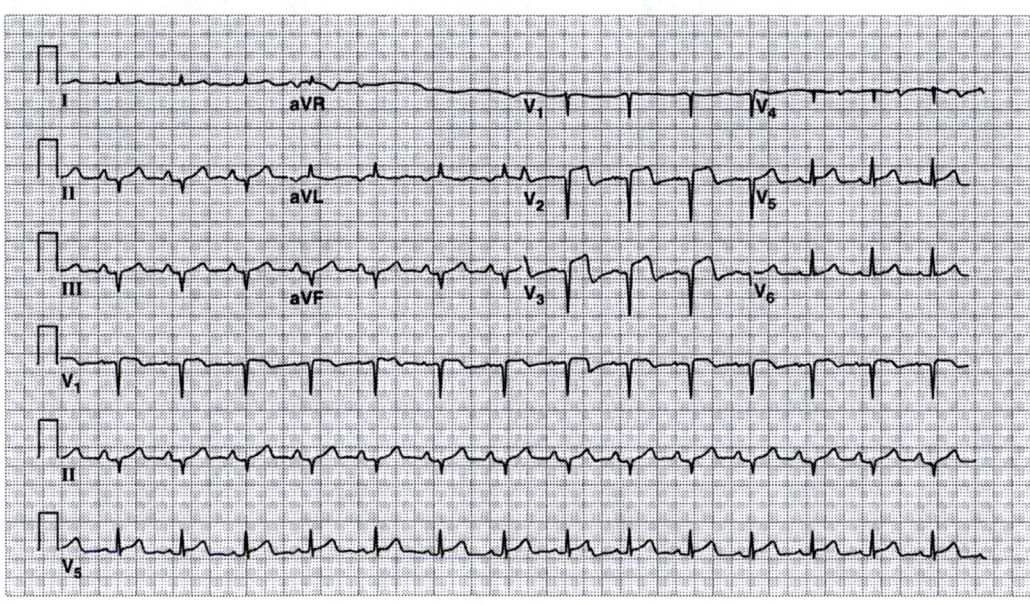

1. **What is the underlying rhythm?**
   Underlying rhythm is sinus at 86/minute
2. **What are the acute changes?**
   Acute changes are rS or QS in II, III, and aVF (no reciprocal changes in I or aVL). Q wave, ST ↑ V_2, V_3, and V_5.

3. **What is your interpretation?**
   Interpretation is sinus at 86/minute; acute anteroseptal MI; need serial ECG to clarify presence of Q waves in leads II, III, and aVF.
4. **What can happen next?**
   Observe for AV and/or BB conduction defects.

CHAPTER 7 INTRAVENTRICULAR CONDUCTION DEFECTS

ECG Rhythm Identification Practice

Figure 7-9

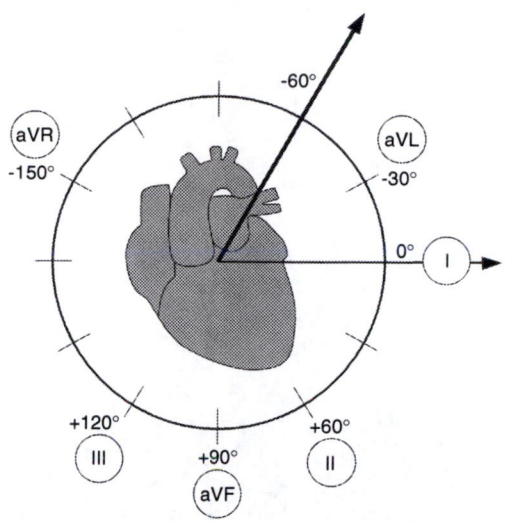

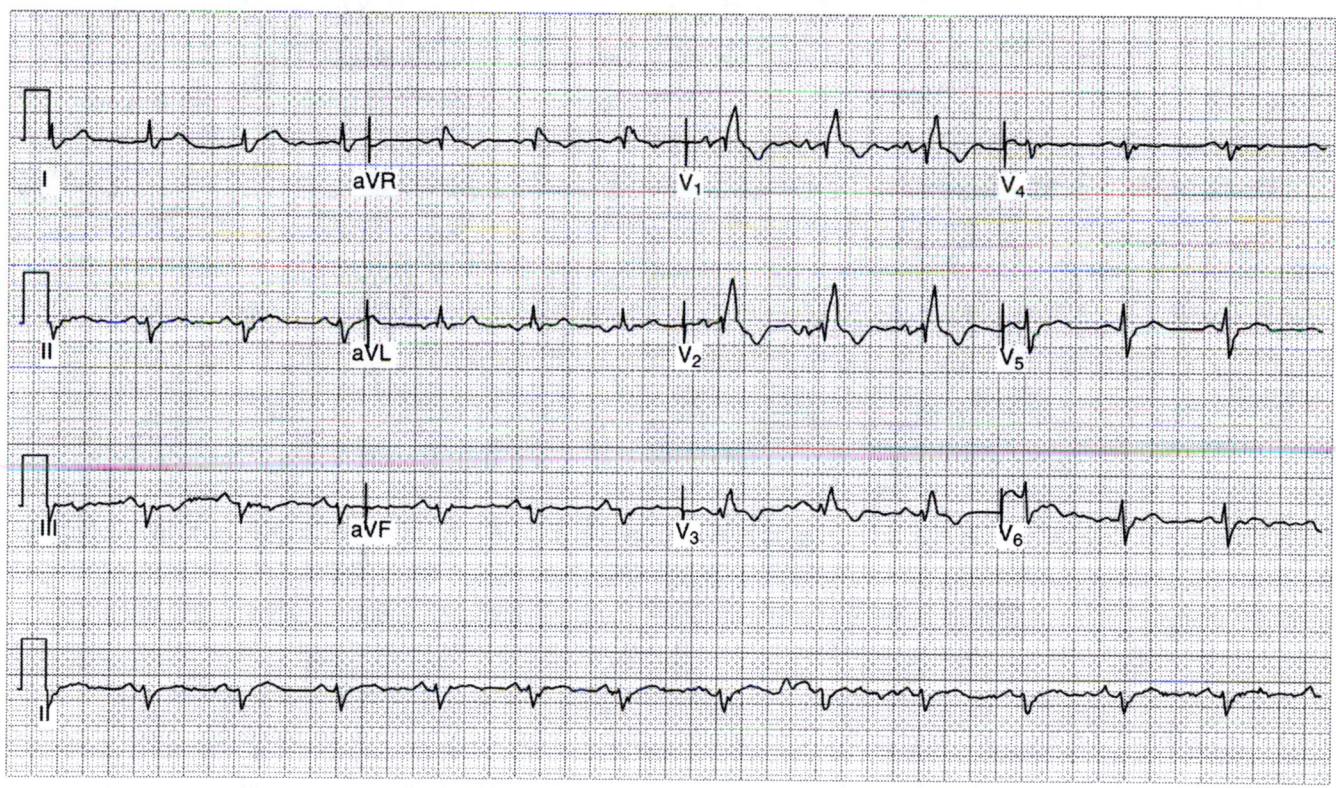

1. **What is the underlying rhythm?**
   Underlying rhythm is sinus at 77/minute

2. **What are the acute changes?**
   Acute changes are rS in leads II, III, and aVF; rsR' in V_1, V_2, and V_3. There are broad S waves in leads I, II, aVF, V_5, and V_6. Axis is at -60°, RBBB.

3. **What is your interpretation?**
   Interpretation is sinus at 77/minute; left axis deviation at -60°.

4. **What can happen next?**
   Observe for complete left anterior fascicular block.

Figure 7-10

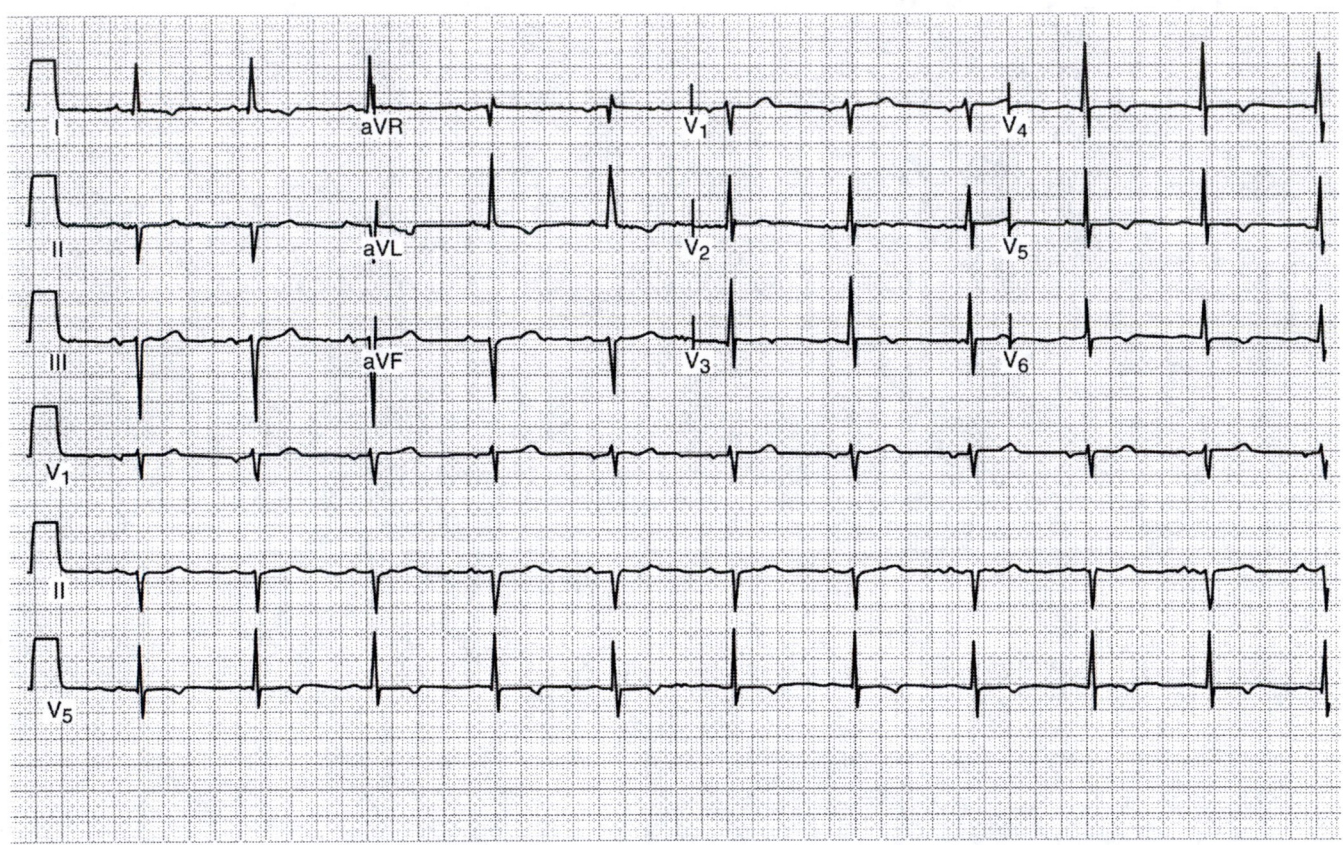

1. What is the underlying rhythm?

   Underlying rhythm is sinus at 63/minute.

2. What are the acute changes?

   rS configuration in leads II, III, and aVF. Lead III is the greatest negative deflection. Axis is at -60°. There are inverted T waves in leads I, aVL, V_3-V_6. The R wave in lead I and the S wave in lead III are greater than 21 mm and the height of the R wave in aVL is greater than 13 mm. Consider ventricular hypertrophy (see Chapter 8).

3. What is your interpretation?

   Interpretation is sinus rhythm at 63/minute; left anterior fascicular block (LAFB); consider lateral ischemia; consider ventricular hypertrophy

4. What can happen next?

   Observe for V_1 RBBB. Observe for s/s failure.

Figure 7-11

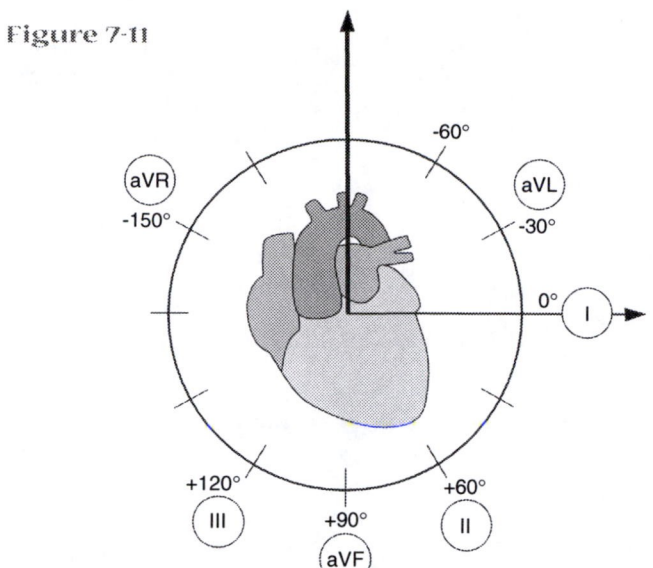

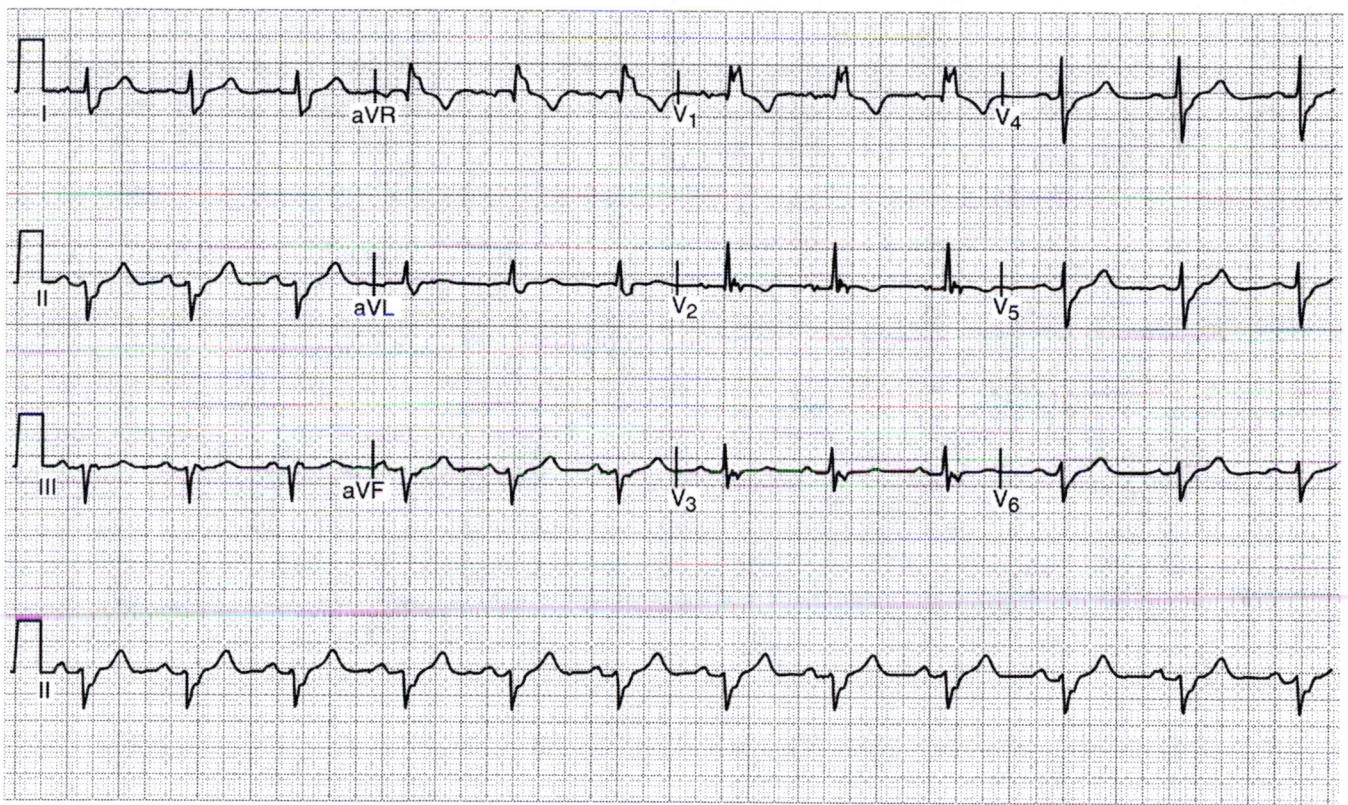

1. **What is the underlying rhythm?**
   Underlying rhythm is sinus approximately 70/minute

2. **What are the acute changes?**
   QRS is 0.12-0.16 second with broad S waves in leads I and aVL; terminal deflections in leads II, V₃, V₄, V₅, and V₆. rS configuration in leads II, III, and aVF. Equiphasic deflection in lead I; lead aVF is negative, axis is abnormal at 90°. The R wave in V₁ is notched and the QRS measures 0.12 second. The overall QT is 0.40-0.44 second.

3. **What is your interpretation?**
   Interpretation is sinus rhythm at 70/minute with right bundle branch block (RBBB); consider left anterior fascicular block (LAFB).

4. **What can happen next?**
   Observe for AV conduction defects; s/s failure.

Figure 7-12

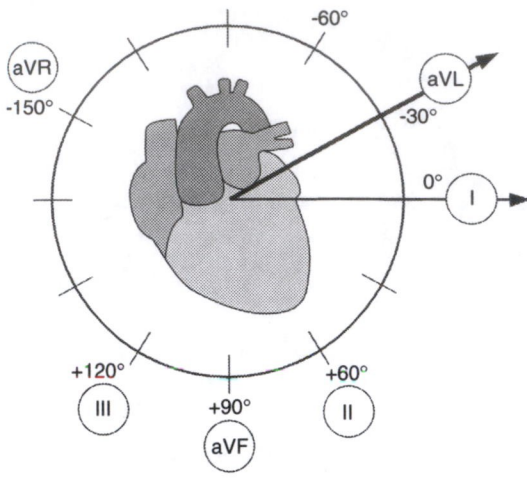

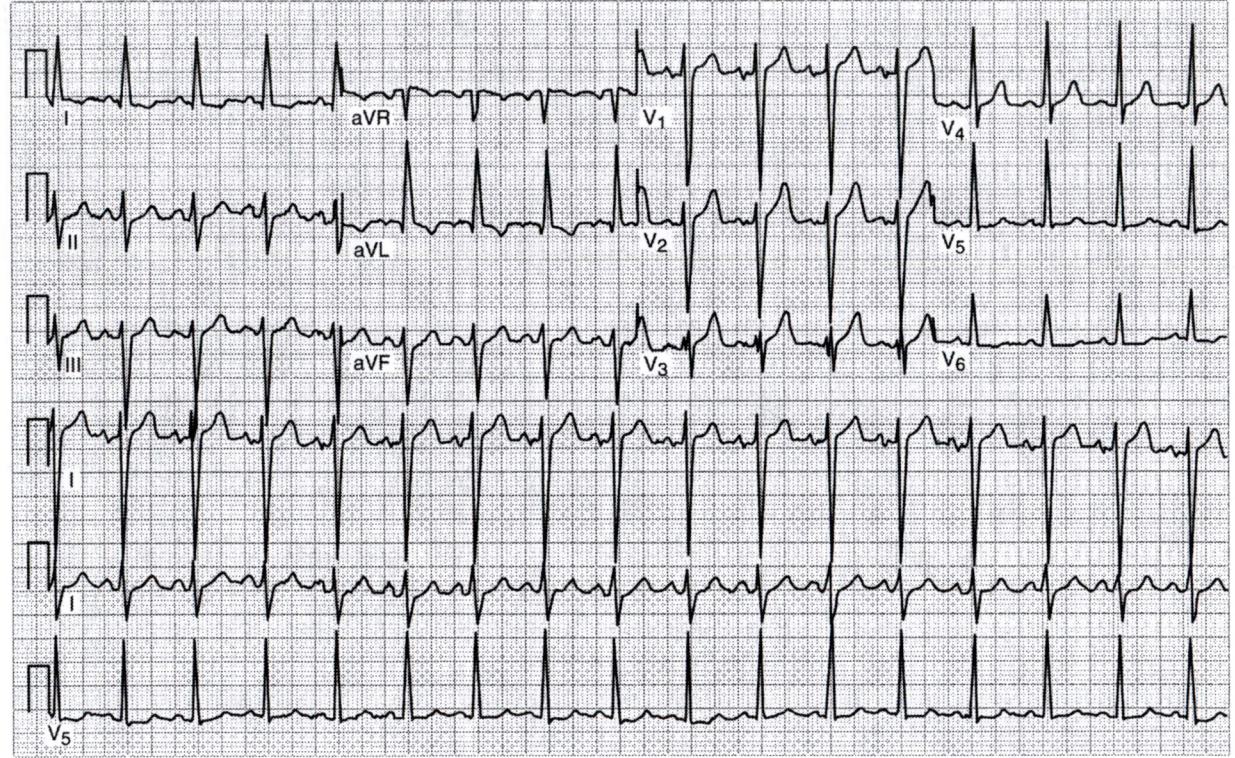

1.
Underlying rhythm is sinus at 100/minute

2. What are the acute changes?
Acute changes are QRS is 0.10-0.12 second with rS configuration in only leads III and aVF. Equiphasic deflection in lead II; lead aVL is positive, so the axis is at -30°. The overall QT is 0.36-0.40 second. The R wave in lead I plus the S wave in lead III is greater than 21 mm and the height of the R wave in aVL is greater than 13 mm. Consider ventricular hypertrophy (see Chapter 8).

Interpretation is sinus rhythm at 100/minute; abnormal QRS, consider rate-dependent LAFB; consider ventricular hypertrophy

4. What can happen next?
Observe for alterations in QRS if rate decreases. Observe for AV conduction defects; s/s failure

CHAPTER 8 CHAMBER ENLARGEMENT AND HYPERTROPHY
ECG Rhythm Identification Practice

Figure 8-9

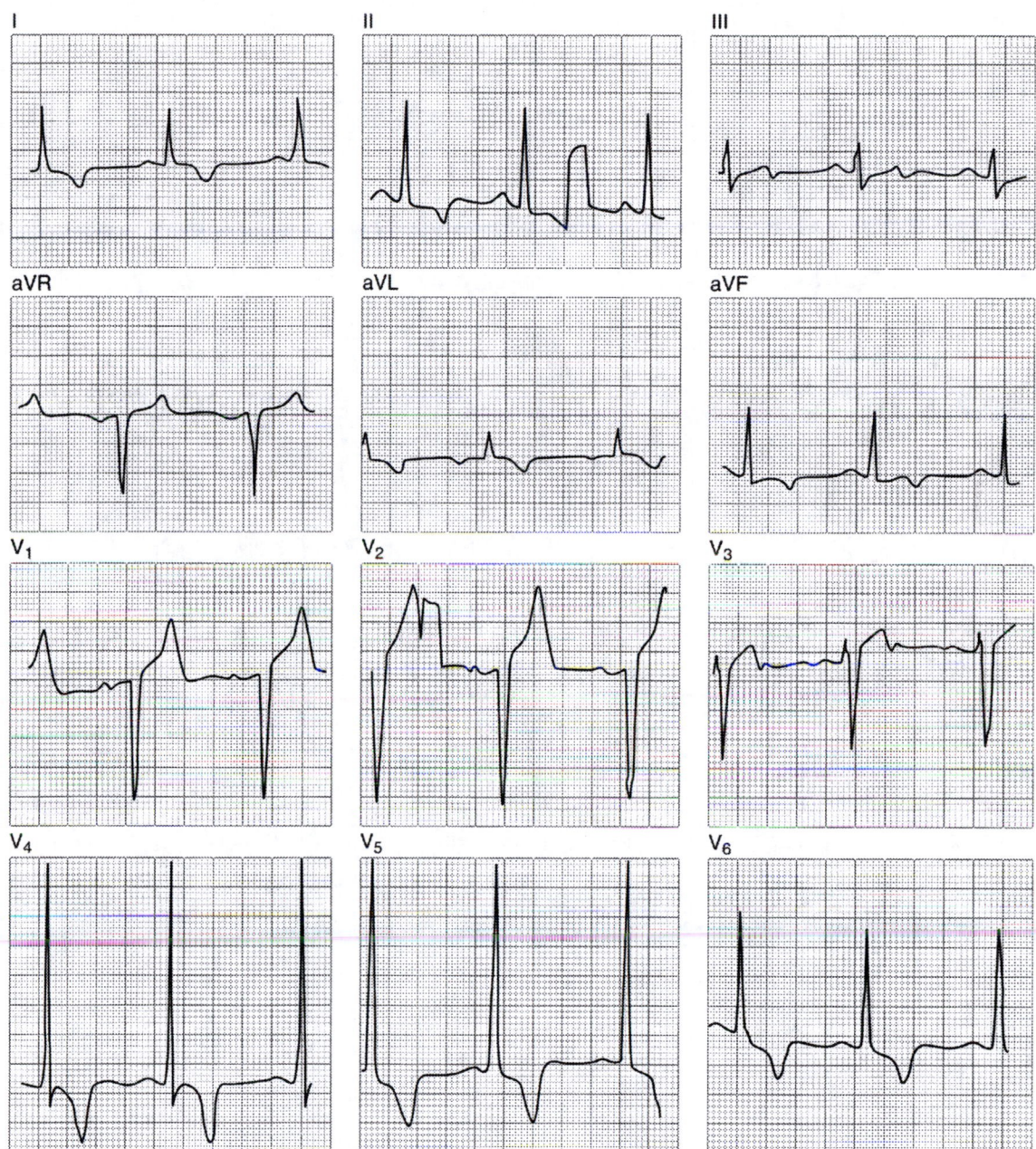

1. What is the underlying rhythm?

   Underlying rhythm is sinus at 68/minute

2. What are the acute changes?

   Acute changes are inverted T waves in I, aVL and aVF, V₄, V₅, and V₆. There are sagging (-) T waves in every lead with a tall R wave in V₄, V₅, and V₆. There are rising ST segments and upright T waves in every lead with a deep S wave in V₁, V₂, and V₃. Axis is (+)60°. (SV₁)20 mm (+) (RV₅)(35 mm) = 55 mm.

3. What is your interpretation?

   Interpretation is sinus rhythm at 68/minute; LVH by R/S voltage criteria and secondary ST-T changes.

4. What can happen next?

   Observe for s/s ischemia, injury, any type of conduction defect.

Figure 8-10

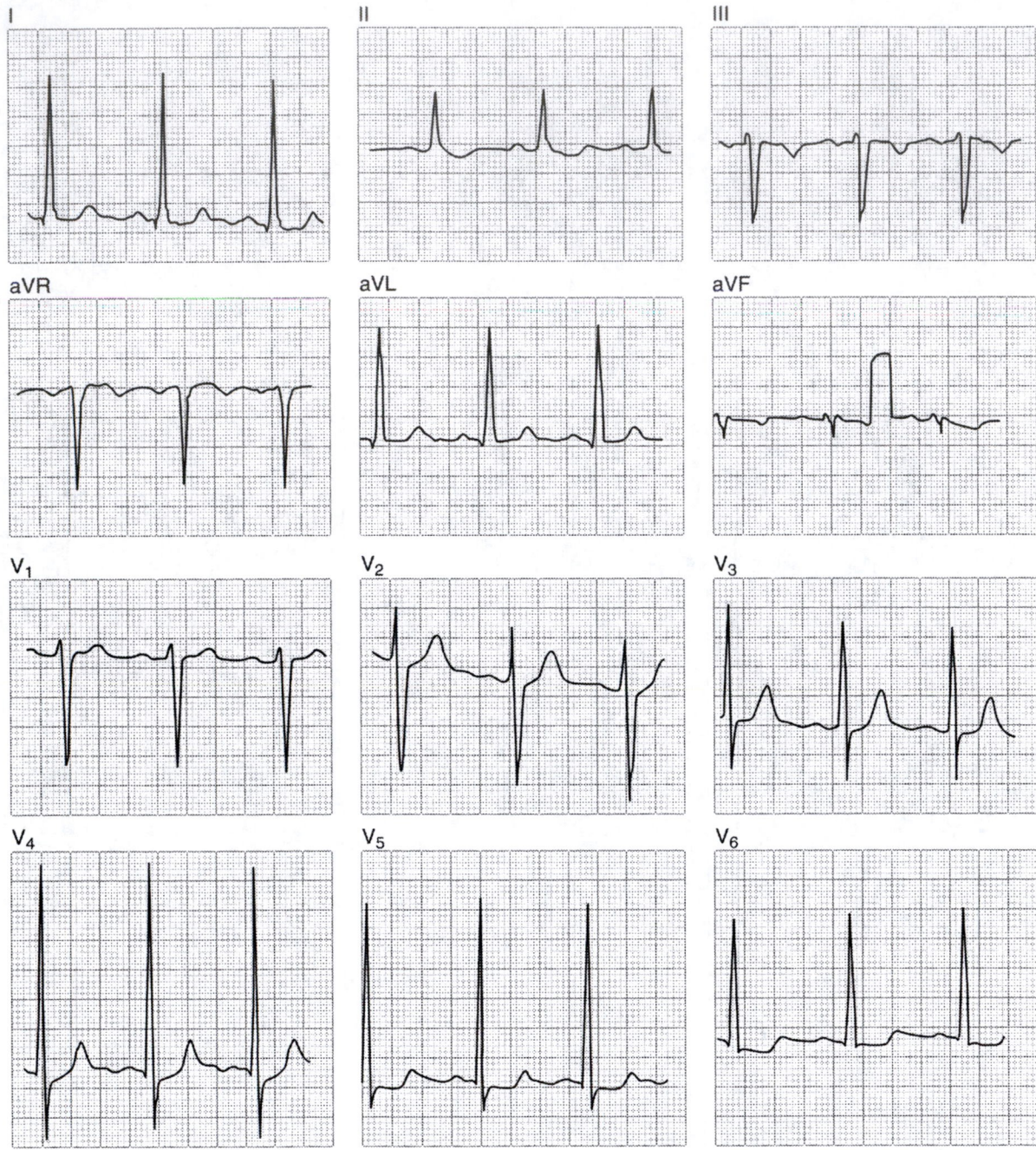

1. What is the underlying rhythm?

   Underlying rhythm is sinus at 78/minute; 1 mm ST depression in II; T wave inversion in III and aVF.

2. What are the acute changes?

   Axis is (+)0° (SV₁)29 mm (+) (RV₅)(31 mm) = 60 mm.

3. What is your interpretation?

   Interpretation is sinus rhythm at 78/minute; LVH by R/S voltage criteria

4. What can happen next?

   Observe for s/s ischemia, injury, any type of conduction defect.

Figure 8-11

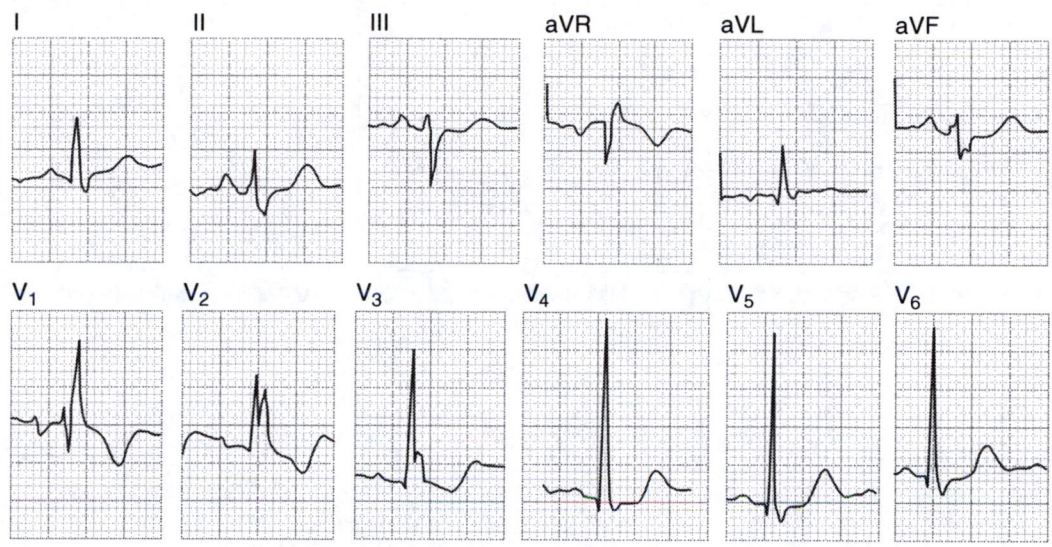

1. **What is the underlying rhythm?**
   Sinus at an undetermined rate

2. **What are the acute changes?**
   Acute changes are rS configuration in leads II, III, and aVF. Lead III is the greatest negative deflection. Axis is at -60°. There are inverted T waves in leads V_1-V_3. There is a broad S wave in leads I and II; rSR' in V_1; tall, notched R waves in V_2 and V_3.

3. **What is your interpretation?**
   Interpretation is sinus with RBBB.

4. **What can happen next?**
   Observe leads II, III, and aVF for LAFB. Observe for s/s failure.

Figure 8-12

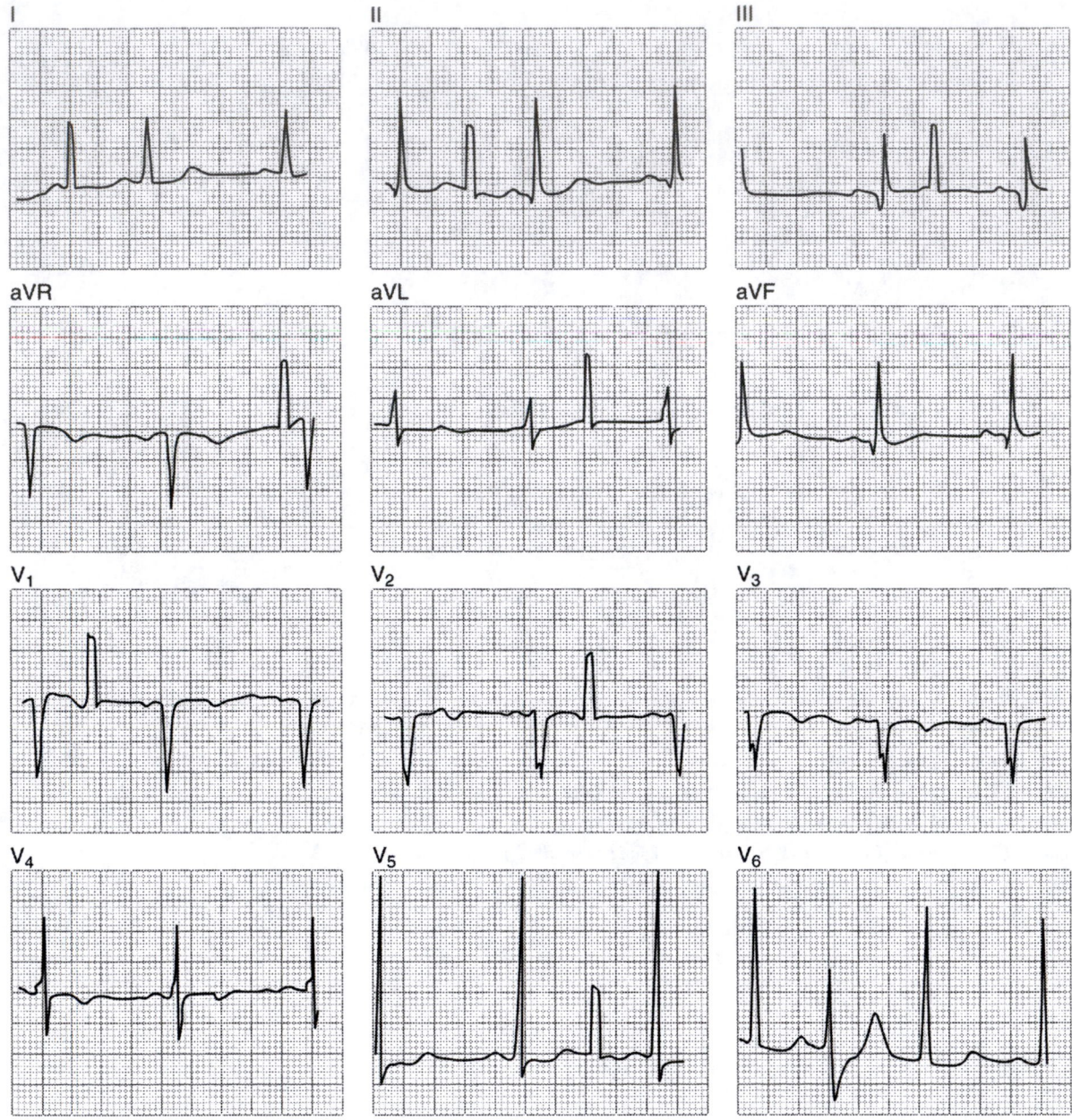

1. What is the underlying rhythm?

   Underlying rhythm is sinus at 67/minute; 1 mm ST elevation in II and III; Q wave in leads II, III, and aVF. It appears the leads are not simultaneous; PACs appear in leads I, ?II, and V₆ (with aberration).

2. What are the acute changes?

   Axis is (+)60° (SV₁)14 mm (+) (RV₅)(29 mm) = 43 mm.

3. What is your interpretation?

   Interpretation is sinus rhythm at 67/minute with PACs; LVH by R/S voltage criteria; possible inferior MI; if so, age undetermined.

4. What can happen next?

   Observe for s/s ischemia, injury, any type of conduction defect.

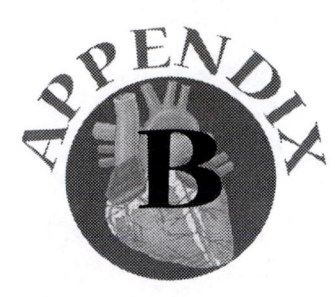

Normal Ranges and Variations in Adults in a 12-Lead ECG

The following table can serve as a guide to a patient's medical condition but must be interpreted only as a tool. Like any other sign, the ECG must be judged within the context of patient history and presentation.

LEAD	P	Q	R	S	ST	T
I	upright	<.04 seconds <25% of the R wave	largest deflection of the QRS complex	< R or none	isoelectric; may vary 1 mm (+) or (-)	upright
II	upright	small or none	dominant	< R or none	isoelectric; may vary 1 mm (+) or (-)	upright
III	(+) or (-) flat, or diphasic. (depends on frontal plane axis)	small or none 0.04–0.05 seconds or >25% of the R wave (depends on frontal plane axis)	none to dominant depending on frontal plane axis	none to dominant depending on frontal plane axis	isoelectric; may vary 1 mm (+) or (-)	upright, flat diphasic or inverted depending on frontal plane axis
aVR	inverted	small, none, or large	small or none depending on frontal plane axis	dominant; may appear as a QS configuration	isoelectric; may vary 1 mm (+) or (-)	inverted
aVL	upright, flat or diphasic; inverted depending on frontal plane axis	small, none, or large	small, none or dominant depending on frontal plane axis	none to dominant, depending on the frontal plane axis	usually isoelectric; may vary from +1 to -0.5 mm	upright, flat or diphasic; may be inverted depending on frontal plane axis
aVF	upright	small or none	small, none or dominant depending on frontal plane axis	none to dominant, depending on the frontal plane axis	usually isoelectric; may vary from +1 to -0.5 mm	upright, flat or diphasic; may be inverted depending on frontal plane axis
V$_1$	inverted, flat, upright or diphasic	none, may be a QS	less than S, or none, (QS) small R' may be present	dominant, may be a QS	0 to (+) 3 mm	upright, flat, diphasic, or inverted
V$_2$	upright, less commonly diphasic or inverted	none, may be a QS	less than S, or none, (QS) small R' may be present	dominant, may be a QS	0 to (+) 3 mm	upright, less commonly flat; diphasic or inverted
V$_3$	upright	small or none	R<S or R>S or R=S	S>R or S<R or R=S	0 to (+) 3 mm	upright
V$_4$	upright	small or none	R>S	S<R	usually isoelectric; (+)1 to (-)0.5 mm	upright
V$_5$	upright	small	dominant, less than 26 mm	S less than SV$_4$	usually isoelectric; (+) 1 to (-) 0.5 mm	upright
V$_6$	upright	small	dominant, less than 26mm	S less than SV$_4$	usually isoelectric; (+) 1 to (-) 0.5 mm	upright

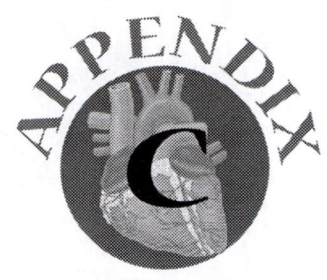
The Lewis Circle

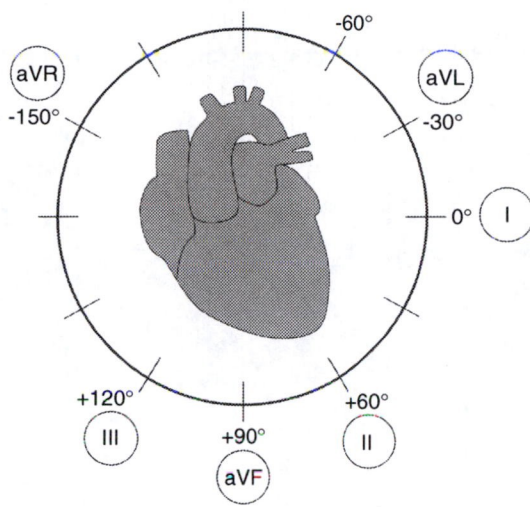

Designed for quick reference, the Lewis circle has degree values assigned to the limb and augmented leads as they reflect the heart's surface. Any of the methods for calculating axis can be applied by drawing an arrow according to the (+) or (-) configuration of the QRS complex in the limb leads.

HOW TO INTERPRET THE 12-LEAD ECG

1. What is the underlying rhythm?

2. Look for the acute changes, according to the surfaces of the heart: Qs, ST segment changes, T-wave inversion.
   a. Leads II, III, aVF: the inferior wall
   b. Leads I, aVL, V$_6$: left lateral wall
   c. V$_1$ → V$_4$: anterior walls
   d. V$_{3R}$ → right anterior wall

3. Look for ventricular conduction disturbances.
   a. Leads II, III, aVF: left anterior fascicle
   b. Leads I, aVL, V$_6$: left posterior fascicle
   c. Lead V$_1$ for RBBB
   d. What is the axis?

4. What can happen next? Which lead to observe?

Glossary

abberancy: QRS distortion that occurs with abnormal impulse transmission; often used when referring to a PAC or SVT with abnormal ventricular conduction; the QRS complex, instead of being narrow, is wide and distorted.

absolute refractory period: Period of time in which cells cannot respond to a stimulus.

accessory pathway: An extra bundle composed of ventricular tissue that exists outside the normal specialized conduction tissue.

action potential: Term that describes the electrolyte exchanges that occur across the cell membrane of the heart during depolarization and repolarization.

acute coronary syndrome: A group of signs and symptoms associated with myocardial ischemia and injury in compromised, and hopefully salvageable, tissue.

akinesis: Lack of motion in the muscle wall of the heart.

arrhythmia: Abnormalities in heart rate or rhythm.

augmented leads: Leads that are automatically set to increase in size by 50 percent without any change in the configuration of the electrodes by the machine's property; leads aVL, aVR, and aVF.

automaticity: The property of cardiac muscles that describes the ability of a cell to spontaneously generate an impulse without being externally stimulated. Cells that possess automaticity at a predictable rate serve as pacemakers.

axis: The direct path between two electrodes or between an electrode and the reference point; the direction of flow of depolarization.

bifascicular block: Right bundle branch block that occurs concomitantly with left anterior fascicular block.

biphasic: Having positive and negative components.

bipolar leads: Leads that comprise one positive and one negative electrode; leads I, II, and III.

bradycardia: Heart rate less than 60 beats per minute.

bundle branch block: A conduction disorder in one or more of the bundle branches.

complete AV block: Independent beating of the atria and ventricles due to complete refractoriness in the AV junction, at the level of the AV node or infranodal.

conductivity: The property of cardiac muscle that describes the ability to transmit an impulse from cell to cell.

contractility: The property of cardiac muscle that describes the ability of the heart to react to electrical conduction with an organized mechanical response.

delta wave: Initial slurring of the QRS complex. A premature upstroke to the QRS complex due to activity of an atrial-ventricular bypass tract. This is seen in preexcitation states such as the Wolff-Parkinson-White pattern. As a result, the PR interval is shortened. It does not have to be seen in all leads.

depolarization: Electrical activation of myocardial cells due to the spread of an electrical impulse.

digitalis effect: A negative scooping or slurring of the ST segment seen in patients on a digitalis preparation; not to be interpreted as digitalis toxicity.

dyskinesia: The paradoxical bulging of the heart wall during ventricular systole.

ectopy: Cells that possess automaticity in competition with pacemakers.

escape rhythm: The development of alternate pacemakers to stimulate the heart when there is sinus node slowing or arrest. The atria, AV junction, or ventricles may be the site of a single escape complex or a sustained escape rhythm.

excitability: The property of cardiac muscles that describes the capacity of a cell to respond to a stimulus.

fascicles: Bundles of fibers; left anterior and left posterior fascicles extend from the left main bundle branch.

fascicular block: Disruption in conduction within one or more of the extensions of the bundle branches.

fibrillation: Chaotic activity due to multiple ectopic foci.

first-degree AV block: A delay in AV conduction reflected in a consistently prolonged PR interval greater than 0.20 second.

fixed atherosclerosis obstruction: Localized accumulations of lipid-containing material (atheromas) within or beneath the intimal surfaces of blood vessels.

frontal plane leads: Leads that visualize current flow that is right, left, inferior, and posterior; the limb leads.

fusion beat: An abnormal QRS complex that occurs when the ventricles are activated partly by sinus, atrial, or junctional impulse, and partly by the PVC.

hemiblock: Fascicular block.

horizontal plane: Plane perpendicular to the chest and frontal plane.

horizontal plane leads: Leads that visualize current flow that is right, left, anterior, or posterior; the precordial leads.

hypercalcemia: Condition in which there is an excessive amount of calcium in the blood; serum levels greater than 3.5 mEq/L

hyperkalemia: Condition in which there is an excessive amount of potassium in the blood; serum levels greater than 6.0 mEq/L.

hypertrophy: A condition in which there is an increase in left ventricular muscle mass as a result of increased workload on the heart.

hypocalcemia: Condition in which there is abnormally low levels of calcium in the blood; serum levels less than 3.5 mEq/L.

hypokalemia: Condition in which there is an extreme lack of potassium in the blood; serum levels less than 3.0 mEq/L.

infarction: Necrosis to heart muscle; usually the result of occlusion of a coronary artery.

injury: Damage to tissue; may be reversible.

intrinsicoid deflection: The deflection made during the time from the beginning of the initial inscription of the QRS to the point where the impulse arrives under a particular electrode of a lead; used to measure ventricular activation time.

ischemia: Deficiency in perfusion of oxygenated blood.

isoelectric line: Flat ECG line found between wave forms or cycles, for example between the T wave and the next wave.

J point: The point where the QRS ends.

junctional rhythm: When the role of pacemaker is sustained by the bundle of His.

lack of R wave progression: The loss of R waves in the precordial leads when anterior forces are lost.

left axis deviation: When the flow of depolarization is superior and toward the left of normal.

low-voltage: Lower than normal amplitude (less than 5 mm) for a given wave form at normal standard calibration.

myocardial cells: The bulk of the heart's muscle; the contractile units of the heart.

nadir T waves: Symmetrical, negative T waves, greater than 5 mm in depth. Considered an acute sign with a high degree of suspicion of coronary artery deficit.

necrosis: Deadening of tissue as a result of occlusion with no oxygenated blood being perfused.

nonrefractory period: Period of time when all cells are repolarized and ready to respond in a normal fashion.

nontransmural: Myocardial infarction that does not involve all 3 layers of the heart

normal axis: The flow of electrical current downward from right to left in the heart.

P mitrale: Notched abnormal P waves.

P Prime (P′): P wave that is from other than a sinus impulse.

P pulmonale: Peaked abnormal P waves.

P wave: The wave form representing atrial depolarization; can be positive (+) when generated by a sinus and most atrial ectopic foci; is usually negative (-) when the atria are depolarized in a retrograde fashion from the AV junction.

pacemaker: A cell or group of cells that generates an impulse at a predictable rate of speed.

paroxysm: An abrupt start or stop.

pericardial effusion: Condition in which there is abnormal accumulation of fluid within the pericardial sac.

pericarditis: Inflammation of the pericardial sac.

poor R wave progression: The change of amplitude in the R waves. The R wave does not increase in size as the anterior forces diminish and the positive electrode gets closer to the current flow.

positive ST segment coving: ST segment elevations that are convex or curved in appearance as a result of myocardial injury.

precordial leads: Those leads in which the exploring electrode is on the chest overlying the heart or in its vicinity.

precordium: The area of the anterior chest overlying the surface of the heart.

PR interval: Period of time from the beginning of atrial depolarization (P wave) to ventricular activation (the QRS).

premature atrial complex (PAC): An ectopic atrial focus that propagates an impulse before the next normal sinus beat.

premature junctional complex (PJC): A discharge of a junctional ectopic focus that causes earlier than normal retrograde atrial depolarization. Represented on the ECG by a negative (-) P′; can occur before, during, or after the QRS complex.

Q wave: Initial negative deflection of the QRS complex shown on the ECG. Q waves are considered pathologic when they are new to the patient, and/or greater than 0.04 second.

QRS complex: That portion of the cardiac cycle corresponding to depolarization of the ventricles; made of any combination of the Q, R, and S wave forms.

QT interval: The period from the start of the QRS complex until the end of the T wave; the time from ventricular depolarization to ventricular repolarization.

R wave: The first positive deflection of the QRS complex shown on the ECG.

R′: The second (+) R in a QRS complex.

R wave progression: The increase in amplitude of the R waves in the precordial leads. If the anterior forces are intact and as the positive electrode gets closer to the current flow, the R wave becomes taller.

reciprocal leads: Leads that are in the same plane but show a reflection or mirror image

reentry: Ability of an impulse to reexcite some region of the atria through which it has already passed.

reflecting leads: Leads that are facing the affected surface of the heart

refractoriness: The property of cardiac muscle that describes the cell's ability to reject an impulse.

relative refractory period: Period of time when only a strong stimulus can cause depolarization.

repolarization: The process by which a cell, after being discharged, returns to its state of readiness.

right axis deviation: When the flow of depolarization is inferior and toward the right of normal.

RR interval: Period of time between consecutive QRS complexes.

S wave: The last negative deflection of the QRS complex shown on the ECG. Represents completion of ventricular depolarization. Usually less than 0.04 second in duration and less than 5 mm in depth.

second-degree AV block: Condition in which one or more sinus impulses are blocked and are unable to stimulate the ventricles.

sinoatrial (SA) block: A disorder where the atria are unable to respond to the sinus stimulus, resulting in a missed PQRST complex; sinus cadence is usually undisturbed

sinus arrest: A sudden failure of the SA node to initiate a timely impulse.

specialized cells: Cells that make up the heart's electrical conduction system.

ST segment: The line between the QRS and the T wave that represents early ventricular repolarization.

supraventricular: Site above the ventricles, that is, the SA node, atria, or AV junction.

T wave: The wave form corresponding to ventricular repolarization.

tachycardia: Heart rate greater than 100 beats per minute.

thrombolysis: Use of medication to dissolve components of vascular occlusion.

trending: Repeated ECG recording with comparison to allow for diagnosis and evaluation of interventions.

trifascicular block: Condition in which a block is located in each of the three main fascicles on the bundle branch system.

U wave: An ECG wave sometimes observed following the T wave; thought to be related to late repolarization of the ventricles.

unipolar leads: Leads that measure the electrical voltages at one location relative to a zero potential, rather than relative to the voltages of another extremity; leads aVL, aVR, aVF, and V_1 through V_6.

vector: The direction of force of electrical energy within the heart.

ventricular activation time: The time from the beginning of the initial inscription of the QRS to the point where the impulse arrives under a particular electrode of a lead.

Index

Note: Page numbers in **bold type** reference non-text material.

A

Aberrancy, defined, **95**
Aberrant ventricular conduction, 93-95, **96**
Absolute refractory period, defined, 5
Accelerated idioventricular rhythm (AIVR), 93, **94-95**
Accelerated junctional rhythm, 73
Accessory pathway, defined, 106
ACS (Acute coronary syndrome), 127, 128
Action potential, described, 3
Acute coronary syndrome (ACS), 128
Acute heart failure
  left bundle branch block and, 170
  right bundle branch block and, 167
Acute myocardial infarction
  left bundle branch block and, 170
  nonclassic ECG wave forms and, 151
  pathophysiology of, 126-129
Akinesis, defined, 134
Aneurysm
  ventricular, 134
    ECG wave forms ad, 42, **43**
Anterior myocardial infarction, right bundle branch block
    and, 167
Anterior wall myocardial infarction, 140-142
  clinical implications of, 142
Anterolateral myocardial infarction, 142-143
Anteroseptal myocardial infarction, 142
Antidromic tachycardia, 109
Aortic valve disease, right atrial enlargement and, 188
Arrest, sinus, 68-69
Arrhythmias
  due to abnormal conduction pathways, 104-113
  with preexcitation, 107-110
  sinus, 67, **68**
Arterial perfusion, bundle branches and, 164-165
Artery occlusion, coronary, consequences of, 128-129
Asystole, 95, 97
Atrial activation. *See* P waves
Atrial complex, premature, 74-76
Atrial enlargement
  left, 188
  right, 187-188
Atrial fibrillation, 79-80, **81**
Atrial flutter, 78-79, **80**
Atrial mechanisms, 73-80
Atrial tachycardia, 76, 77
Augmented leads, 11

Automaticity, of specialized cells, 5
AV block
  ECG configurations for, **105**
  second-degree, 99-101
  sinus rhythm with,
    complete, 102-104
    first-degree, 98, **99**
    high-grade, 102, **103**
AV conduction defects, 94-104
AV junction, described, 2, **3**
AVIR (Accelerated idioventricular rhythm), 93, **94-95**
Axis
  calculating, 50-53, **54**
  defined, **48**
  deviation, 49-50
  of lead, 10
  normal, 48, **49**
  values of, 54-55

B

Bifascicular block, 175
Bipolar leads, 10
Blocked PAC, 75
Bradycardia
  defined, **21**
  sinus, 67
Bundle branch block, 164
  ECG changes in, 166-174
  left, complete, 179, **180**
  types of, **180**
Bundle branch system, described, 2
Bundle branches, arterial perfusion and, 164-165

C

Cardiac cycle, phases of, 3-4
Cardiomyopathy
  left bundle branch block and, 170
  right bundle branch block and, 167
Chagas' disease, right bundle branch block and, 167
Chest leads, 12-13
  MCL, 15
Chronic obstructive pulmonary disease, pseudo-infarction
    patterns and, 150
Chronic pulmonary disease, right atrial enlargement and, 188
Complete AV block
  defined, **102**
  ECG configuration for, **105**
Conduction, abnormalities, of the left bundle, **180**
Conduction defects, AV, 94-104

Conduction pathways, 104-113
Conduction system, electrical, 1-2
Congenital defects, right ventricular hypertrophy and, 189
Congenital heart disease, right ventricular hypertrophy and, 189
Congenital lesions
    left bundle branch block and, 170
    right bundle branch block and, 167
Contractility, of specialized cells, 5
Cornell voltage test, left ventricular hypertrophy and, 193
Coronary artery occlusion, consequences of, 128-129
Coronary artery perfusion, 125-126
    myocardial infarction sites and, **153**
Current of injury pattern, described, 131

D

Delta wave
    defined, 106
    QRS complex and, 33
Depolarization, defined, 3
Digitalis, ECG wave forms and, 36
Digitalis effect, defined, 36
Drugs, ECG wave forms and, 35-36
Dyskinesia, defined, 134

E

Early repolarization
    described, 131
    pseudo-infarction patterns and, 151
Early transition, defined, 14
ECG wave forms
    affected by preexcitation, 106-107
    changes in,
        from bundle branch block, 166-174
        drug induced, 35-36
        from ischemia/injury/infarction, 131-138
    configurations for AV blocks, **105**
    described, 9
    indicating perfusion deficits, 138
    labeling, 64-65
    leads, 10-15
    monitoring, myocardial ischemia/injury/necrosis, 129-138
    myocardial infarction and, 151
    see also Wave forms
Ectopic rhythm, defined, 6
Ectopy, defined, 5
Eisenmenger's Syndrome, right ventricular hypertrophy and, 189
Electrical conduction, 6
    of the heart system, 1-2
Electrocardiogram (ECG). *See* ECG
Electrophysiology, of the heart, 3-5
Embolism, pulmonary, ECG wave forms and, 44-45
Escape rhythm, described, 6
Excitability, of specialized cells, 5

F

Fascicles, described, 164-165
Fascicular block, defined, **174**
Fascicular blocks, 174-179
Fibrillation, **79**
    atrial, 79-80, **81**
    ventricular, 90-92, **93**

First-degree AV block
    defined, **98**
    ECG configuration for, **105**
Fixed atherosclerotic obstruction, 127
Fixed-rate second-degree AV block, 102
Flutter, atrial, 78-79, **80**
Frontal plane, defined, 10
Fusion beat, defined, 88

H

Handal-Lewis method, axis calculation by, 52-53, **54**
Heart
    electrical conduction system of, 1-2
    electrophysiology of, 3-5
    posterior surface of, monitoring the, 14-15
Hemiblock, defined, **174**
Hexaxial reference system, 50
Horizontal plane, described, 12
Hypercalcemia, ECG wave forms and, 36
Hyperkalemia, ECG wave forms and, 36
Hypertrophic cardiomypoathy, ECG wave forms and, 42, **43**
Hypocalcemia, ECG wave forms and, 38, **39**
Hypokalemia, ECG wave forms and, 36

I

Idioventricular rhythm (IVR)
    accelerated, 93, **94-95**
    ventricular escape, 92-93, **94**
Incomplete left bundle branch block, 173
Incomplete right bundle branch block, 169
Infarction
    acute myocaridal, pathophysiology of, 126-129
    defined, **124**
    see also specific type of infarction
Inferior wall myocardial infarction, clinical implications in, 140
Injury
    defined, **124**
    monitoring, 129-138
Intermittent ventricular tachycardia, 88, **89**
Intracranial pressure, increased, ECG wave forms and, 42, 44
Intraventricular conduction deficit, described, 163-164
Intrinsicoid defection, defined, 173
Ischemia, defined, **124**
Ischemic LCA disease, left bundle branch block and, 170
Ischemic RCA disease, right bundle branch block and, 167
Isoelectric line, defined, 26
IVR (Idioventricular rhythm), ventricular escape, 92-93, **94**

J

J point, defined, 26
Junctional complex, premature, 71, **72**
Junctional mechanisms, 69-73
Junctional rhythm, 70, **71**
Junctional tachycardia, 73

L

Labeling, ECGs, 64-65
LAFB (Left anterior fascicular block), 174-176
    myocardial infarction and, 177
LAH (Left anterior hemiblock), 174
Lateral wall myocardial infarction, 143-144

Lead aVF, described, 11
Lead aVL, described, 11
Lead aVR, described, 11
Lead I, described, 10
Lead II, described, 11
Lead III, described, 11
Lead V₁, described, 12
Lead V₁R, described, 13
Lead V₂, described, 12
Lead V₂R, described, 13
Lead V₃, described, 12
Lead V₃R, described, 13
Lead V₄, described, 12
Lead V₄R, described, 13
Lead V₅, described, 12
Lead V₅R, described, 13
Lead V₆, described, 13
Lead V₆R, described, 13
Leads
  improper placement hazards, 15
  reflecting/reciprocal, 129
Left anterior fascicular block (LAFB), 174-176
  myocardial infarction and, 177
Left anterior hemiblock (LAH), 174
Left atrial enlargement, 188
Left axis deviation, 50
Left bundle branch block, 170-174
  complete, 179, **180**
Left posterior fascicular block (LPHB), 174, 177, **178-179**
Left posterior hemiblock (LPH), 174
Left ventricular failure, right atrial enlargement and, 188
Left ventricular hypertrophy, 190-195
  with right bundle branch block, 195
Legnegre's disease
  left bundle branch block and, 172
    right bundle branch block and, 167
Lev's disease
  left bundle branch block and, 172
  right bundle branch block and, 167
Lewis circle, calculating axis with, 55
Limb leads, 10-11
Lown-Ganong-Levine syndrome, 110-111
Low-voltage, described, 39
LPH (Left posterior hemiblock), 174
LPHB (Left posterior fascicular block), 174, 177, **178-179**

M
MCL leads, 15
Mitral insufficiency, right ventricular hypertrophy and, 189
Mitral stenosis, right ventricular hypertrophy and, 189
Mitral valve disease, right atrial enlargement and, 188
Monitor pattern, assessing, 65
Myocardial cells, described, 1
Myocardial infarction
  acute,
    ECG wave forms and, 151
    left bundle branch block and, 170
    pathophysiology of, 126-129
  anterior wall, 140-142
    clinical implications of, 142
  anterolateral, 142-143

  anteroseptal, 142
  coronary artery perfusion and, **153**
  inferior wall, clinical implications in, 140
  interior wall, 138-140
  lateral wall, 143-144
  left anterior fascicular block and, 177
  left bundle branch block and, 174
  non Q-wave, 148-150
  posterior wall, 144-146
  pseudo patterns of, 150-151
  right bundle branch block and, 169-170
  right ventricular, 146-148
Myocardial ischemia, monitoring, 129-138

N
Nadir T wave, described, 28
Narrow complex PVCs, 84-85
Necrosis
  defined, **124**
  monitoring, 129-138
Non Q-wave myocardial infarction, 148-150
Nonconducted PAC, 75
Non-refractory period, defined, 5
Nontransmural infarction, 137

P
P mitrale, defined, 29
P prime (P') wave, 70
P pulmonale, 187
  defined, 29
P' wave, 70, **71**
P waves, 24
  abnormal, 29-30
  monitoring, 65
PAC (Premature atrial complex), 74-76
Pacemaker cells
  described, 2
  sinus node as primary, 66
Perfusion
  coronary artery, 125-126
    myocardial infarction sites and, **153**
Perfusion deficits, ECG indicators of, 138
Pericardial effusion, ECG waveforms and, 42
Pericarditis, ECG wave forms and, 40-41
Pneumothorax, pseudo-infarction patterns and, 150
Polymorphic ventricular tachycardia, 88-90
Poor-R-wave progression, defined, 14
Positive ST segment coving, described, 133
Posterior wall myocardial infarction, 144-146
PR interval, 25
  abnormal, 30
Precordial leads, 12-13
Preexcitation
  arrhythmias with, 107-110
  defined, 106
  degrees of, 107, **108**
  ECG wave forms affected by, 106-107
Preexcitation syndrome, 106
Premature atrial complex (PAC), 74-76
Premature junctional complex, 71, **72**
Pseudo-infarction patterns, 150-151

Pulmonary emboli
  right atrial enlargement and, 188
  right ventricular hypertrophy and, 189
Pulmonary embolism
  ECG wave forms and, 44-45
  pseudo-infarction patterns and, 150
Pulmonary hypertension
  right atrial enlargement and, 188
  right ventricular hypertrophy and, 189
Pulmonary stenosis, right ventricular hypertrophy and, 289
Pulmonary valve disease, right atrial enlargement and, 188
Pulmonary vascular hypertension, right ventricular hypertrophy and, 189
Purkinje's fibers, described, 2
PVCs
  narrow complex, 84-85
  variations in, 85-87, **88**

Q
Q waves
  defined, **25**
  ischemia/injury/infarction and, 136-137
QRS complex, 25-26
  abnormal, 32-33
  notching, 33
  slurring, 33
  left ventricular hypertrophy and, 191
  low-voltage, ECG changes caused by, 39
  second-degree AV block and, 101-102
QRS vector, normal sequence of, 165-166
QT interval
  abnormal, 33-34
  described, 28-29
Quadrant method, axis calculation by, 51

R
R waves, described, 26
R/S voltage criteria, left ventricular hypertrophy and, 193
Ramus intermedius, 125
Rate, calculating, 20-23
Rate-related left bundle branch block, 172-173
Rate-related right bundle branch block, 167-168
RBBB. *See* Right bundle branch block
Reciprocal leads, 129
Reentry, defined, 77
Reflecting leads, 129
Refractoriness, of specialized cells, 5
Relative refractory period (RRP), defined, 5
Repolarization, defined, 3
Rheumatic heart disease
  left bundle branch block and, 172
  right bundle branch block and, 167
Rhythm, calculating, 20-23
Right atrial enlargement, 187-188
Right axis deviation, 49
Right bundle branch block, 167-170, **171-172**
  myocardial infarction and, 169-170
Right ventricular
  hypertrophy, 289-290
  ventricular myocardial infarction, 146-148

RR intervals, described, 23
RRP (Relative refractory period), defined, 5
R-wave progression, defined, 14

S
S wave, described, 26
Second-degree AV block, 99-101
  with 2:1 conduction, 102
  defined, **98**
  ECG configuration for, **105**
  with wide QRS complex, 101-102
Septal perforating arteries, 125
Sinoatrial (SA) block, 68
Sinus arrest, 68-69
Sinus arrhythmia, 67, **68**
Sinus bradycardia, 67
  defined, 21
Sinus mechanisms, 66-69
Sinus node
  described, 2
  as primary pacemaker, 66
Sinus rhythm
  with complete AV block, 102-104
  with first-degree AV block, 98, **99**
  with high-grade AV block, 102, **103**
  interpreting, 64
  second-degree, with AV block, 98, 100
Sinus tachycardia, 66, **67**
  defined, 21, 66
Sokolow-Lyon criteria, left ventricular hypertrophy and, 193
Specialized cells
  described, 2
  properties of, 4-5
ST segment
  continuous monitoring, 151-152
  depression, 131
  described, 26-27
  elevation, 131-134
ST-T abnormalities, 134
Supraventricular tachycardia, 76-78
Syphilis
  left bundle branch block and, 172
  right bundle branch block and, 167
Systemic hypertension, right atrial enlargement and, 188

T
T waves
  changes in, ischemia/injury/infarction and, 134-136
  described, 27-28
Tachycardia
  antidromic, 109
  atrial, 76, **77**
  defined, **21**, 66
  junctional, 73
  sinus, 66, **67**
  supraventricular, 76-78
  ventricular, 88, **89**
    intermittent, 88, **89**
    polymorphic, 88-90

Tetralogy of Fallot,
    right bundle branch block and, 167
    right ventricular hypertrophy and, 189
Thrombolysis, defined, **127**
Time is muscle, described, 129
Tosade de Pointes (TdP), 89
Transmural infarctions, 137
Trauma
    left bundle branch block and, 172
    right bundle branch block and, 167
Trending, defined, 125
Tricuspid valve disease, right atrial enlargement and, 188
Trifascicular block, 179, 181
Tumors
    left bundle branch block and, 172
    right bundle branch block and, 167
Type I AV block, 99-101

U

U waves
    abnormal, 34
        ischemia/injury/infarction and, 136
    described, 29-30
Unipolar leads, 10

V

VAT (Ventricular activation time), defined, 173
Vector, defined, 50

Ventricular activation time (VAT), defined, 173
Ventricular aneurysm, 134
    ECG wave forms and, 42, **43**
Ventricular conduction, aberrant, 93-95, **96**
Ventricular depolarization, normal sequence of, 165-166
Ventricular ectopic, characteristics of a, 83
Ventricular escape, idioventricular rhythm, 92-93, **94**
Ventricular fibrillation, 90-92, **93**
Ventricular hypertrophy, 188-189
    left, 190-195
        with right bundle branch block, 195
    right, 189-190
Ventricular mechanisms, 83-98
Ventricular strain pattern, 195-197
Ventricular tachycardia, 88, **89**
    intermittent, 88, **89**
    polymorphic, 88-90
Voltage criteria, left ventricular hypertrophy and, 191-195

W

Wave forms, 23-29
    abnormal, 29-34
    affected by preexcitation, 106-107
    alternations of, 35-45
    see also ECG wave forms
Wenckebach phenomenon, 99-101
Wolff-Parkinson-White syndrome, 111-113
    pseudo-infarction patterns and, 150